EXERCISES IN
ORAL RADIOLOGY
and
INTERPRETATION

EXERCISES IN ORAL RADIOLOGY and INTERPRETATION

FOURTH EDITION

Robert P. Langlais, DDS, MS, FRCD (C)
Professor, Department of Dental Diagnostic Science
University of Texas Health Science Center Dental School
   San Antonio, Texas
Diplomate, American Board of Oral and Maxillofacial Radiology

SAUNDERS
An Imprint of Elsevier

SAUNDERS

An Imprint of Elsevier

11830 Westline Industrial Drive
St. Louis, Missouri 63146

Notice

Oral radiology is an ever-changing field. Standard safety precautions must be followed, but as new research and clinical experience broaden our knowledge, changes in treatment and drug therapy may become necessary or appropriate. Readers are advised to check the most current product information provided by the manufacturer of each drug to be administered to verify the recommended dose, the method and duration of administration, and contraindications. It is the responsibility of the licensed prescriber, relying on experience and knowledge of the patient, to determine dosages and the best treatment for each individual patient. Neither the publisher nor the author assumes any liability for any injury and/or damage to persons or property arising from this publication.

ISBN-13: 978-0-7216-0025-3
ISBN-10: 0-7216-0025-5

Publishing Director: Linda L. Duncan
Executive Editor: Penny Rudolph
Senior Developmental Editor: Jaime Pendill
Publishing Services Manager: John Rogers
Project Manager: Helen Hudlin
Designer: Amy Buxton

Printed in USA

Last digit is the print number: 9   8   7   6   5   4

To my students. It is they who stimulate me to learn and therefore teach me to be the best I can be.

Preface

For this fourth edition, the original writing style was preserved, the language kept simple, and the questions clear and succinct. More little "humorous asides" or "out takes" such as "OK take a break" in which the author speaks to the student were added. The book is well known for this feature, which was pioneered by the author. It can be very helpful for students to know the author has thought about what their moods or feelings might be as the material is studied. The question and answer format was also maintained. Where possible, the many arrows, numbers, and letters that littered many of the cases were eliminated. Instead, matching diagrams for the normal anatomy have been added so the radiographs can be studied free of clutter, simulating the realistic clinical situation where images are not assessed with arrows. In some questions the reader is directed to the pertinent part of the figure with words rather than arrows to preserve the integrity of the images. On the other hand, the reader will find some arrows, numbers, and letters where it was deemed advantageous or unavoidable. An Answer Key is provided at the back of the book as with previous editions.

Another important improvement to the book is the addition of 300 new multiple choice questions to better prepare the student for final school, state, and national board examinations in the areas of radiation physics, biology, and health. These questions include a complete review of the basic principles of dental radiology, covering many new areas such as intraoral and panoramic principles, all aspects of digital radiology, infection control in dental radiology, film processing, and quality assurance procedures. The answers to these questions have been verified by Dr. John Preece, board-certified oral and maxillofacial radiologist and long-time educator and national and state examiner for dental, dental hygiene, and dental assisting students. Additionally the material has been reviewed by Dr. Doss McDavid, nationally certified radiation physicist and long-time teacher and researcher in dental radiology.

A further improvement to the book includes an expansion of most of the chapters to include a broader scope of material and more practice opportunities for answering questions, preparing for examinations, and ultimately using this aid to learning as a method to finally master the subject. In conjunction with these expanded areas, a concerted effort was made to improve the quality of the printed illustrations. This was done in two ways. First more representative and better original radiographs were selected to clearly illustrate the features. After 30 years of collecting cases, a huge inventory was perused to obtain the most current content. Second every single figure in this fourth edition was reprinted from original radiographs or digital images.

One of the more subtle additions to the content is the actual giving away of certain diagnoses for certain illustrations, which are not the subject of the question. In this way the student reviews material while reading the current question. Also the history given in each case is usually pertinent to the diagnosis. Information such as age, race, sex, laboratory findings, signs and symptoms should be evaluated carefully by the reader. In many cases the correct answer is found by correlating the information observed in the radiograph with the pertinent background history given. On a lighter note, and, hopefully to break the tension a little, the really subtle clues supplied by the patient's fictitious name or other seemingly unrelated details should hopefully bring a smile when these clues are recognized. In other less frequent circumstances, false clues are given that are plausible but which might lead an uncertain student away from the correct answer. For questions that are not multiple choice, the short answer format is retained. This way the student must recall information, process it, work out the problem, and come up with the correct answer in the absence of any check list. Also many of the questions are case based and are worded in such a way that the student must solve one or several related problems in order to obtain the correct answer.

Unlike previous editions, this book is not limited to radiographs. New chapters, diagrams, clinical photographs, and questions that include clinical material pertaining to normal anatomy, intraoral and panoramic clinical technique errors, infection control, radiation protection, and digital imaging have been added. The new clinical scenarios presented are even more important than recognizing errors in the image. Remember retakes double the dose of radiation to the patient and

increase costs; thus they are worth recognizing and avoiding in the first place before exposing the radiograph.

"The eye cannot see what the mind does not know."
Sir William Osler, Late 1800s

"You can't be good at what you don't know; you can only be good at being no good."
Robert Paul Langlais, 2003

Robert Paul Langlais
March, 2003

Acknowledgments

First I would like to recognize and thank Dr. Myron Kasle on the occasion of his retirement from co-authorship of this book. He was my mentor at Indiana University and was instrumental in having our first edition published. During the earlier years of my academic career, he was very helpful to me and gave me encouragement and support. I will always be grateful for the things Myron has done for me personally and for the special relationship we shared as coauthors. Our many former students also owe Dr. Kasle a debt of gratitude for the help he gave them in learning this often dry and difficult subject. I wish him a healthy and happy retirement. Once again, Myron, thank you.

The material on digital imaging in this text could not have been developed without Dr. Diane Flint, whose help was invaluable. In addition, much of the material in this text was reviewed by Drs. John Preece and William "Doss" McDavid. Dr. McDavid supplied some of the text and questions.

A special thank you is also due to Elsevier, particularly executive editor Penny Rudolph who had confidence in the future potential of this book. For this 25th silver anniversary edition, the publisher pulled out all the stops and gave me the support and the preparation time needed to completely redo the book to meet the needs of the next millennium. We looked at what the book does well and kept that; we then identified areas requiring improvement and finally recognized new material was also needed. I am also grateful to Jaime Pendill and Helen Hudlin who took care of the many publication details and were instrumental in the production process.

At UTHSCSA, Al Julian, director of photography, and Albert Preciado, interim director of photography, along with April Cox and Thurman Hood, generated some 3 to 5 prints of each radiograph, using varying densities and contrast so only perfect prints demonstrating all of the features were selected. Many of these illustrations had to be reprinted with Thurman's special tricks to get the features out of the radiograph and into the print. Some whole sections contain digitally generated prints. Many of the photographs are the work of photographer extraordinaire, Lee Bennack. The artwork featured in Chapters 1 and 7 is the creation of the incredibly talented David Baker, a medical illustrator and artist to the Bush first family of the United States. Words cannot adequately express his boundless patience or my debt of gratitude to him.

Acknowledgments

Contents

PART One

Principles and Interpretation

Chapter 1

Normal Anatomy

Goal

To learn to recognize normal anatomic structures as they appear in various radiographs

Learning Objectives

1. Recognize anatomic structures on labeled diagrams
2. Learn by correlating diagrammatic information and the structure on the radiograph
3. Identify anatomic structures in intraoral radiographs
4. Recognize anatomic structures in panoramic radiographs
5. Begin to correlate anatomic distortions and panoramic technique errors

Instructions

Look at the figure(s) and identify the indicated anatomic structures. First try to identify the structure from memory. If that does not work, go to the answer page at the end of the book for the answer.

NOTE TO STUDENTS: At this time, some of these structures may not seem relevant. Remember, we will be looking at not only intraoral images but also panoramic radiographs.

ANATOMIC DIAGRAMS

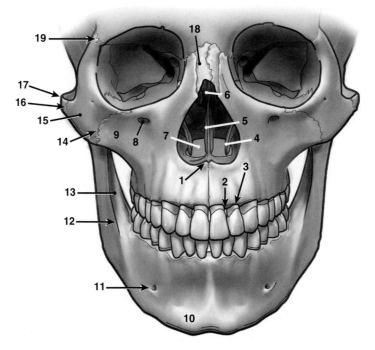

FIGURE **1-1** Identify the indicated anatomic structures.

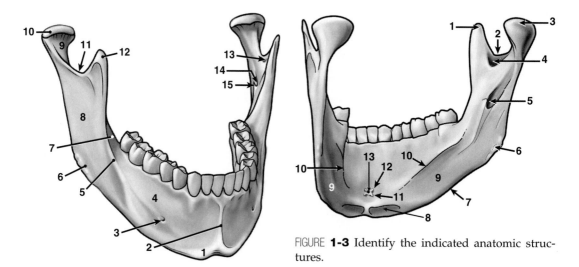

FIGURE **1-2** Identify the indicated anatomic structures.

FIGURE **1-3** Identify the indicated anatomic structures.

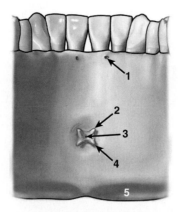

FIGURE **1-4** Identify the indicated anatomic structures.

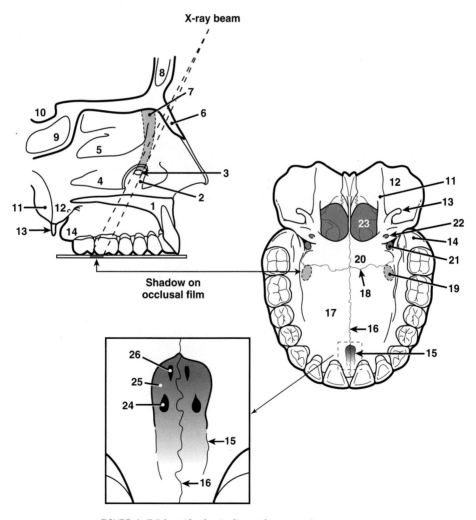

FIGURE **1-5** Identify the indicated anatomic structures.

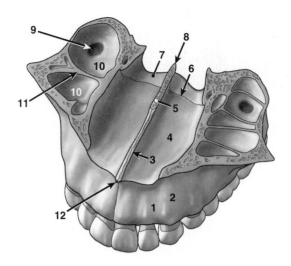

FIGURE **1-6** Identify the indicated anatomic structures.

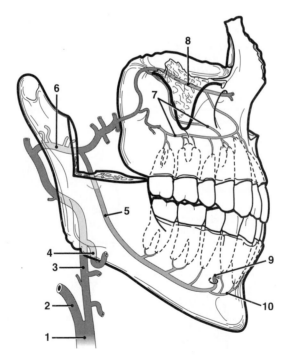

FIGURE **1-7** Identify the indicated anatomic structures.

OSTEOLOGY

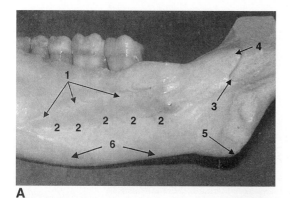

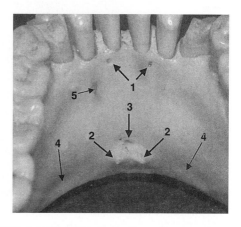

FIGURE **1-9** Identify the indicated anatomic structures.

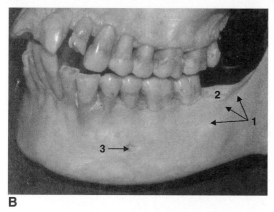

FIGURE **1-8** Identify the indicated anatomic bony landmarks.

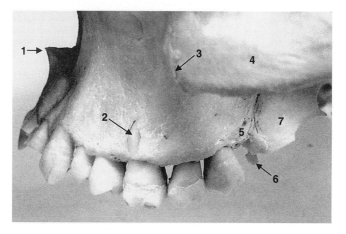

FIGURE **1-10** Identify the indicated anatomic structures.

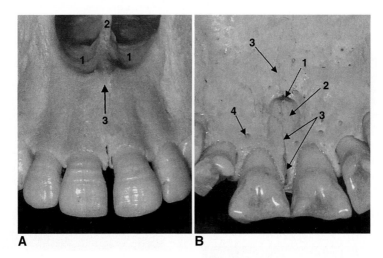

FIGURE **1-11** Identify the indicated anatomic structures.

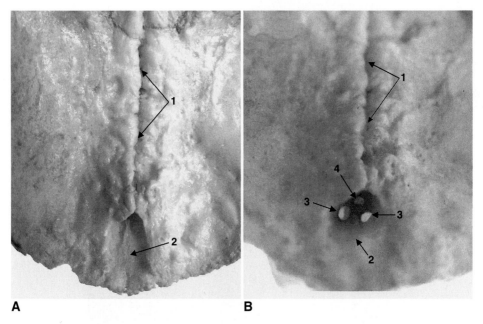

FIGURE **1-12** *A* and *B* illustrate an edentulous anterior maxilla. Identify the indicated anatomic structures.

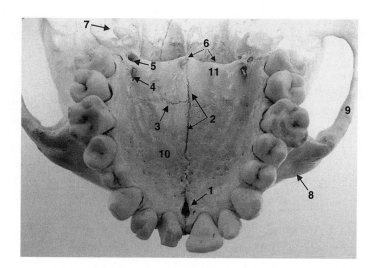

FIGURE **1-13** Identify the indicated anatomic structures.

INTRAORAL RADIOGRAPHIC ANATOMY WITH MATCHING DIAGRAMS

Each of these figures consists of a custom drawing on the left (part *A*) and the corresponding intraoral radiograph on the right (part *B*). These drawings have been created to avoid placing arrows and numbers on the radiograph itself. Because in the clinical situation the radiographs do not come with the clutter, distraction, or obscurity of structures caused by arrows, the author and the artist David Baker have created this format to enhance the learning process.

Examples with film sizes both #1 and #2 are included for some areas such as the anterior regions. Variations, including children with developing and erupting teeth and edentulous patients, are illustrated. .

Numerous examples of the same anatomic region have been included to habituate the student to the various combinations of presentations in which these anatomic structures appear. Also, repetition enhances the learning process and progressively instills confidence in the student.

For Figures 1-14 through 1-59, identify the indicated structures. Figure 1-16 begins in the maxillary anterior area; the remainder of the figures proceed posteriorly, then to the mandibular anterior area, and end in the posterior region.

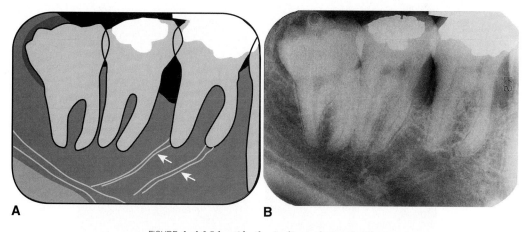

A   **B**

FIGURE **1-14** Identify the indicated structures.

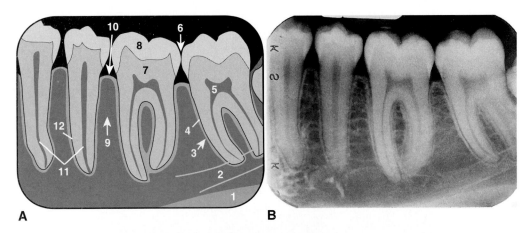

FIGURE **1-15** Identify the indicated structures.

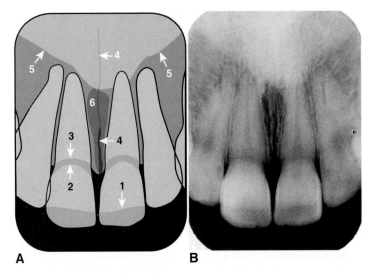

FIGURE **1-16** Identify the indicated structures.

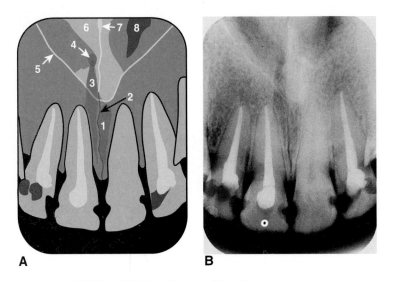

FIGURE **1-17** Identify the indicated structures.

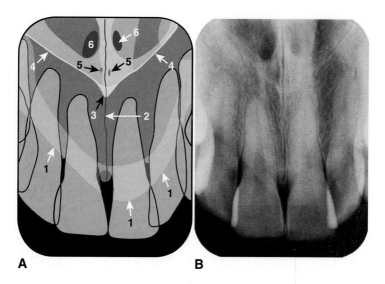

FIGURE **1-18** Identify the indicated structures.

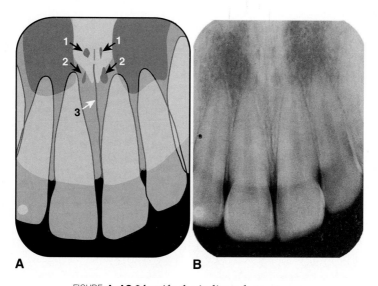

FIGURE **1-19** Identify the indicated structures.

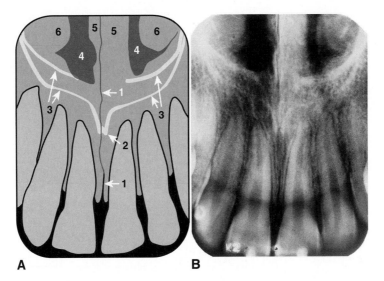

FIGURE **1-20** Identify the indicated structures.

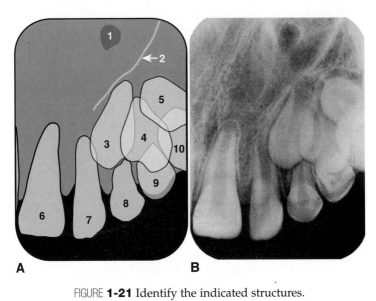

FIGURE **1-21** Identify the indicated structures.

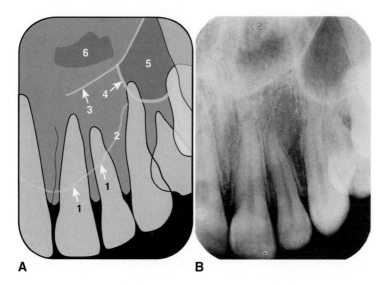

FIGURE **1-22** Identify the indicated structures.

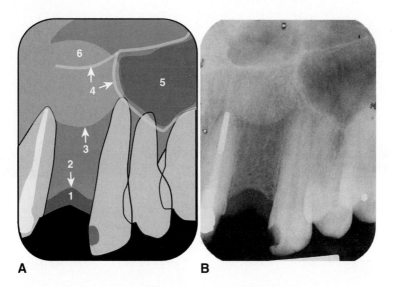

FIGURE **1-23** Identify the indicated structures.

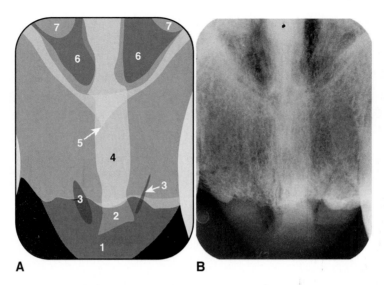

FIGURE **1-24** Identify the indicated structures.

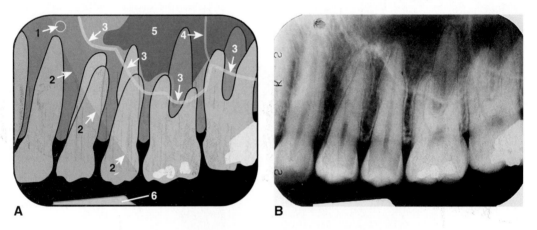

FIGURE **1-25** Identify the indicated structures.

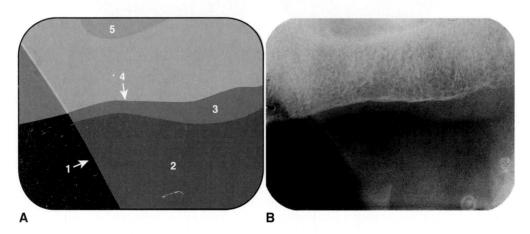

FIGURE **1-26** Identify the indicated structures.

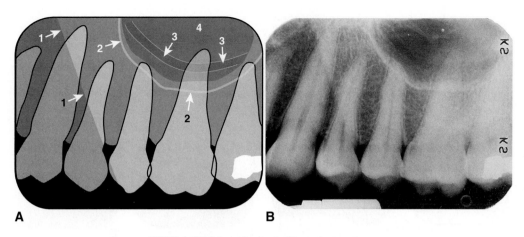

FIGURE **1-27** Identify the indicated structures.

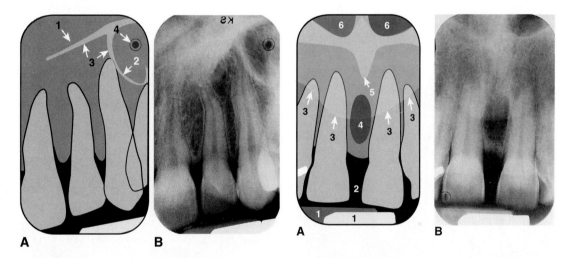

FIGURE **1-28** Identify the indicated structures.

FIGURE **1-29** Identify the indicated structures.

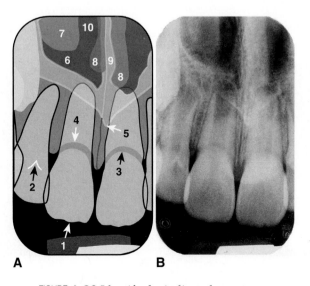

FIGURE **1-30** Identify the indicated structures.

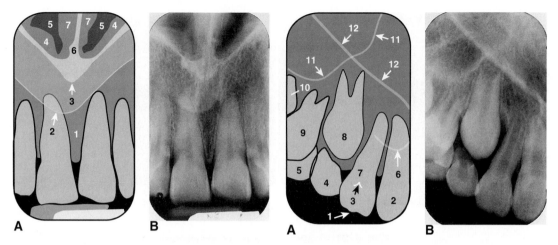

FIGURE **1-31** Identify the indicated structures.

FIGURE **1-32** Identify the indicated structures.

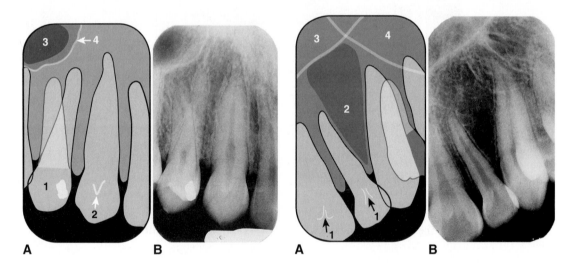

FIGURE **1-33** Identify the indicated structures.

FIGURE **1-34** Identify the indicated structures.

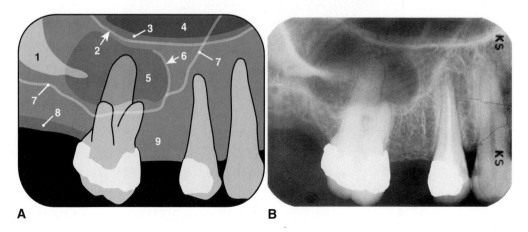

FIGURE **1-35** Identify the indicated structures.

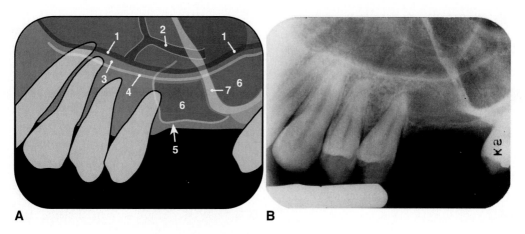

FIGURE **1-36** Identify the indicated structures.

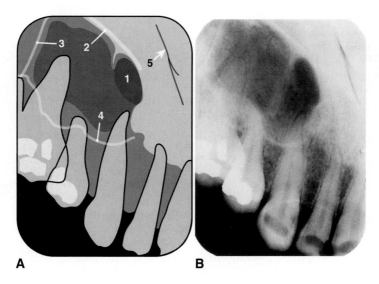

FIGURE **1-37** Identify the indicated structures.

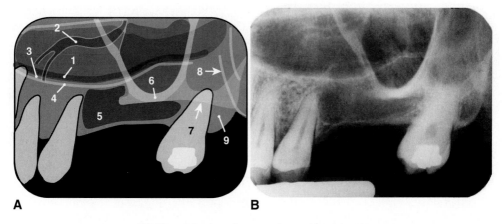

FIGURE **1-38** Identify the indicated structures.

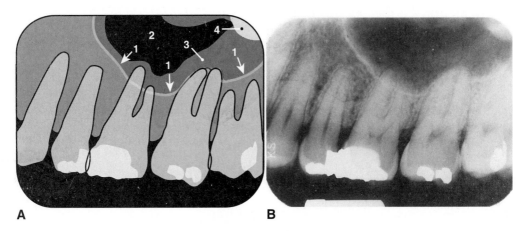

FIGURE **1-39** Identify the indicated structures.

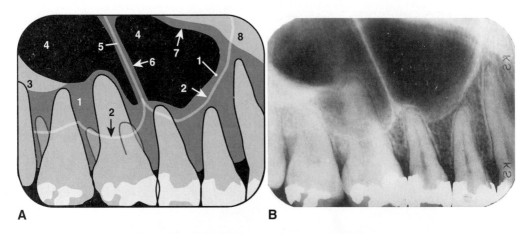

FIGURE **1-40** Identify the indicated structures.

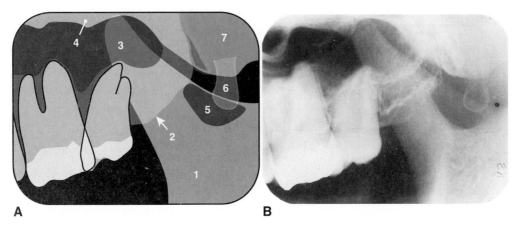

FIGURE **1-41** Identify the indicated structures.

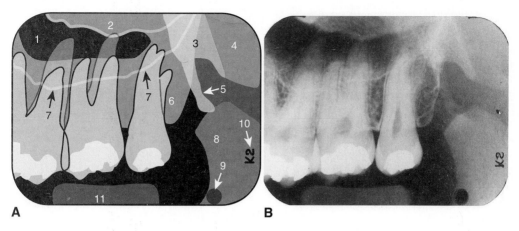

FIGURE **1-42** Identify the indicated structures.

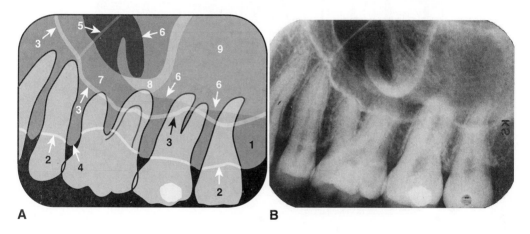

FIGURE **1-43** Identify the indicated structures.

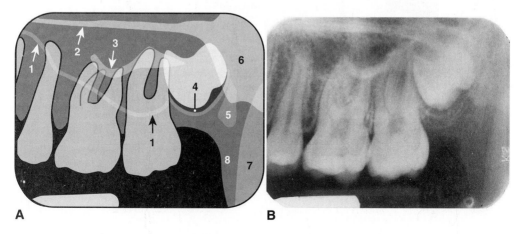

FIGURE **1-44** Identify the indicated structures.

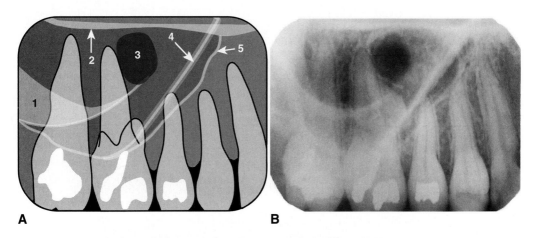

A   B

FIGURE **1-45** Identify the indicated structures.

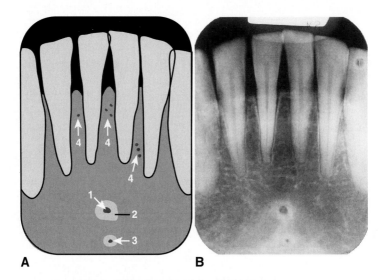

A   B

FIGURE **1-46** Identify the indicated structures.

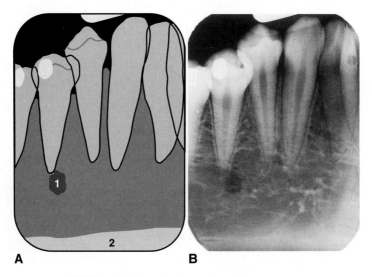

A   B

FIGURE **1-47** Identify the indicated structures.

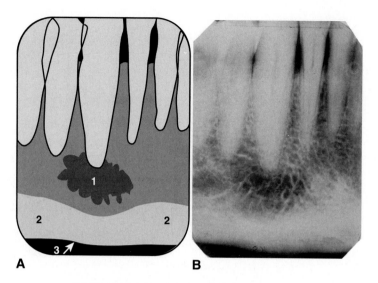

FIGURE **1-48** Identify the indicated structures.

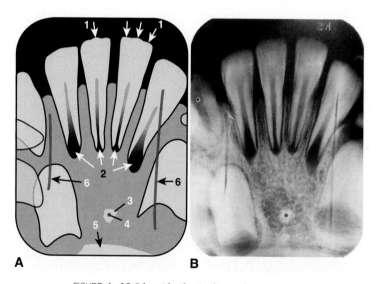

FIGURE **1-49** Identify the indicated structures.

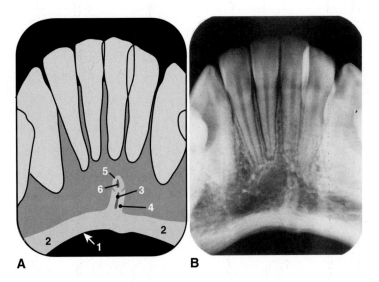

FIGURE **1-50** Identify the indicated structures.

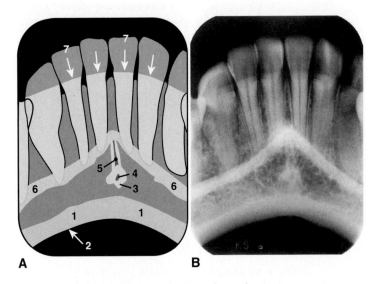

FIGURE **1-51** Identify the indicated structures.

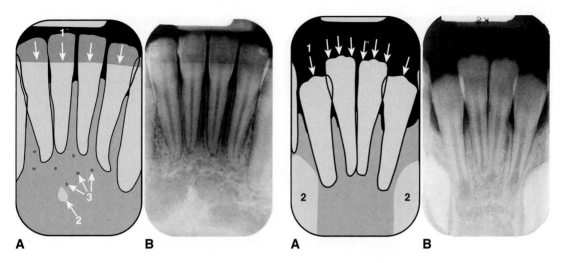

FIGURE **1-52** Identify the indicated structures.

FIGURE **1-53** Identify the indicated structures.

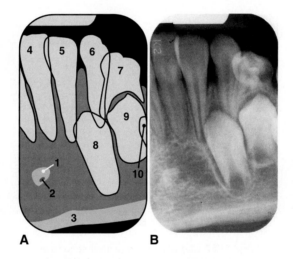

FIGURE **1-54** Identify the indicated structures.

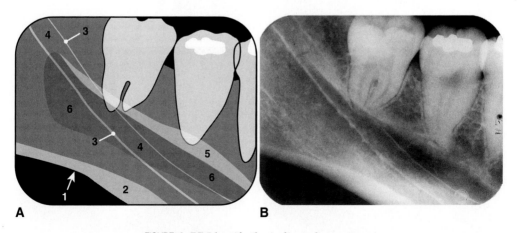

FIGURE **1-55** Identify the indicated structures.

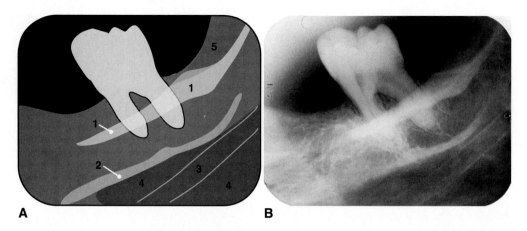

FIGURE **1-56** Identify the indicated structures.

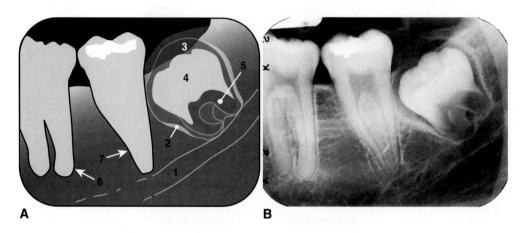

FIGURE **1-57** Identify the indicated structures.

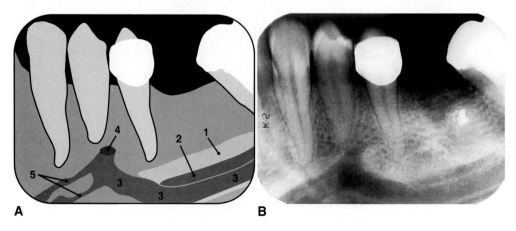

FIGURE **1-58** Identify the indicated structures.

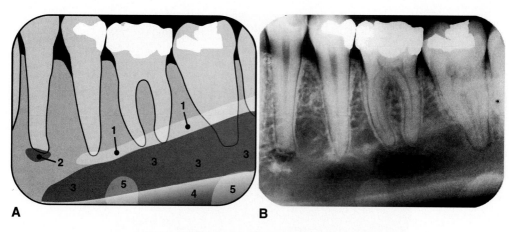

A **B**

FIGURE **1-59** Identify the indicated structures.

INTRAORAL ANATOMIC STRUCTURES

In spite of the many diagrams and radiographs, several anatomic structures have not yet been seen. In other instances important variations or edentulous cases are included. The following cases are in no particular order.

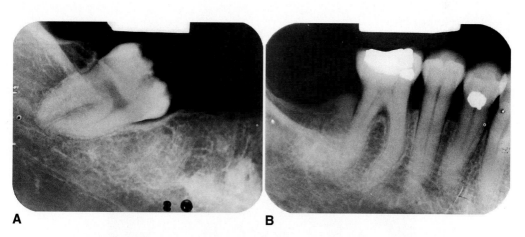

A **B**

FIGURE **1-60** Parts *A* and *B* are variants of the same anatomic structure (crest of ridge distal to molar).
1. Name the structure.
2. Can you explain the difference between situations *A* and *B*?

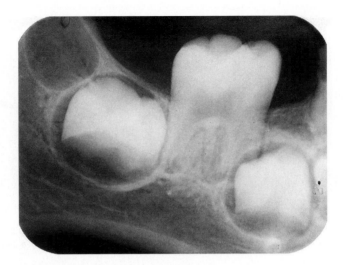

FIGURE **1-61** This patient is a 6-year-old male.
1. Identify the radiolucent area distal to the developing 2nd molar.

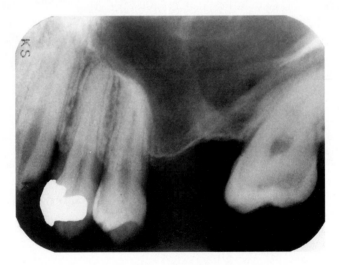

FIGURE **1-62** Here we see that several molars have been extracted. As a result, the sinus has enlarged to where the floor of the sinus is at the crest of the alveolar ridge.
1. What term is used to describe the sinus enlargement?

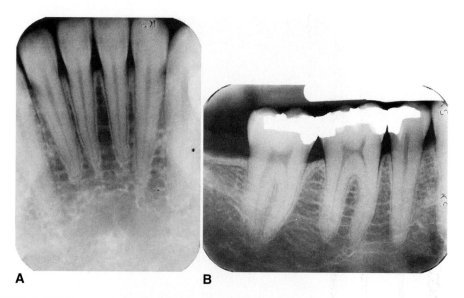

A   **B**

FIGURE **1-63** This question is about a specific trabecular pattern seen in parts *A* and *B*. In part *A* it is between the central incisors, and in part *B* it is between the 1st molar roots.
1. What term best describes this trabecular pattern?
2. Is this of any significance?

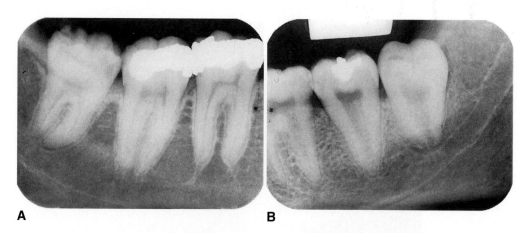

A   **B**

FIGURE **1-64** This question is about trabecular patterns in general as seen in parts *A* and *B*.
1. What term best describes the trabecular pattern in part *A*?
2. What term best describes the trabecular pattern in part *B*?
3. In which part of the alveolar bone is the trabecular pattern? (Cortex vs. spongiosum or marrow space.)

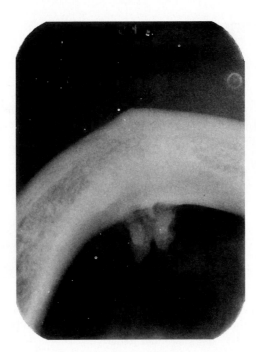

FIGURE **1-65** Here you see a #2 film oriented like an occlusal view.
1. What structures do we see at the lingual midline?
2. Of what significance (if any) are these?

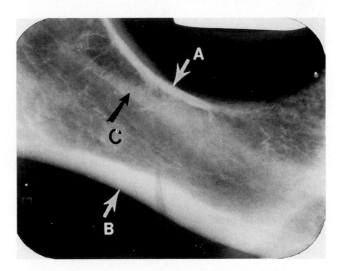

FIGURE **1-66** Here you see an edentulous mandible.
1. To what structures are *arrows A, B,* and *C* pointing?

NORMAL PANORAMIC ANATOMY

Instructions

Figures 1-67 through 1-72 illustrate structures indicated by a *letter, arrow* or *arrowhead*, or *series of arrowheads*. When the letter appears without an arrow, name the structure the letter is on; *single arrows* indicate a structure immediately in front of the arrow, and a *group of arrowheads* indicates the margin of a structure to be identified. Most of the structures are indicated in Figures 1-1 to 1-13.

Remember, some "structures" are soft tissue, suture lines, air spaces such as the meatuses or nasopharynx, canals, foramina, bony sinus walls, or bone margins as well as the major parts of a bone such as the ramus or pterygoid plates.

Remember also, in panoramic radiographs we see ghost images that tend to be on the opposite side and above the real image (e.g., the real and ghost images of the hard palate and ramus). There are also real double images where midline objects like the hard palate or hyoid bone can be seen twice in the image—one being the mirror image of the other. Note that the hard palate can have both ghost and real double images in the same radiograph, whereas the soft palate is always only a real double image.

Some of the most important structures for the recognition of technique errors or for the localization of disease have been selected.

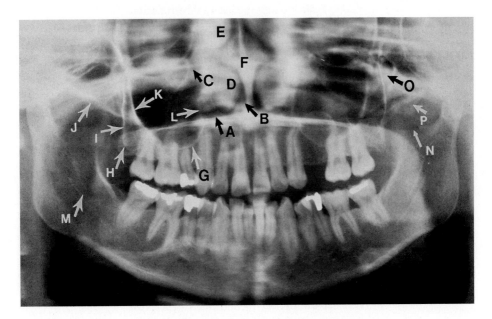

FIGURE **1-67** Identify the indicated structures.

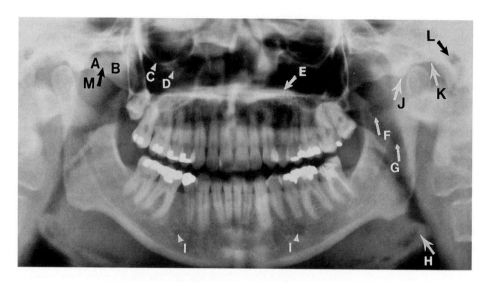

FIGURE **1-68** Identify the indicated structures.

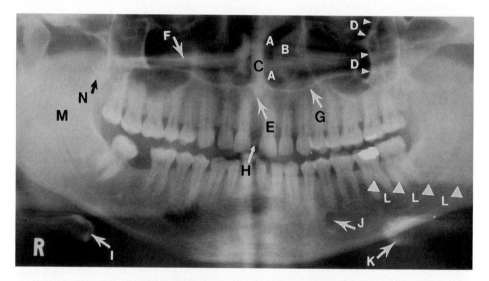

FIGURE **1-69** Identify the indicated structures.

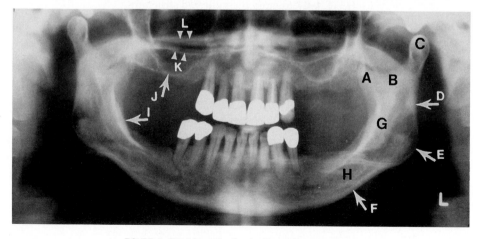

FIGURE **1-70** Identify the indicated structures.

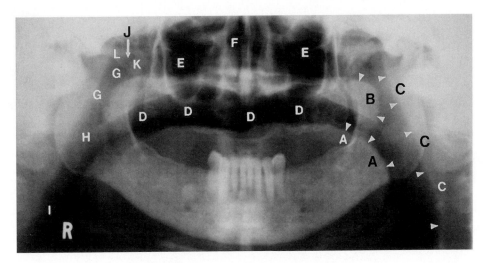

FIGURE **1-71** Identify the indicated structures.

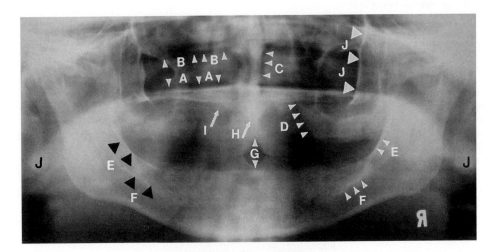

FIGURE **1-72** Identify the indicated structures.

Chapter 2

Materials and Foreign Objects

Goal

To recognize materials and foreign objects in radiographs

Learning Objectives

1. Recognize the appearance of dental materials in the radiographs
2. Identify foreign objects in the radiographs
3. Know the features as seen in intraoral radiographs
4. Know the features as seen in panoramic radiographs

Instructions

Look at the figures and identify the materials, foreign objects, or case-related information in the following questions.

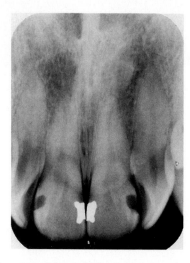

FIGURE **2-1** What materials could have been used to restore the:
1. Mesial of the central incisors?
2. Distal of the central incisors?

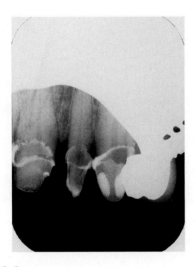

FIGURE **2-2**
1. With what metals might this patient's prosthesis be made?
2. With what materials are the crowns of the anterior teeth restored?
3. What are the radiopaque lines seen in the cervical area of these teeth?

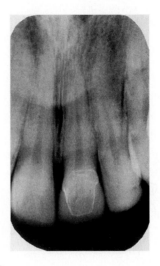

FIGURE **2-3**
1. What type of crown has been placed on the left central incisor?
2. What is the radiopaque line within the crown area?

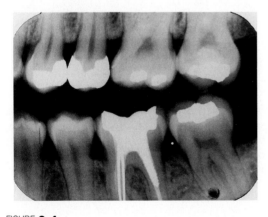

FIGURE **2-4**
1. What materials can we see in the lower 1st molar?
2. What is the radiolucent area on the distal cervical of the lower 1st molar?

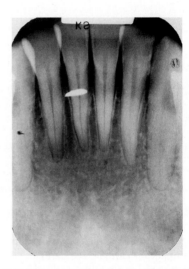

FIGURE **2-5** This is a 23-year-old. The radiograph revealed a radiopaque area on the right central incisor. There was no restoration on this tooth, but she had been in an auto accident several months previously.
1. What do you think this radiopacity might represent?
2. What else could look like this?

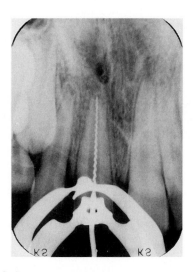

FIGURE **2-6**
1. Name two metallic objects seen in this radiograph.

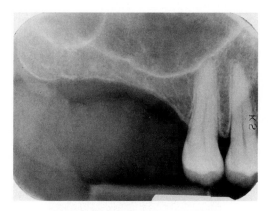

FIGURE **2-7** Here we can see three different materials associated with taking this radiograph.
1. Can you enumerate them?

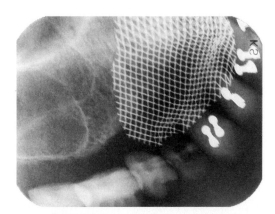

FIGURE **2-8** This patient wears a complete upper denture against his natural lowers and keeps breaking the denture while masticating food.
1. What materials can you see here?
2. What material can you not see?

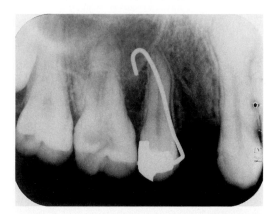

FIGURE **2-9** This patient is 13 years old and needs several carious lesions restored. She is also missing both central incisors, which were extracted for caries.
1. What do you think this radiopaque object superimposed on the premolar represents?

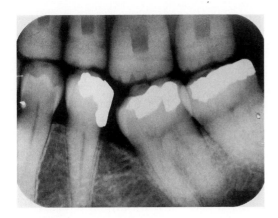

FIGURE **2-10**
1. Can you account for the strange appearance of the maxillary teeth?

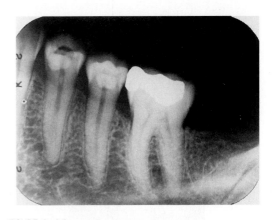

FIGURE **2-11**
1. With what material are the premolars restored?
2. With what material is the molar restored?

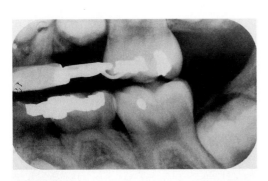

FIGURE **2-12**
1. What type of appliance do we see in the maxilla of this 10-year-old boy?

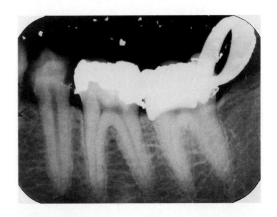

FIGURE **2-13**
1. What materials do you see in this radiograph?
2. What material do you not see?

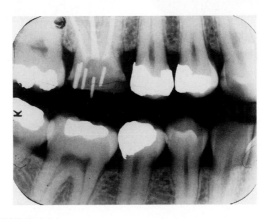

FIGURE **2-14**
1. What materials do we see in the upper 1st molar?

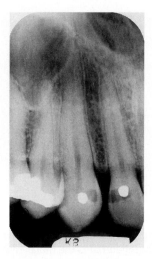

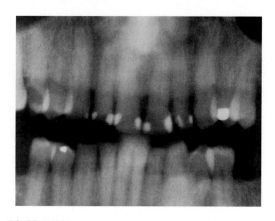

FIGURE **2-16**
1. What material do we see in these anterior
   teeth?

FIGURE **2-15** Look at the lateral incisor and canine
teeth. Each tooth has a radiopaque and a radiolucent restoration in proximity to each other. Ignore
the restoration on the distal of the canine.
1. What materials were used, and where on the
   teeth are they?

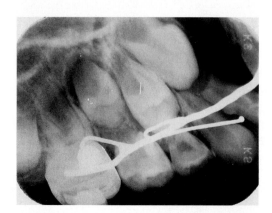

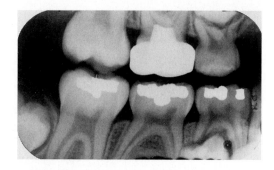

FIGURE **2-17** This is a 6-year-old girl with a habit
that is contributing to a developing orthodontic
problem.
1. What is this appliance?

FIGURE **2-18**
1. Compare and contrast the treatment and
   materials in the upper and lower primary 2nd
   molars.

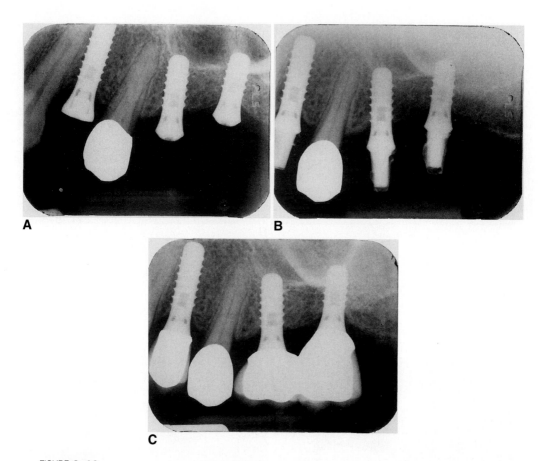

FIGURE **2-19**

1. This case illustrates three different phases in the treatment of this patient. Apart from the crown on the 2nd premolar, which appears to be all gold, what materials do we see in parts *A, B,* and *C*?

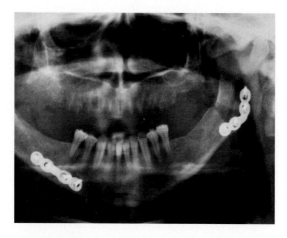

FIGURE **2-20**

1. What materials do you see in this patient?
2. What happened to this patient?

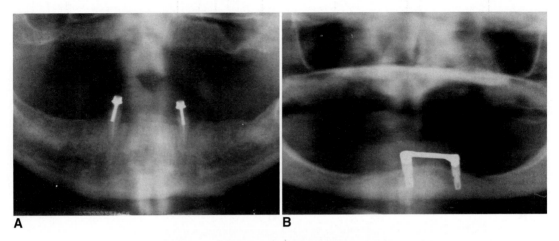

FIGURE **2-21**
1. Compare and contrast the materials seen in parts *A* and *B*.
2. What types of prostheses are these two patients wearing?

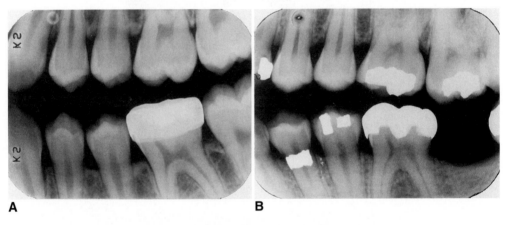

FIGURE **2-22**
1. Compare and contrast the restorative materials for the lower 1st molars in patients *A* and *B*.
2. Which one has the amalgam tattoo?

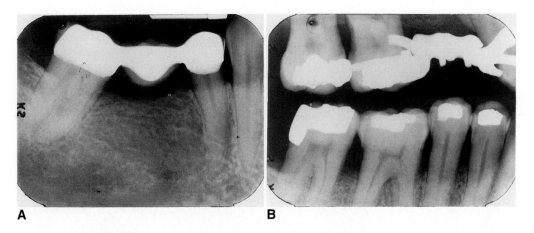

A   B

FIGURE **2-23**

1. Compare and contrast the two prostheses seen in patients *A* and *B*.

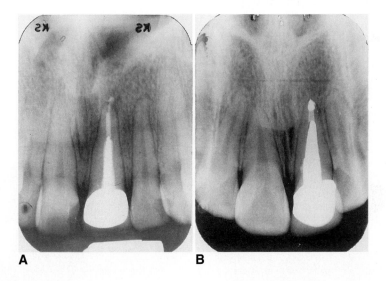

A   B

FIGURE **2-24**

1. Compare and contrast the restorative materials in the left central incisors of patients *A* and *B*.

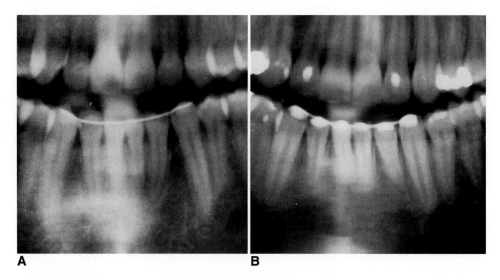

FIGURE **2-25** Patients *A* and *B* both have had orthodontic treatment.
1. What orthodontic appliance does each have?
2. Compare and contrast the two appliances.

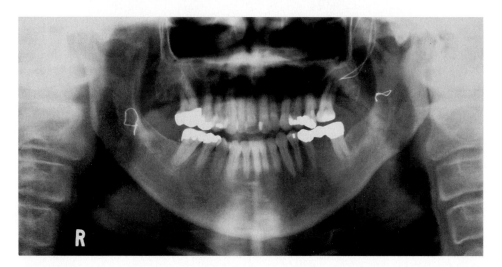

FIGURE **2-26**
1. List the restorative materials and types of restorations in this patient.
2. What else do you see? Explain.

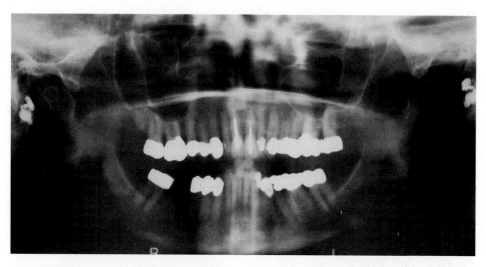

FIGURE **2-27** This is one time you will not need to look at the dental materials or even the jawbones.

1. What else can you see?

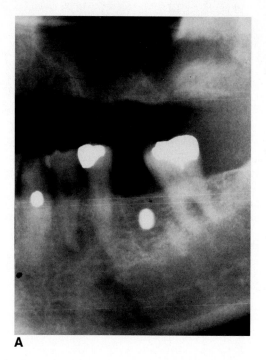

A

FIGURE **2-28** Here's the history of this case: part *A*, the panoramic radiograph, was taken first.

Continued

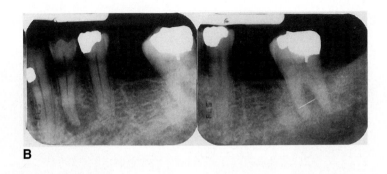

B

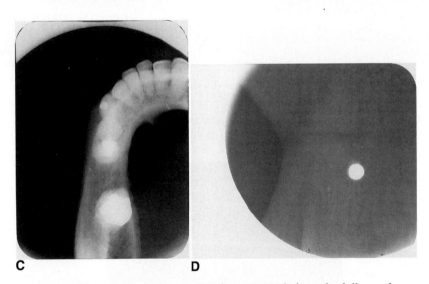

C   D

FIGURE **2-28 cont'd** On the same day part *B*, the periapicals from the full mouth survey, also taken that day, revealed a mystery. To solve the mystery, part *C*, the occlusal, was taken but with no further solution to the mystery. Finally, part *D* was taken and the mystery was solved. Now you also will have a chance to solve the mystery.

1. Part *D* is a radiograph of what area? How was this taken?
2. What is the solution to the mystery, and what and where is the foreign object seen in *A* and *D*?

Chapter 3

Intraoral Radiography: Clinical Technique

Goals

To become familiar with intraoral radiography equipment and supplies
To recognize and correct intraoral technique errors before exposing the radiograph

Learning Objectives

1. Recognize the parts of the x-ray machine
2. Be familiar with the machine controls
3. Understand how to use an exposure chart
4. Know about film and film packets
5. Recognize different film mounts
6. Understand basic patient and operator protection
7. Recognize which patient items must be removed
8. Identify errors in setting up the bite-block, film, and positioning ring
9. Recognize film-handling errors
10. Identify beam alignment problems

Instructions

Look at each figure and answer the following questions regarding intraoral clinical technique with a short answer.

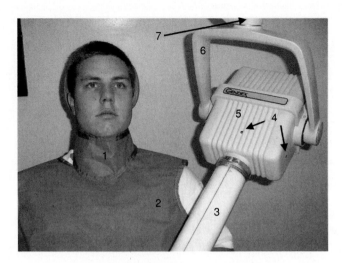

FIGURE **3-1** Name the labeled items.

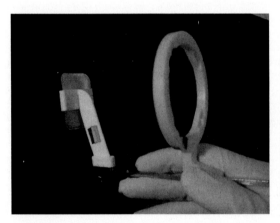

FIGURE **3-2**
1. Name this instrument.
2. For exactly what purpose is it used?
3. What error has occurred in this setup?

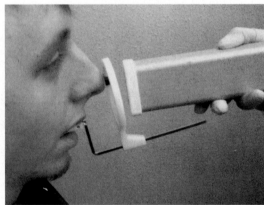

FIGURE **3-3** Here we see the XCP instrument in use.
1. Which teeth are being radiographed?
2. What type of BID is in use?
3. What error is about to happen?
4. What will this do to the image of the teeth?

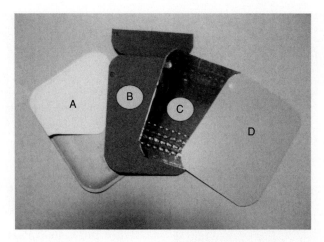

FIGURE **3-4** This picture demonstrates the contents of an intraoral film packet.
1. Name the labeled items.
2. From front to back, in which order are the items found in the packet?

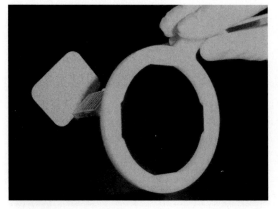

FIGURE **3-5**
1. What is wrong with this setup?

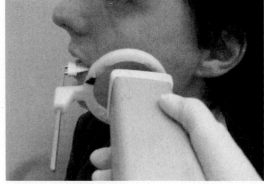

FIGURE **3-6**
1. What type of intraoral radiograph is being taken?
2. What error is occurring?
3. What will this look like on the radiograph?

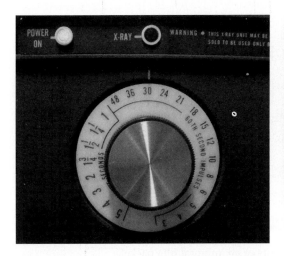

FIGURE **3-7** This is a part of the control panel of the x-ray machine. List what part(s) or function(s) can be seen in this photo.

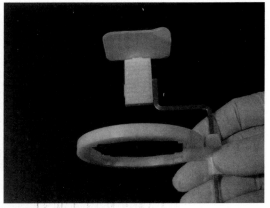

FIGURE **3-8** This is an XCP setup.
1. For exactly which quadrants is it set up?
2. What size of film is being used?
3. What (if any) error has occurred in this setup?
4. How will this appear in the processed image?
5. When using an automatic processor, what can happen to this film?

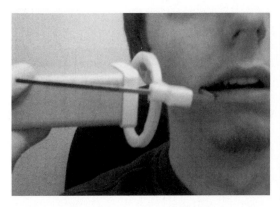

FIGURE **3-9** A posterior intraoral radiograph is being taken on this patient.
1. Which posterior quadrant is being radiographed?
2. What error is occurring?
3. How will this appear in the processed image?
4. In what situations is it important to avoid this error?
5. In what situations (if ever) is this error desirable?

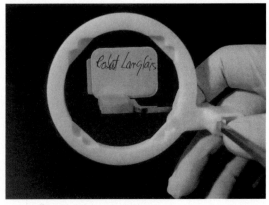

FIGURE **3-10** Here you can see a setup with a ring-positioning instrument.
1. For what technique (paralleling or bisecting angle) is this setup being used?
2. For what posterior quadrants is the instrument setup?
3. What error(s) do you see here?
4. What will this look like in the processed radiograph?

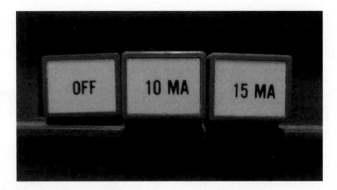

FIGURE **3-11** Here we see a portion of the control panel of an x-ray machine. List and explain the functions of these controls.

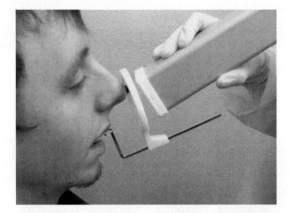

FIGURE **3-12** Here you can see that the anterior maxillary central incisors are being radiographed.
1. What error is occurring?
2. What will this look like in the processed radiograph?

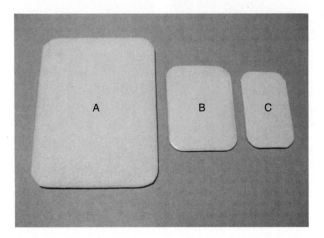

FIGURE **3-13** Here we see three commonly used film sizes designed for use primarily in adults.
1. Name the sizes of film depicted in this photograph.
2. Specify what each size is used for.

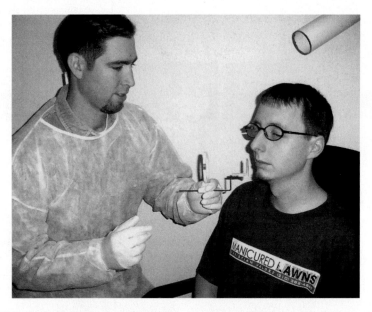

FIGURE **3-14** Here we see one or more errors about to happen. Name the error(s).

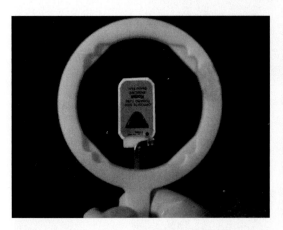

FIGURE **3-15** This is a setup for the XCP paralleling instrument.
1. For what teeth is this setup?
2. What error has occurred?
3. How will this look on the processed radiograph?
4. If the image can be seen, should this film be retained or retaken? Explain why.

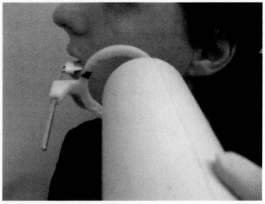

FIGURE **3-16**
1. Uh-oh! An error is in progress! Can you identify the error?

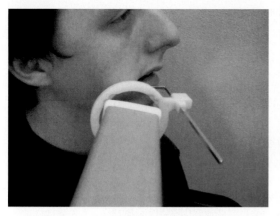

FIGURE **3-17** Here we see a lower right posterior periapical radiograph about to be taken.
1. What error has occurred?
2. How will this appear on the processed radiograph?

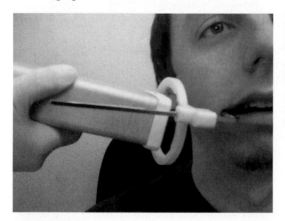

FIGURE **3-19** Here we see the maxillary right posterior quadrant being set up for an exposure.
1. What error is about to happen?
2. What will it look like in the processed radiograph?

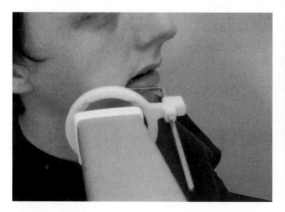

FIGURE **3-21** Here we see a lower posterior periapical radiograph about to be taken.
1. What error is about to occur?
2. Describe what would be seen on the processed radiograph.

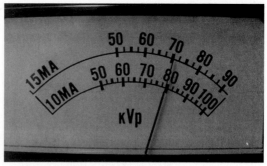

FIGURE **3-18** What part of the control panel are we looking at here? Explain.

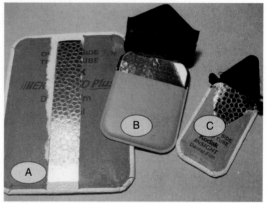

FIGURE **3-20** Here we are looking at the partially opened film packets of the three most common film sizes used in intraoral radiography.
1. What part of the film packet is immediately behind the back side of the outer envelope?
2. What is the purpose of this item?
3. How would you describe the three embossed patterns seen in the item?

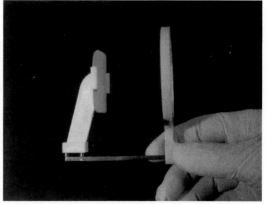

FIGURE **3-22** This is an incorrect bitewing setup.
1. What is wrong here?
2. What phrase can be used to help remember the correct bitewing setup when viewing the XCP instrument from this angle?

Exposure Chart 3rd Floor, **Cubicle 3.**

Film Type: **Speed Group F**
Kilovoltage = **70 kVp;**   Milliamperage = **15 mA**
BID Length = **LONG** Rectangular or Open
Patient ADULT: **Average** = 120 to 170 lbs.

Max. & Mand.	Adult	Pedo
		(includes erupted 1ˢᵗ perm.
Anterior:	18 imp	15 imp
Premolar:	24 imp	18 imp
Molar:	30 imp	

FIGURE **3-23** This is an actual exposure chart. Use the chart to answer the questions regarding how you will adjust the machine settings (Part 1).

1. What BID length is specified?
2. What is the mA setting?
3. Will the settings be okay for an adult weighing 150 pounds?
4. What speed of intraoral film must we use for these settings?
5. What should we set the kVp at?
6. What will the exposure time be for the maxillary anterior periapicals?

Now you must do a little bit of thinking to answer these more difficult questions about this exposure chart (Part 2). Assume the patient is an average adult unless otherwise specified and that all exposure factors are to remain the same as specified on the chart except those needing modification to answer the questions.

1. If you wanted to use a short, 8-inch BID, what would the exposure time be for a premolar periapical radiograph?
2. If the patient weighs 200 pounds, what exposure time would you use for the premolar periapicals? (Select from the settings on the chart.)
3. If you have only "D" speed film available, what exposure time would you use for a child with erupted 1st permanent molars for a periapical radiograph of the maxillary anterior region. (Select one of the exposure times from the chart.)
4. Let's say you wished to use 10 mA for a molar periapical radiograph. How many impulses would you need to use? Explain.
5. If you are directed to use 85 kVp for a molar periapical view in a 165-pound adult, how many impulses would you have to reset the timer to? Explain. (Select from any of the settings on the chart.)
6. If you wanted to use the fastest available speed of intraoral film, what (if any) modifications would you make to the exposure times on this chart?
7. Say you wanted to switch from a long, 16-inch, round, open-ended cone to a long, 16-inch, rectangular cone, what modifications (if any) would you need to make to this exposure chart?
8. If the patient is a small adult weighing 100 pounds, what exposure time would you use for the molar periapicals? (Select from the settings on the chart.)
9. If 1 impulse is 1/60 of a second, what fraction of a second is an exposure time of 30 impulses?
10. Someone indicates you must use an exposure time of three fourths of a second (3/4 sec), but the timer settings are in impulses; so how many impulses will you set the timer to?

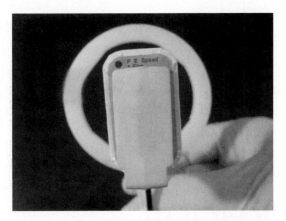

FIGURE **3-24** Note the view of the operator as she studies this XCP setup.
1. What is wrong with this anterior periapical setup?
2. What will it look like in the processed radiograph?

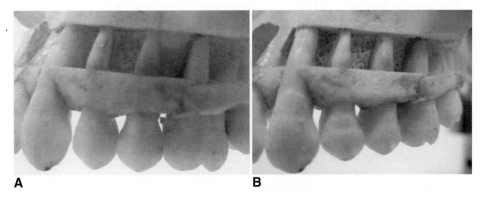

A   **B**

FIGURE **3-25** Study carefully parts *A* and *B* of this picture. Answer the following questions:
1. Which periapical region does this represent?
2. Using the chart in Figure 3-23, what would the exposure time be for cubicle 3 on the 3rd floor?
3. Which view represents an error in positioning the BID?
4. What BID positioning error is pictured?

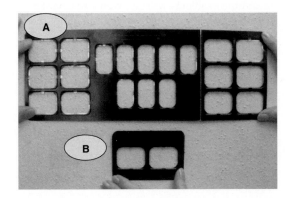

FIGURE **3-26** We see two items in this photograph.
1. What is item *A* called?
2. What is item *B* called?
3. What film numbers (how many of each) and sizes are used in item *A*?

Chapter 4

Intraoral Radiography: Errors Seen in Radiographs

Goals

To understand intraoral technique errors as seen in radiographs
To understand darkroom and film-processing problems

Learning Objectives

1. Recognize items needing to be removed
2. Identify exposure problems
3. Know film-handling errors
4. Understand beam-alignment problems
5. Troubleshoot film-placement problems
6. Recognize patient-related problems
7. Know how to correct intraoral technique errors
8. Recognize safe lighting problems
9. Identify manual processing errors
10. Learn to troubleshoot automatic processor troubles
11. Know how to correct darkroom and processing problems

BASIC CONCEPTS

Refer to the following tables in the Answer Key: Table 4-1 (*Intraoral Projection or Technique Errors*), Table 4-2 (*Intraoral Exposure and Manual Processing Errors*), and Table 4-3 (*Automatic Processor Troubleshooting Guide*).

Although digital imaging is here to stay, digital exposure errors are pretty much the same as those in radiographic imaging. However, there are some differences. Digital imaging also gives rise to problems unique to the new technology. Digital imag-

ing and the problems will be covered in Chapter 5. There is one certainty with digital imaging: there are no darkroom (processing) problems! It is estimated that some 7% to 15% of dental offices in the USA use digital imaging in 2004.

Instructions

Identify the errors found in each image. In some questions, you are asked to explain how to correct the error or why the error occurred.

TECHNIQUE ERRORS IN ADULT DENTATE PATIENTS

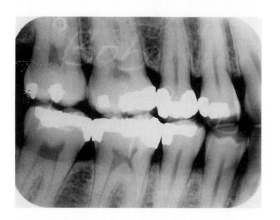

FIGURE **4-1** It looks like ole Bob got a radiograph taken.
1. What happened here?

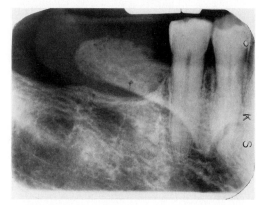

FIGURE **4-2** Here we see a bone not usually found in intraoral images.
1. What happened here?
2. What term describes this situation?

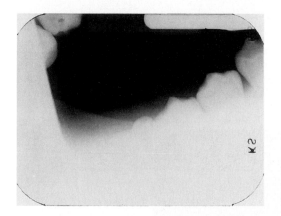

FIGURE **4-3** Note the partial image of the teeth.
1. What technique error was made here?

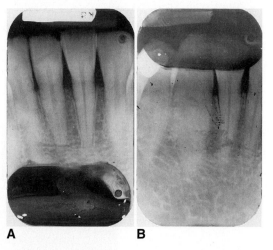

A   B

FIGURE **4-4** These two films (A and B) were part of a full-mouth survey developed in an automatic processor.
1. What happened to these two films?
2. How can this be corrected?

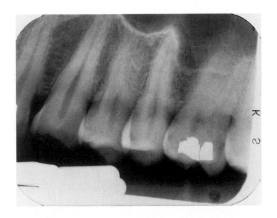

FIGURE **4-5**
1. Why do the 1st premolar roots appear "fuzzed out"?
2. When may this error be used to advantage?

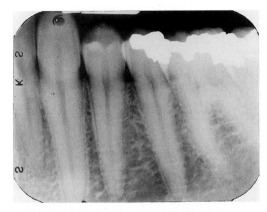

FIGURE **4-6**
1. Would you call this an acceptable premolar periapical radiograph?
2. In any case, how could you increase the area of periapical coverage?

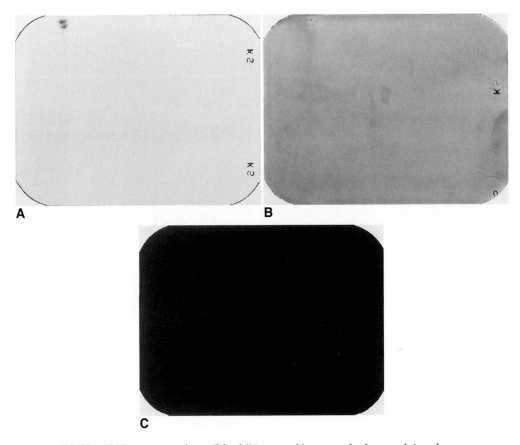

A

B

C

FIGURE **4-7** Here we see three "blank" images. You are asked to explain why...
1. Image *A* is completely clear.
2. Image *B* is somewhat grayish.
3. Image *C* is completely black.

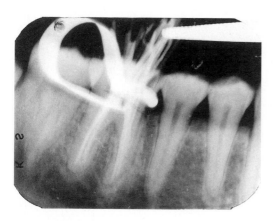

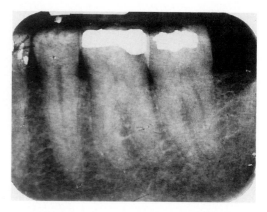

FIGURE **4-8** There is a certain "fuzziness" to this image.
1. What exposure error(s) was (were) made here. List several possibilities if you are unsure exactly what happened.

FIGURE **4-9** This was the student's first opportunity to process a film. She was a little excited and nervous. This film was fed into the automatic processor; the student waited and waited but to no avail. The film just was not coming out. The processor was turned off and opened, and the roller sections were removed. The "lost" film was found in the bottom of the processor.
1. How would you describe the overall appearance of this film?
2. What do you think happened?

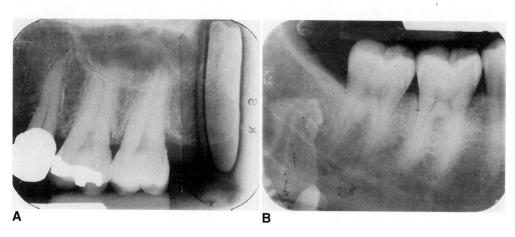

A   B

FIGURE **4-10** Radiographs *A* and *B* each have a different processing solution stain that can be seen.
1. What processing solution produced the dark, radiolucent stain?
2. What processing solution caused the whitish, radiopaque stain?

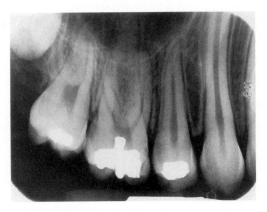

FIGURE **4-11**
1. What film-handling error was made here?

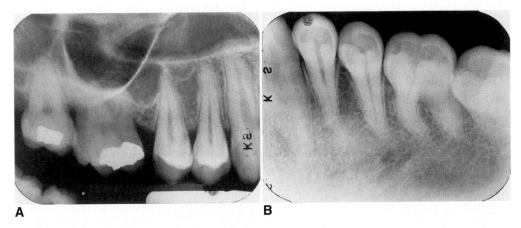

A   B

FIGURE **4-12** In images *A* and *B,* the same exposure error was made. Part *A* represents the maxillary posterior region and *B* the mandibular posterior area.
1. State what error was made.
2. What features in *A* and *B* allow you to identify the error?
3. In some situations could this error be used to advantage or on purpose?

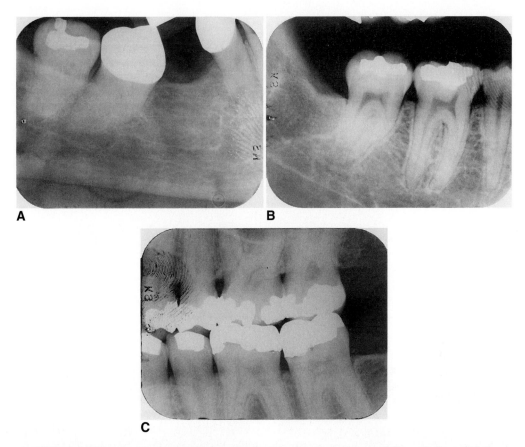

A

B

C

FIGURE **4-13** Sloppy film handling has resulted in chemical stains on films *A, B,* and *C.* In each case, contaminated fingers marred the films.
1. Which one of three different chemicals produced each of the errors?

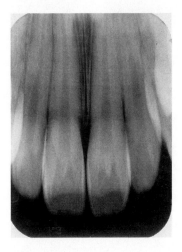

FIGURE **4-14**
1. What term best describes what has happened to these teeth?
2. Explain how this occurred.

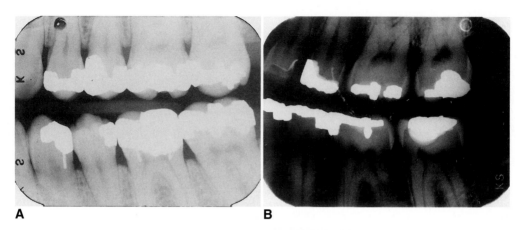

A   **B**

FIGURE **4-15** These are two bitewing radiographs. Example *A* is too light, and the other is too dark.
1. List some reasons film *A* is too light.
2. List some reasons film *B* is too dark.

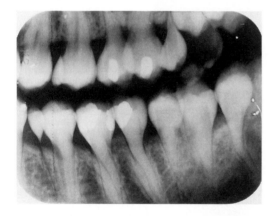

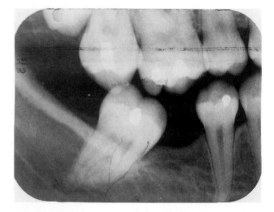

FIGURE **4-16** Strange looking teeth...
1. What exposure error was made here?

FIGURE **4-17** This radiograph was processed in an automatic processor in Alaska during the coldest part of winter.
1. List two processing errors seen here.
2. Explain how each can be corrected.

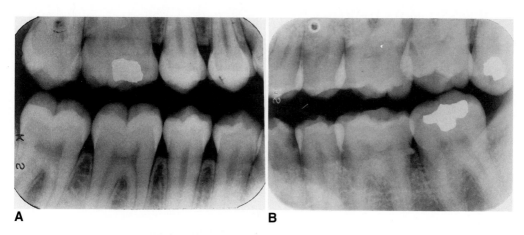

A   B

FIGURE **4-18** Here are two bitewings: *A* (premolar) and *B* (molar).
1. What is wrong with bitewing *A*?
2. What is wrong with bitewing *B*?
3. Which (if any) need(s) retaking?

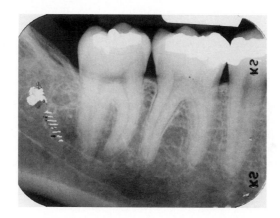

FIGURE **4-19**
1. What film-handling error produced this radiopaque artifact distal to the 2nd molar?

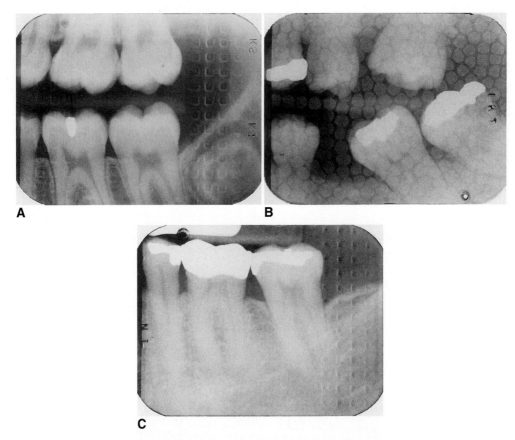

FIGURE **4-20** Examples *A, B,* and *C* have all occurred as a result of the same error.
1. What error has occurred here?
2. Example *C* (and possibly the others) seems quite readable. Why is it better to retake all three of these radiographs?
3. Notice the patterns are a bit different from each other. Could this have to do with film type?

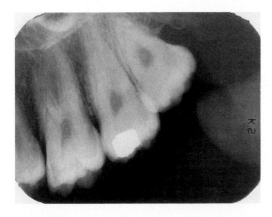

FIGURE **4-21**
1. Why was the apical region of the 2nd and 3rd maxillary molars missed?
2. What is the radiopaque object with the embossed KS mark superimposed?

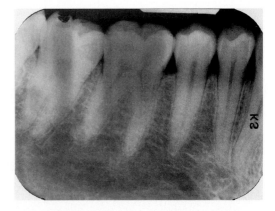

FIGURE **4-22** Clinically this radiograph looked a little greenish and lacked translucency.
1. What processing error was made?

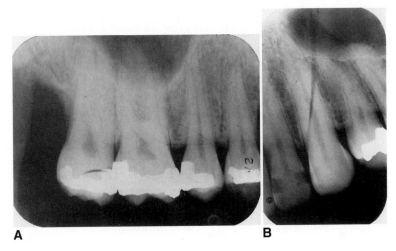

FIGURE **4-31** Examples *A* and *B* have a similar but not identical error. Both are the result of mishandling the film.

1. State what errors you are being asked to identify.

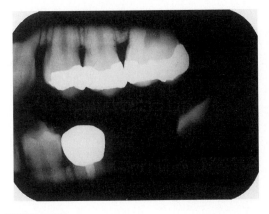

FIGURE **4-32**

1. What happened to this radiograph?

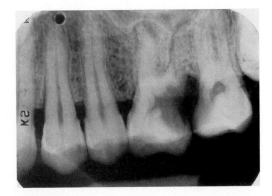

FIGURE **4-33** This film involves inadequate apical coverage in general and specifically at the apex of the 1st premolar.

1. In general, how could you increase the apical coverage?
2. What happened at the apex of the 1st premolar?

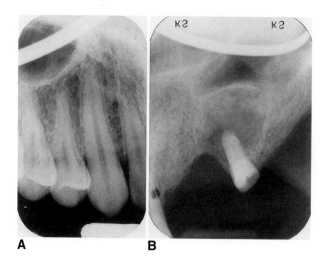

A   B

FIGURE **4-29** In examples *A* and *B,* one error is common to both images and involves some sort of foreign body or material. Both *A* and *B* are views of just about the same anatomic region though the film size is different.

1. State what error has occurred.
2. From what material(s) is the foreign object made?
3. What film sizes do we see here?

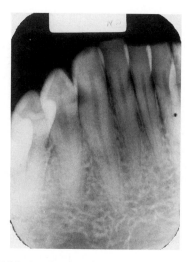

FIGURE **4-30** Notice the distal of the mandibular canine.

1. What error does the radiolucent area represent?
2. Why would you not think it is caries?
3. Would you repeat this view?

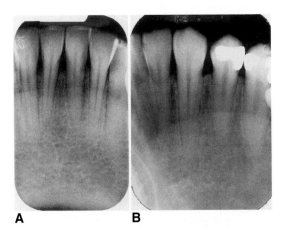

A   B

FIGURE **4-26** This patient was really cooperative though the bite-block was uncomfortable when she bit down.
1. What error occurred in both examples *A* and *B*?
2. What further error occurred in example *B*?

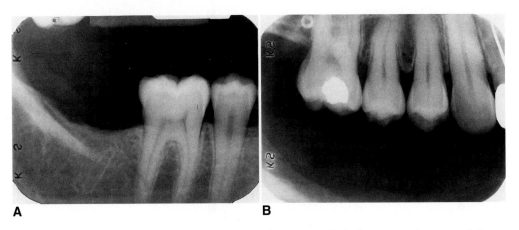

A   B

FIGURE **4-27** In examples *A* and *B* we see inadequate periapical coverage because of the exact same error.
1. What error occurred here?

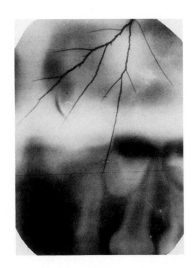

FIGURE **4-28** Okay. You asked for it, and here it is...but look closely because there may be more than one problem!
1. What problems do you see? Ignore the background image quality.

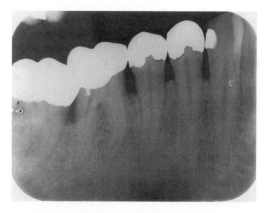

FIGURE **4-23** This is a fogged film.
1. List possible reasons for this problem.

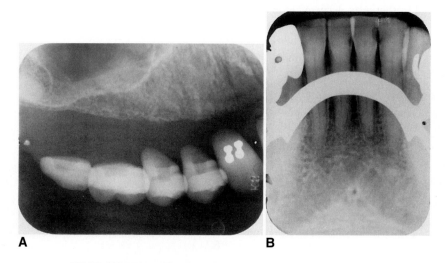

A   **B**

FIGURE **4-24** From the "stuff left in or on" department:
1. What happened here?
2. Do both examples *A* and *B* represent technique errors?

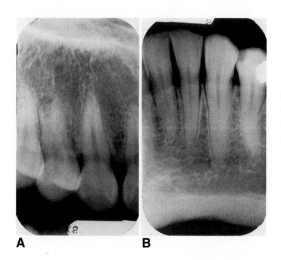

FIGURE **4-25** Examples *A* (maxillary canine) and *B* (mandibular canine) both illustrate the same two errors.
1. Name the two errors.

A   **B**

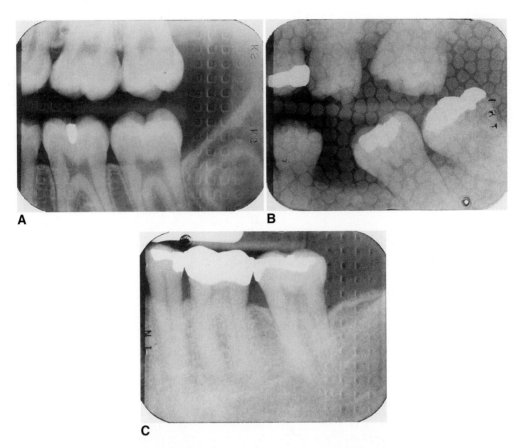

A B

C

FIGURE **4-20** Examples *A*, *B*, and *C* have all occurred as a result of the same error.
1. What error has occurred here?
2. Example *C* (and possibly the others) seems quite readable. Why is it better to retake all three of these radiographs?
3. Notice the patterns are a bit different from each other. Could this have to do with film type?

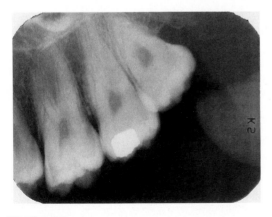

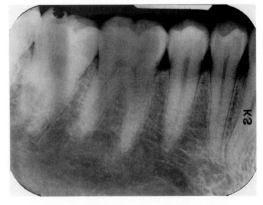

FIGURE **4-21**
1. Why was the apical region of the 2nd and 3rd maxillary molars missed?
2. What is the radiopaque object with the embossed KS mark superimposed?

FIGURE **4-22** Clinically this radiograph looked a little greenish and lacked translucency.
1. What processing error was made?

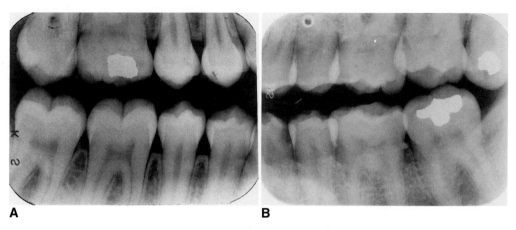

A   **B**

FIGURE **4-18** Here are two bitewings: *A* (premolar) and *B* (molar).
1. What is wrong with bitewing *A*?
2. What is wrong with bitewing *B*?
3. Which (if any) need(s) retaking?

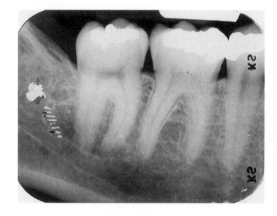

FIGURE **4-19**
1. What film-handling error produced this radiopaque artifact distal to the 2nd molar?

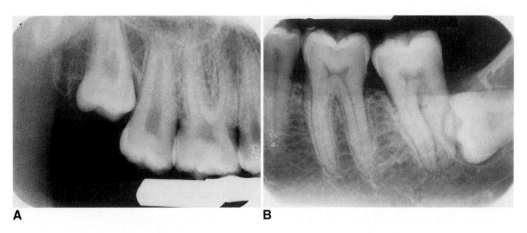

A   **B**

FIGURE **4-34** Both of these 3rd molars lack apical coverage.
1. In examples *A* and *B*, what could you do to correct this?

TECHNIQUE ERRORS IN ADULT EDENTULOUS PATIENTS

NOTE: This short section may also serve as a review because many of the errors are repeated for these edentulous patients.

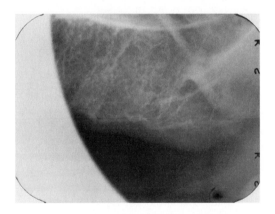

FIGURE **4-35** What error(s) occurred here?

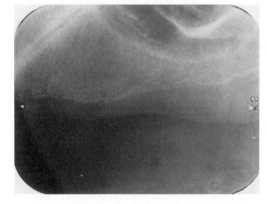

FIGURE **4-36** What error(s) occurred here?

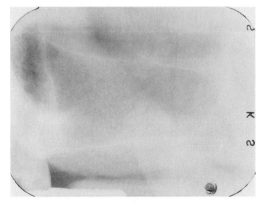

FIGURE **4-37** What error(s) occurred here?

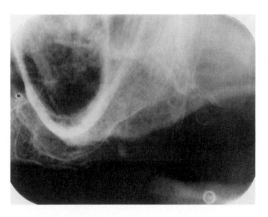

FIGURE **4-38** What error(s) occurred here?

TECHNIQUE ERRORS IN CHILDREN

NOTE: This short section will serve to introduce several new errors.

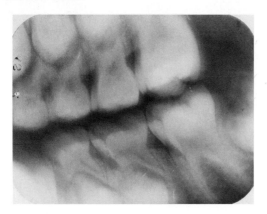

FIGURE **4-39** What error(s) occurred here?

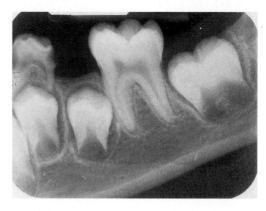

FIGURE **4-40** What error(s) occurred here?

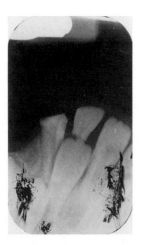

FIGURE **4-41** What error(s) occurred here?

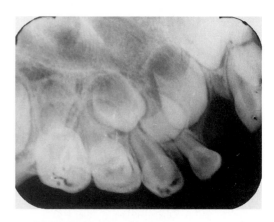

FIGURE **4-42** What error(s) occurred here?

Intraoral Digital Imaging

Goals

To understand digital image acquisition
To understand the basics of intraoral digital image processing

Learning Objectives

1. Explain basic sensor differences
2. Recognize clinical technique errors in digital image acquisition procedures
3. Know how to use ring locator devices with sensors
4. Learn how PSP scanners are used
5. Explain PSP erasure procedures
6. Identify various digital image processing tools
7. Recognize the effects of image processing on the original image
8. Analyze digital image acquisition and processing errors

Instructions

Review each image, and answer the following questions accordingly. Before proceeding with the questions, carefully read the introductory information on digital imaging. This consists of a minimum of information on digital imaging after which the student may be able to either answer the question or refer back to the introductory information to find the answer. If that fails, the student may then go to the Answer Key and read the answer. Textbooks are only beginning to include information on digital imaging. However, students should expect to see more and more of the national examinations and state certifying tests with questions on this subject matter.

BASIC CONCEPTS

1. **The computer:** A computer with digital imaging software is needed. Its function is to receive and view the digital image, identify the image as to orientation and patient/date data, process the image if needed, store the image, and transmit the image to other offices or third party payers. Safeguards must be in place to protect the patient's privacy as outlined by the Health Insurance Portability and Accountability Act (HIPAA) law that came into effect April 14, 2003. The computer can be a laptop, a wall-mounted type, a display-only monitor connected to a computer by a wire or wireless networking, or a full computer setup in the treatment room. To get a fast, flawless imaging setup, the computer will need at least 512 megs of RAM (random access memory) and a fast processor with 2.5 gigahertz (GHz) speed, as well as adequate temporary storage in the 80 gigabyte (GB) range. Further high capacity hard drive storage and a server will be needed for later storage, archiving, and retrieval of the images.

2. **The sensor:** Sensors are either wired or not wired. The wired type can be a CCD (charge coupled device) or a CMOS (complementary metal oxide sensor), which transfers the image instantaneously to the computer at the moment of image acquisition (analogous to exposing the film and developing it). The CMOS type is now available in a wireless format. The film-like wireless type is called the *PSP (photostimulable phosphor)* plate. The exposed plate or sensor (looks a lot like a piece of film) must then be scanned in a laser scanner, which then transfers the image into the computer.
3. **The scanner:** A laser scanner is needed only for PSP-type sensors. There are currently three brands: DenOptix, Digora, and Scan-x. The Scan-x scanner has significantly faster scanning times.
4. **The imaging software:** Once the image is in the computer, the software allows the user to process the image. This means the original image can be altered. For security, most software systems do not allow the user to process the original image so it can be later retrieved if needed by third parties such as insurance carriers or courts of law.
5. **Image processing:** The original image can be copied then altered by processing to enhance its appearance for diagnostics or to highlight a feature for patient education. Some basic processing options (algorithms) include: rotate or flip the image to get it properly oriented on the computer screen because the sensor cannot distinguish left, right, up, or down; lighten/darken the image (histogram shift); change the contrast (histogram stretch); use filters to sharpen the image, smooth edges, or remove noise; zoom, which magnifies a selected area; reverse the image so that it looks like a negative (everything black becomes white, and the whites become black) (histogram reverse); emboss, which produces a 3-D–like look; colorize all or a portion (e.g., a carious lesion or the inferior alveolar canal); and many other options, including some of those just mentioned that are known by different terms to make the individual brands appear different or unique.
6. **Image characteristics:**
   - **Spatial resolution** is really how clean and sharp the image is. It is a function of having small pixels in the 20- to 40-micron size and lots of them (megapixels). Spatial resolution is expressed in line pairs per millimeter (lp/mm). Digital intraoral x-ray systems are capable of image resolution in excess of 20 lp/mm. The human eye can discern somewhere between 12 and 14 lp/mm. Most intraoral films are in the 11- to 12-lp/mm range. Most high-definition monitors are limited to 8 to 10 lp/mm. Most software systems keep only the best 8 lp/mm. The more lp/mm, the greater is the need for storage room. Resolution is limited to the lowest common denominator in the system; thus a system of 8 to 10 lp/mm represents the most current practical system.
   - **Gray scale resolution** is how many shades of gray are in the image; also known as *contrast or bit depth.* The imaging system is capable of capturing and separating literally thousands of shades of gray. Contrast is expressed in bits. A 1-bit image has only 2 shades (pure black and white—the darkest and lightest shades of gray in the imaging scale) and is expressed as "1 to the power of 1." A 2-bit image is expressed as "1 to the power of 2," or $1 \times 2 = 2 \times 2 = 4$ shades of gray. A 3-bit image has 8 shades of gray, or $1 \times 2 = 2 \times 2 = 4 \times 2 = 8$. A 4-bit image has 16 shades of gray, and so on. In an 8-bit image, there are 256 shades of gray and this is the standard. However, systems capable of up to 12 bits or 4098 shades of gray presently exist. The more bits in the image, the greater are the storage needs for the images. The human eye of the person in the street can commonly separate 16 shades of gray, a photographer or radiologist can separate about 25 shades of gray, and under laboratory conditions the maximum for the unaided eye to separate is somewhere around 64 shades of gray. The image itself usually does not occupy the entire gray scale as can be seen by viewing the histogram. The image may be confined to about 30 shades of gray. For best results it is desirable to have a system capable of at least 256 shades of gray. This way there is space on the scale to lighten or darken the image (histogram shift) or spread the shades of gray over a bigger part of the scale (histogram stretch). Remember, 8 bits or 256 shades of gray represents the limit of most monitors.
7. **Image viewing:** The image can be viewed on a monitor, printed on photo quality paper, or printed on a film-like acetate sheet.
8. **Sensor reuse:** All sensor types can be reused almost indefinitely. However, the PSP types need to be "erased" by exposing them to a bright light for a few minutes before reuse.
9. **X-ray equipment:** Because of the shorter exposure times needed in digital imaging, the constant potential DC-type x-ray machine with exposure increments in 1/100 seconds is the most desirable. PSP sensors are the most adaptable to older AC machine designs because they are not very sensitive to exposure variations. CCD and CMOS sensors can also be used; however, noise from too

little exposure and blooming from too much exposure will be more prone to occur as timer increments will be in impulses at 60 impulses per second. Sometimes the first 1 to 3 impulses produce varying amounts of radiation, especially in older machines, and older machines cannot have an exposure time in increments of less than 1/60 of a second.

10. **The next generation:** *You saw it here first.* There will be more use of wireless CCD or CMOS sensors that are currently on the market. These were first developed in Israel for gastrointestinal imaging with the so-called "pill cam." You will use a lightweight, hand-held, miniature x-ray machine configured much like a digital camera. This product is now ready to be marketed. The wireless sensor will send the image to the back of the camera, as with current digital cameras, or to a palm-held computer to see if it is okay. The image will then either be saved in the portable x-ray machine itself or be sent electronically to the palm-held mini-computer currently on the market. At this point and using the wireless network, the image can be downloaded to any of the wall-mounted, flat plasma computer screens, which will also display any photographs and the chart

information, all of which are currently available. Further chart entries will be made by voice recognition software right in the operatory or anywhere else in the office where a microphone pick-up is installed... and of course you knew that. During all phases of treatment, the patient will have in place virtual reality goggles and will be able to choose from menus by locking on to an icon in the screen with the gaze of the retina of the eye; this feature exists right now in some video cameras. In this way, the patient can randomly access HIPAA chart information during treatment, or he or she can tune in to the video camera mounted on the handpiece to watch the procedure; watch a movie, a cartoon, or the news; or simply tune in to the virtual Carnegie Hall and listen to favorite music selections. Just about everything exists now, and it's coming soon to the dental office! Who can be anything but excited about these probabilities! Yep, it's great to be able to see into the future, though such writings may cause the author to be ridiculed and even publicly challenged by more near-sighted colleagues. Oh and by the way... protective aprons and "D" speed film will be a thing of the past!

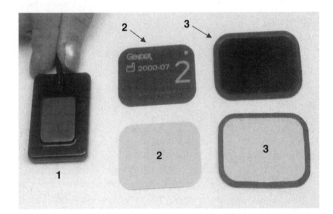

FIGURE **5-1** This illustration shows 3 types of sensors. Number *1* illustrates the back side only; numbers *2* and *3* demonstrate both the front and back sides. Answer the following questions:

1. What basic sensor type does number *1* represent?
2. What basic sensor type do numbers *2* and *3* represent?
3. For numbers *2* and *3*, which side faces the radiation (dark or light side)?
4. What corresponding adult film size do these sensors match?
5. Which sensor(s) will have an image size the same as the corresponding film size?
6. Which sensor(s) is (are) the most susceptible to damage by dropping on floor or disinfection?
7. Which sensor(s) is (are) the most expensive? Name approximate prices.
8. Which sensor(s) produce(s) the fastest image?
9. Which sensor(s) is (are) the most like film with respect to clinical techniques?
10. Which sensor(s) is (are) the most forgiving regarding exposure times?
11. Which sensor(s) has (have) the best resolution?
12. Which sensor(s) require(s) a laser scanner?
13. Which sensor(s) must be erased?

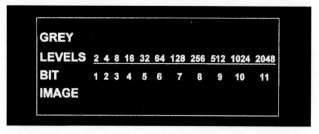

GREY											
LEVELS	2	4	8	16	32	64	128	256	512	1024	2048
BIT	1	2	3	4	5	6	7	8	9	10	11
IMAGE											

FIGURE **5-2** Using the table, answer the following questions:
1. How many gray levels does a 3-bit image have?
2. How many gray levels in a 6-bit image?
3. If 256 gray levels are in the image, how would you express this in bits?
4. How many shades of gray would be in a 13-bit image?
5. In this table, which bit level image would require the most storage space in the computer hard drive?
6. How many bits can the ordinary person distinguish?
7. What is the bit limit of most standard monitors?
8. What type of digital image resolution is illustrated in the table?

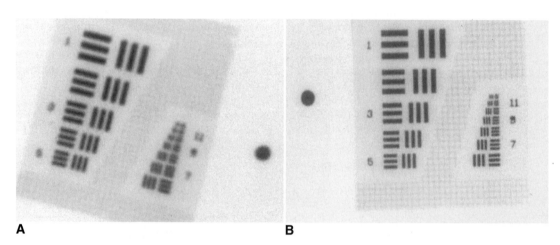

A   **B**

FIGURE **5-3** Images *A* and *B* are the actual line-pair values for an older and a newer x-ray machine, which are otherwise identical. These images were obtained by exposing an occlusal film to a standardized testing/measuring device. We can also use these film images to help to understand line pairs in digital imaging. Number *1* in the images represents 1 lp/mm, 5 equals 5 lp/mm, and so on. In other words, each pair of lines remains separate in horizontal and vertical orientations in 1 mm of space. Therefore 1 lp/mm means one pair of lines are seen as separate images in 1 mm of space, whereas 9 lp/mm means that the equivalent of nine line pairs are squeezed into 1 mm of space and can still be separated as individual lines. These values are standardized much like pounds and ounces of weight or millimeters and meters of distance.

Referring to images *A* and *B*, answer the following questions:
1. Which is the "best" image to your eye just by quickly looking at it?
2. What is the maximum lp/mm capability of the device seen in images *A* and *B*?
3. In digital imaging, what image characteristic are we studying here?
4. What is the resolution of image *A*?
5. What is the resolution of image *B*?
6. Referring back to answer 1, explain why you selected *A* or *B* as the best image.
7. What is the resolving limit of the human eye?
8. What is the resolving limit of the computer monitor?
9. What is this standardized device used for?
10. Back to the x-ray machines, what is the difference between the two machines as tested in *A* and *B*?

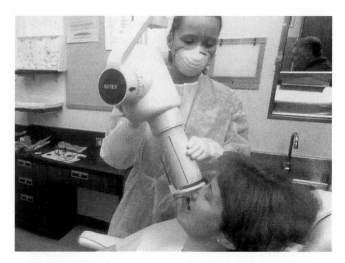

FIGURE **5-4** Here you can see a digital image being taken with a PSP. This is an older Intrex machine, which preceded the current Keystone CDX machine. It is a constant potential machine with a recessed tube head. The timer has been updated.

1. What is the advantage of constant potential machines in general?
2. What was their traditional disadvantage?
3. Why are constant potential machines now most desirable for digital intraoral imaging?
4. How long is the BID of this machine? (8 or 16 inches)
5. Can technique errors such as cone cutting, elongation, foreshortening, improper horizontal angulation, double exposure, no exposure, improper setup of the ring positioning device, and improper sensor placement produce the same effects as for film in digital imaging?
6. Can technique errors such as overexposure, underexposure, leaving film packets exposed to room light, film bending and crimping, scratched emulsion, film reversed, and "dot not in the slot" produce the same effects in digital imaging?
7. Can other errors like fog, chemical spills, depleted developer or fixer, cold solutions, dirty rollers, over-development, or inadequate fixation also occur in digital imaging?
8. Are there unique errors or problems with digital imaging? If so, can you name and describe some?
9. What is the difference between processing film-based x-ray images and processing digital images?
10. How many people are in this picture? What item is not needed in digital imaging?

NOTE TO STUDENTS: You have just gotten through quite a grueling session on digital imaging. You may even have a headache or be tempted to quit and watch a little TV. Take a break, listen to a little music, and come on back. A chocolate snack would be good because it has an excellent taste, makes you feel great, provides energy, and wakes you up (most contain caffeine, which may also ease the headache). Yep, eat chocolate! I promise the rest is a lot easier.

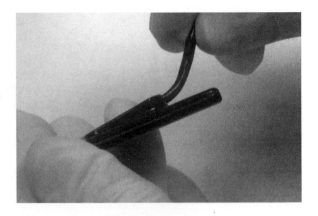

FIGURE **5-5**
1. What basic sensor type do we see here?
2. How is the thickness of this sensor measured?

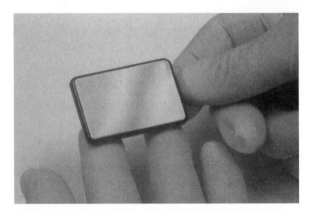

FIGURE **5-6** This is the other side of the sensor seen in Figure *5-5*.
1. Is this the side that captures the image?
2. Does this side go behind the teeth and face the radiation beam?
3. Can this be oriented either vertically or horizontally in the mouth?
4. If this is about the size of a #2 film, how will the size of the two images compare?

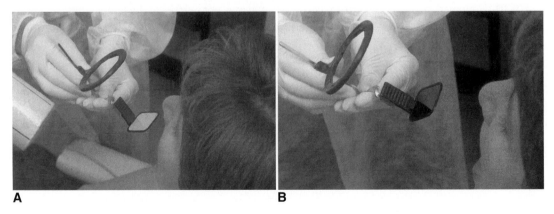

A   B

FIGURE **5-7** Here we see a sensor that has been placed in a ring locator device.
1. What type of sensor do we see here?
2. What brand of sensor is this?
3. Study images *A* and *B*; which demonstrates an error?

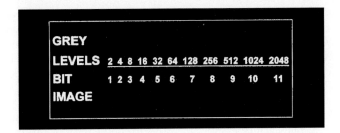

GREY											
LEVELS	2	4	8	16	32	64	128	256	512	1024	2048
BIT	1	2	3	4	5	6	7	8	9	10	11
IMAGE											

FIGURE **5-2** Using the table, answer the following questions:

1. How many gray levels does a 3-bit image have?
2. How many gray levels in a 6-bit image?
3. If 256 gray levels are in the image, how would you express this in bits?
4. How many shades of gray would be in a 13-bit image?
5. In this table, which bit level image would require the most storage space in the computer hard drive?
6. How many bits can the ordinary person distinguish?
7. What is the bit limit of most standard monitors?
8. What type of digital image resolution is illustrated in the table?

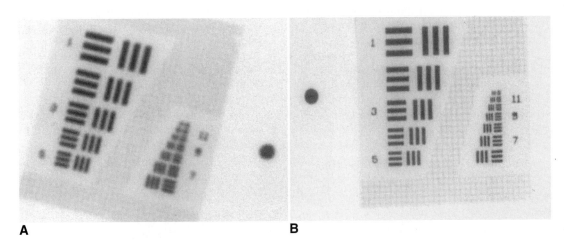

A   B

FIGURE **5-3** Images *A* and *B* are the actual line-pair values for an older and a newer x-ray machine, which are otherwise identical. These images were obtained by exposing an occlusal film to a standardized testing/measuring device. We can also use these film images to help to understand line pairs in digital imaging. Number *1* in the images represents 1 lp/mm, 5 equals 5 lp/mm, and so on. In other words, each pair of lines remains separate in horizontal and vertical orientations in 1 mm of space. Therefore 1 lp/mm means one pair of lines are seen as separate images in 1 mm of space, whereas 9 lp/mm means that the equivalent of nine line pairs are squeezed into 1 mm of space and can still be separated as individual lines. These values are standardized much like pounds and ounces of weight or millimeters and meters of distance.

Referring to images *A* and *B*, answer the following questions:

1. Which is the "best" image to your eye just by quickly looking at it?
2. What is the maximum lp/mm capability of the device seen in images *A* and *B*?
3. In digital imaging, what image characteristic are we studying here?
4. What is the resolution of image *A*?
5. What is the resolution of image *B*?
6. Referring back to answer 1, explain why you selected *A* or *B* as the best image.
7. What is the resolving limit of the human eye?
8. What is the resolving limit of the computer monitor?
9. What is this standardized device used for?
10. Back to the x-ray machines, what is the difference between the two machines as tested in *A* and *B*?

little exposure and blooming from too much exposure will be more prone to occur as timer increments will be in impulses at 60 impulses per second. Sometimes the first 1 to 3 impulses produce varying amounts of radiation, especially in older machines, and older machines cannot have an exposure time in increments of less than 1/60 of a second.

10. **The next generation:** *You saw it here first.* There will be more use of wireless CCD or CMOS sensors that are currently on the market. These were first developed in Israel for gastrointestinal imaging with the so-called "pill cam." You will use a lightweight, hand-held, miniature x-ray machine configured much like a digital camera. This product is now ready to be marketed. The wireless sensor will send the image to the back of the camera, as with current digital cameras, or to a palm-held computer to see if it is okay. The image will then either be saved in the portable x-ray machine itself or be sent electronically to the palm-held mini-computer currently on the market. At this point and using the wireless network, the image can be downloaded to any of the wall-mounted, flat plasma computer screens, which will also display any photographs and the chart information, all of which are currently available. Further chart entries will be made by voice recognition software right in the operatory or anywhere else in the office where a microphone pick-up is installed... and of course you knew that. During all phases of treatment, the patient will have in place virtual reality goggles and will be able to choose from menus by locking on to an icon in the screen with the gaze of the retina of the eye; this feature exists right now in some video cameras. In this way, the patient can randomly access HIPAA chart information during treatment, or he or she can tune in to the video camera mounted on the handpiece to watch the procedure; watch a movie, a cartoon, or the news; or simply tune in to the virtual Carnegie Hall and listen to favorite music selections. Just about everything exists now, and it's coming soon to the dental office! Who can be anything but excited about these probabilities! Yep, it's great to be able to see into the future, though such writings may cause the author to be ridiculed and even publicly challenged by more near-sighted colleagues. Oh and by the way... protective aprons and "D" speed film will be a thing of the past!

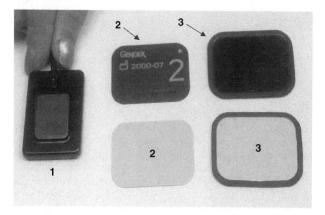

FIGURE **5-1** This illustration shows 3 types of sensors. Number *1* illustrates the back side only; numbers *2* and *3* demonstrate both the front and back sides. Answer the following questions:

1. What basic sensor type does number *1* represent?
2. What basic sensor type do numbers *2* and *3* represent?
3. For numbers *2* and *3*, which side faces the radiation (dark or light side)?
4. What corresponding adult film size do these sensors match?
5. Which sensor(s) will have an image size the same as the corresponding film size?
6. Which sensor(s) is (are) the most susceptible to damage by dropping on floor or disinfection?
7. Which sensor(s) is (are) the most expensive? Name approximate prices.
8. Which sensor(s) produce(s) the fastest image?
9. Which sensor(s) is (are) the most like film with respect to clinical techniques?
10. Which sensor(s) is (are) the most forgiving regarding exposure times?
11. Which sensor(s) has (have) the best resolution?
12. Which sensor(s) require(s) a laser scanner?
13. Which sensor(s) must be erased?

2. **The sensor:** Sensors are either wired or not wired. The wired type can be a CCD (charge coupled device) or a CMOS (complementary metal oxide sensor), which transfers the image instantaneously to the computer at the moment of image acquisition (analogous to exposing the film and developing it). The CMOS type is now available in a wireless format. The film-like wireless type is called the *PSP (photostimulable phosphor)* plate. The exposed plate or sensor (looks a lot like a piece of film) must then be scanned in a laser scanner, which then transfers the image into the computer.

3. **The scanner:** A laser scanner is needed only for PSP-type sensors. There are currently three brands: DenOptix, Digora, and Scan-x. The Scan-x scanner has significantly faster scanning times.

4. **The imaging software:** Once the image is in the computer, the software allows the user to process the image. This means the original image can be altered. For security, most software systems do not allow the user to process the original image so it can be later retrieved if needed by third parties such as insurance carriers or courts of law.

5. **Image processing:** The original image can be copied then altered by processing to enhance its appearance for diagnostics or to highlight a feature for patient education. Some basic processing options (algorithms) include: rotate or flip the image to get it properly oriented on the computer screen because the sensor cannot distinguish left, right, up, or down; lighten/darken the image (histogram shift); change the contrast (histogram stretch); use filters to sharpen the image, smooth edges, or remove noise; zoom, which magnifies a selected area; reverse the image so that it looks like a negative (everything black becomes white, and the whites become black) (histogram reverse); emboss, which produces a 3-D–like look; colorize all or a portion (e.g., a carious lesion or the inferior alveolar canal); and many other options, including some of those just mentioned that are known by different terms to make the individual brands appear different or unique.

6. **Image characteristics:**
   - **Spatial resolution** is really how clean and sharp the image is. It is a function of having small pixels in the 20- to 40-micron size and lots of them (megapixels). Spatial resolution is expressed in line pairs per millimeter (lp/mm). Digital intraoral x-ray systems are capable of image resolution in excess of 20 lp/mm. The human eye can discern somewhere between 12 and 14 lp/mm. Most intraoral films are in the 11- to 12-lp/mm range. Most high-definition monitors are limited to 8 to 10 lp/mm. Most software systems keep only the best 8 lp/mm. The more lp/mm, the greater is the need for storage room. Resolution is limited to the lowest common denominator in the system; thus a system of 8 to 10 lp/mm represents the most current practical system.
   - **Gray scale resolution** is how many shades of gray are in the image; also known as *contrast or bit depth.* The imaging system is capable of capturing and separating literally thousands of shades of gray. Contrast is expressed in bits. A 1-bit image has only 2 shades (pure black and white—the darkest and lightest shades of gray in the imaging scale) and is expressed as "1 to the power of 1." A 2-bit image is expressed as "1 to the power of 2," or $1 \times 2 = 2 \times 2 = 4$ shades of gray. A 3-bit image has 8 shades of gray, or $1 \times 2 = 2 \times 2 = 4 \times 2 = 8$. A 4-bit image has 16 shades of gray, and so on. In an 8-bit image, there are 256 shades of gray and this is the standard. However, systems capable of up to 12 bits or 4098 shades of gray presently exist. The more bits in the image, the greater are the storage needs for the images. The human eye of the person in the street can commonly separate 16 shades of gray, a photographer or radiologist can separate about 25 shades of gray, and under laboratory conditions the maximum for the unaided eye to separate is somewhere around 64 shades of gray. The image itself usually does not occupy the entire gray scale as can be seen by viewing the histogram. The image may be confined to about 30 shades of gray. For best results it is desirable to have a system capable of at least 256 shades of gray. This way there is space on the scale to lighten or darken the image (histogram shift) or spread the shades of gray over a bigger part of the scale (histogram stretch). Remember, 8 bits or 256 shades of gray represents the limit of most monitors.

7. **Image viewing:** The image can be viewed on a monitor, printed on photo quality paper, or printed on a film-like acetate sheet.

8. **Sensor reuse:** All sensor types can be reused almost indefinitely. However, the PSP types need to be "erased" by exposing them to a bright light for a few minutes before reuse.

9. **X-ray equipment:** Because of the shorter exposure times needed in digital imaging, the constant potential DC-type x-ray machine with exposure increments in 1/100 seconds is the most desirable. PSP sensors are the most adaptable to older AC machine designs because they are not very sensitive to exposure variations. CCD and CMOS sensors can also be used; however, noise from too

Intraoral Digital Imaging

Goals

To understand digital image acquisition
To understand the basics of intraoral digital image processing

Learning Objectives

1. Explain basic sensor differences
2. Recognize clinical technique errors in digital image acquisition procedures
3. Know how to use ring locator devices with sensors
4. Learn how PSP scanners are used
5. Explain PSP erasure procedures
6. Identify various digital image processing tools
7. Recognize the effects of image processing on the original image
8. Analyze digital image acquisition and processing errors

Instructions

Review each image, and answer the following questions accordingly. Before proceeding with the questions, carefully read the introductory information on digital imaging. This consists of a minimum of information on digital imaging after which the student may be able to either answer the question or refer back to the introductory information to find the answer. If that fails, the student may then go to the Answer Key and read the answer. Textbooks are only beginning to include information on digital imaging. However, students should expect to see more and more of the national examinations and state certifying tests with questions on this subject matter.

BASIC CONCEPTS

1. **The computer:** A computer with digital imaging software is needed. Its function is to receive and view the digital image, identify the image as to orientation and patient/date data, process the image if needed, store the image, and transmit the image to other offices or third party payers. Safeguards must be in place to protect the patient's privacy as outlined by the Health Insurance Portability and Accountability Act (HIPAA) law that came into effect April 14, 2003. The computer can be a laptop, a wall-mounted type, a display-only monitor connected to a computer by a wire or wireless networking, or a full computer setup in the treatment room. To get a fast, flawless imaging setup, the computer will need at least 512 megs of RAM (random access memory) and a fast processor with 2.5 gigahertz (GHz) speed, as well as adequate temporary storage in the 80 gigabyte (GB) range. Further high capacity hard drive storage and a server will be needed for later storage, archiving, and retrieval of the images.

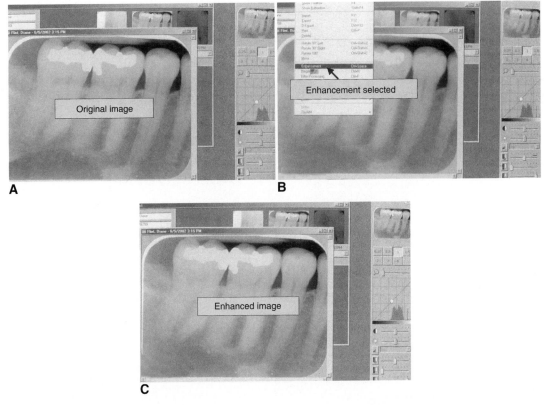

FIGURE **5-16** Here we see three images: *A, B,* and *C. A* is the original image for the beginning of this processing sequence. You can see it is lighter than in Figure 5-15, *A.* By the way, the histogram is the small, twin-peaked, mountain-like graph on the middle far right of the screen. Explain what has happened in images *B* and *C.*

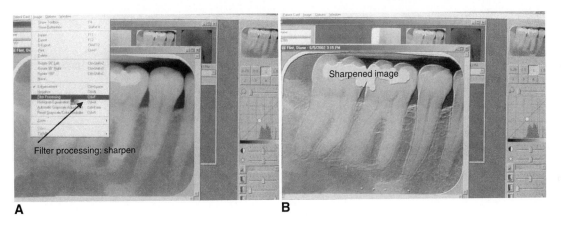

FIGURE **5-17** In image *A* you can see the mildly enhanced image seen in Figure 5-16, *C.* Notice the check mark beside the previous enhancement field in image *A.* Describe what further image processing treatment was done in image *B.*

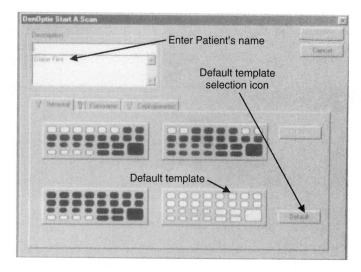

FIGURE **5-14** This is the next DenOptix screen. Explain what must now be done.

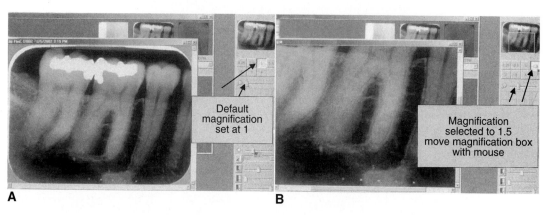

FIGURE **5-15** Here you can see the scanned image. Study images *A* and *B* and try to figure out what was done.

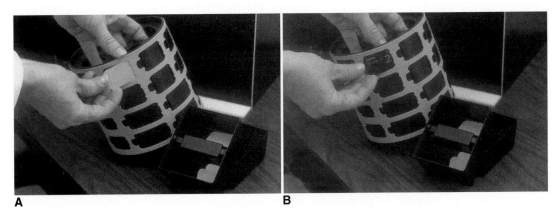

A   B

FIGURE **5-11** Now you can see the DenOptix drum being loaded with the first PSP. The other PSP sensors can be seen in the plastic container that can be divided into contaminated and clean divisions. Study images *A* and *B*. Where is the error being made?

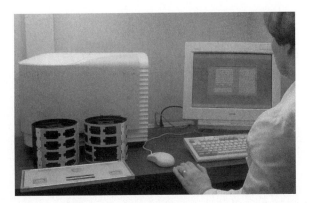

FIGURE **5-12** Here you are looking at a typical DenOptix setup. Try to identify every single item in the picture.

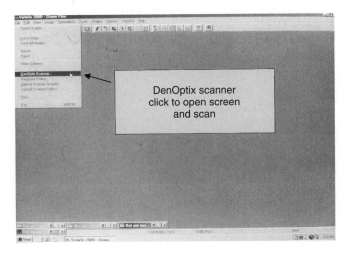

FIGURE **5-13** You have just loaded the drum into the bread box scanner by simply guiding it on the central vertical metal shaft until it reaches the bottom. There is a cover on the top that you open to do this (see Chapter 8). Here you see a close-up picture of the screen on the monitor with a drop box and a highlighted item. Using the information in the picture and, if you were the operator in the picture in Figure 5-12, how would you initiate the scan.

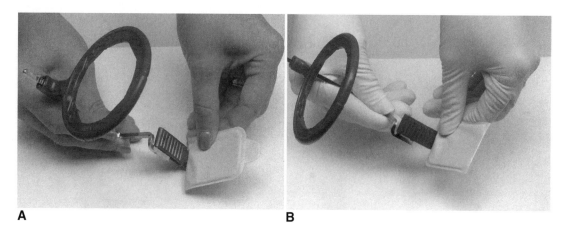

A   B

FIGURE **5-8** Here we see the Digora sensor in the Digora barrier envelope. Study images *A* and *B*; which demonstrates improper technique(s)?

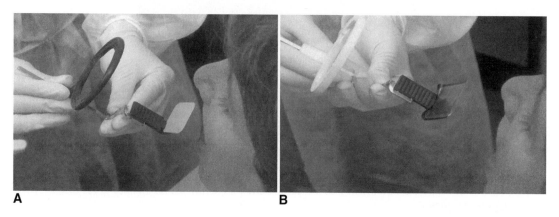

A   B

FIGURE **5-9** Here we see the DenOptix PSP sensor. Study images *A* and *B* carefully and see if you can identify any errors.

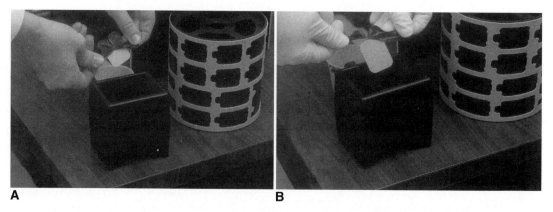

A   B

FIGURE **5-10** Here we see the DenOptix PSP sensor being removed from the barrier envelope after image capture (exposing the sensor in the patient's mouth just like film). This system provides a plastic container into which the PSP is dropped as it is unwrapped. Beside this is the drum for the scanner. Study images *A* and *B*; where is the error being made?

FIGURE **5-5**

1. What basic sensor type do we see here?
2. How is the thickness of this sensor measured?

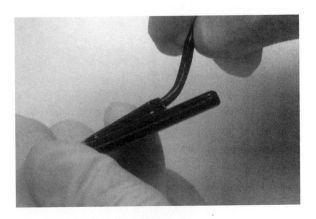

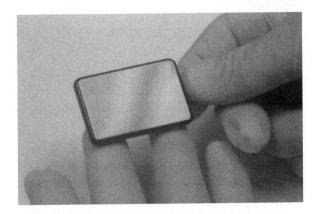

FIGURE **5-6** This is the other side of the sensor seen in Figure *5-5*.

1. Is this the side that captures the image?
2. Does this side go behind the teeth and face the radiation beam?
3. Can this be oriented either vertically or horizontally in the mouth?
4. If this is about the size of a #2 film, how will the size of the two images compare?

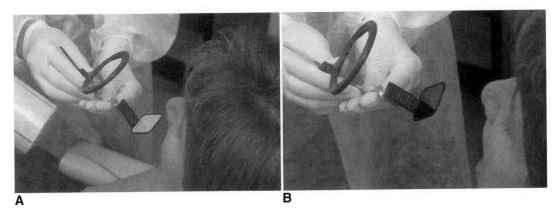

A   **B**

FIGURE **5-7** Here we see a sensor that has been placed in a ring locator device.

1. What type of sensor do we see here?
2. What brand of sensor is this?
3. Study images *A* and *B*; which demonstrates an error?

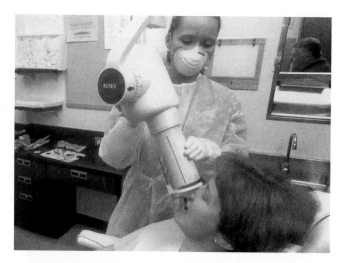

FIGURE **5-4** Here you can see a digital image being taken with a PSP. This is an older Intrex machine, which preceded the current Keystone CDX machine. It is a constant potential machine with a recessed tube head. The timer has been updated.

1. What is the advantage of constant potential machines in general?
2. What was their traditional disadvantage?
3. Why are constant potential machines now most desirable for digital intraoral imaging?
4. How long is the BID of this machine? (8 or 16 inches)
5. Can technique errors such as cone cutting, elongation, foreshortening, improper horizontal angulation, double exposure, no exposure, improper setup of the ring positioning device, and improper sensor placement produce the same effects as for film in digital imaging?
6. Can technique errors such as overexposure, underexposure, leaving film packets exposed to room light, film bending and crimping, scratched emulsion, film reversed, and "dot not in the slot" produce the same effects in digital imaging?
7. Can other errors like fog, chemical spills, depleted developer or fixer, cold solutions, dirty rollers, over-development, or inadequate fixation also occur in digital imaging?
8. Are there unique errors or problems with digital imaging? If so, can you name and describe some?
9. What is the difference between processing film-based x-ray images and processing digital images?
10. How many people are in this picture? What item is not needed in digital imaging?

NOTE TO STUDENTS: You have just gotten through quite a grueling session on digital imaging. You may even have a headache or be tempted to quit and watch a little TV. Take a break, listen to a little music, and come on back. A chocolate snack would be good because it has an excellent taste, makes you feel great, provides energy, and wakes you up (most contain caffeine, which may also ease the headache). Yep, eat chocolate! I promise the rest is a lot easier.

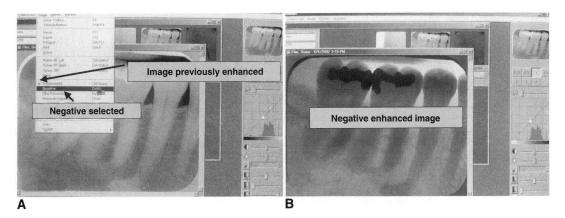

A B

FIGURE **5-18** Here we have gone back to the image before the sharpening. Instead, we want to try the negative image. This time look at the histogram in image *A* and compare it with the histogram in image *B.* What have we done to the image here?

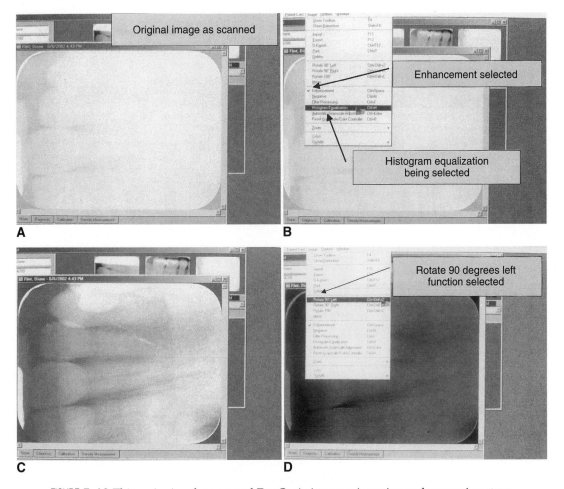

A B

C D

FIGURE **5-19** This series involves several DenOptix image orientation and processing steps. Answer the following questions:

1. This image was captured with a properly oriented PSP sensor with the proper mA, kVp, and exposure time. Why is it so light?
2. In images *A* through *F,* explain what was done. Use all of the information provided.

Continued

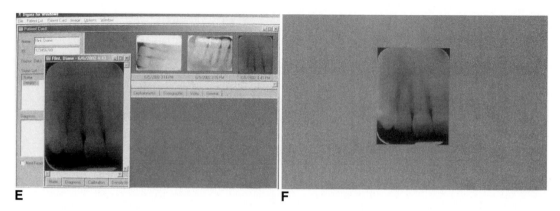

FIGURE **5-19 cont'd**

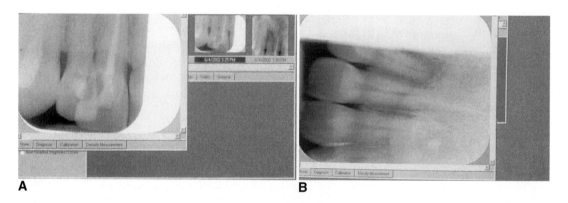

FIGURE **5-20** Compare images *A* and *B*.

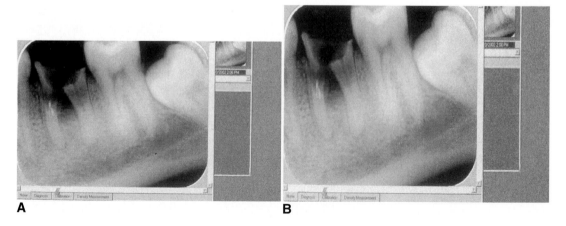

FIGURE **5-21** Compare images *A* and *B*.

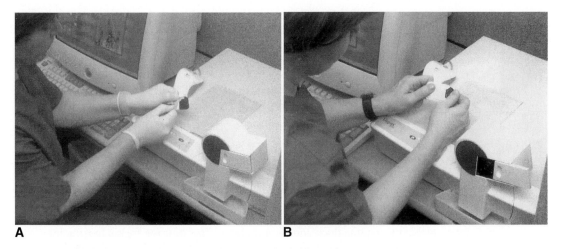

A   B

FIGURE **5-22** Here we see the Digora PSP system. The scanner and loading dock are seen in the right-hand side of the pictures. Study images *A* and *B* and identify the error.

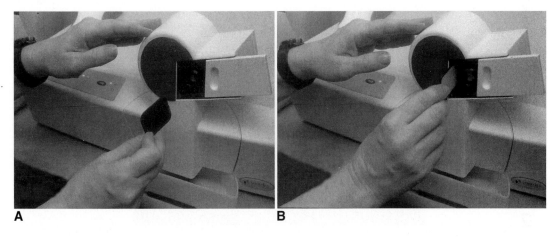

A   B

FIGURE **5-23** The Digora PSP is being inserted into the loading dock. At this stage the gloves should be off and the hands washed. Study images *A* and *B* and identify the error.

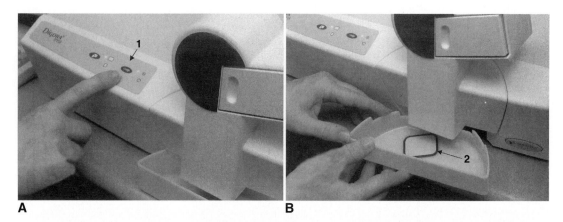

A   B

FIGURE **5-24** Note that the loading dock door is now closed. This time we are not looking for an error. Rather, can you surmise what is happening at *arrow 1* in image *A* and at *arrow 2* in image *B*?

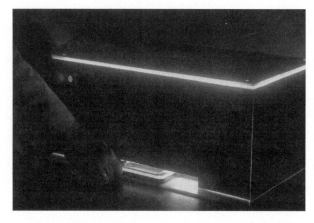

FIGURE **5-25** Here the room lights have been turned off only to demonstrate the procedure more dramatically. Some PSPs have been placed in the bottom slot of this device. What is going on?

Panoramic Radiography: Clinical Technique

Goal

To understand correct clinical techniques in panoramic radiology

Learning Objectives

1. Recognize the parts of the panoramic machine
2. Know how to use the parts of the panoramic machine
3. Identify errors in taking the panoramic radiograph
4. Know how to correct errors in taking the panoramic radiograph

Instructions

Carefully read the introductory information on panoramic techniques. Note that further information on digital panoramic radiography is included, although a separate chapter has been dedicated to digital panoramic imaging. The machines illustrated are several of the newest and most advanced that are available in our dental school. Several other excellent brands are available. Also, many older panoramic machines are in schools and practices, and all of them can be operated basically in the same way. Slight differences in technique exist from one brand or model to another; however, the errors remain the same. The principles for the recognition and correction of errors are pretty well universal. Having said that, some brands or models may be more prone to certain errors or artifacts and some may even produce unique errors. The information here is the basis for understanding, recognizing, and correcting problems for most machines, models, and situations. Once this basic information is mastered, unique problems can be identified and corrected. And . . . by the way, we often forget to refer to the owner's operating manual where most of the answers to common problems can be found.

BASIC CONCEPTS

The panoramic machines illustrated in this and other chapters are the Morita Veraviewepocs in a film-based version and the Planmeca ProMax Pan-Ceph factory digital panoramic machine. Older film-based panoramic machine designs can be converted to digital in two ways: (1) by substituting the film and fluorescent screen and chemical film development for the PSP memory plates and laser scanner; or (2) by substituting the cassette assembly for a CCD sensor. In either case, software and a computer will be needed. The factory-assembled digital panoramic machines come with the CCD sensor and appropriate software; however, a

computer may not always be included. Digital panoramic machines have menus of functions and settings that can be selected on the machine; however, the machine software must also be opened in the computer, patient data entered, and other menus selected before an exposure can be made. All machines (film-based machines, digitally converted machines, and factory digital machines) have the same type of exposure switch that must be continually depressed throughout the exposure; releasing the pressure on the exposure button will abort the exposure cycle.

Also, some new panoramic machines such as the Morita Veraviewepocs can automatically correct for some positioning errors. An example is the automatic patient distance to film/sensor adjustment (autofocus), whereby the layer is shifted to correct for a malpositioned patient. Another example is the auto exposure function, which adjusts for underexposure or overexposure settings or areas of increased or decreased density as a result of malpositioning.

The new panoramic machines are robotic in design and controlled by a computer chip. That is, each moving part can be programmed to move independently of other moving parts by a stepper motor. Thus projections that open the interproximal contacts such as found on the ProMax can eliminate the need for bitewings—a tremendous advantage when all of the extra time, cost of materials, and risk of disease transmission associated with intraoral radiography are considered. Because the ProMax boasts a resolution of nearly 10 lp/mm, the sharpness and detail now approach those of many intraoral machines, especially those that have been in use for a few years. There are no infection control considerations for the operator in panoramic radiology, and the contaminated bite-block or bite-block sleeve is removed by the patient. Typically, most machines are capable of TMJ, sinus, tomography, and multiple panoramic projections such as to open interproximal contacts.

Panoramic radiography has evolved tremendously in the past few years and now offers exciting potential for every dental practitioner. In nearly all instances, positioning errors will be seen regardless of the machine design or brand. However, the operator's careful attention to the minute technique details remains the most essential factor necessary for the dentist to gain the maximum potential from the panoramic machine.

Further chapters deal specifically with other aspects of panoramic radiography including patient protection, operator protection, infection control, digital panoramic radiology, and the recognition of errors on film or in the digital image.

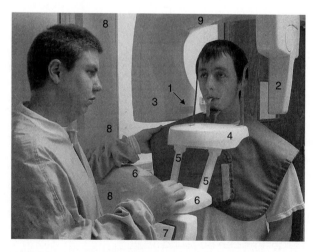

FIGURE **6-1** This is the Planmeca Digital ProMax Pan-Ceph machine. Name or identify the numbered parts.

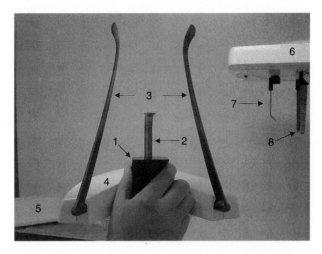

FIGURE **6-2** This is the chin rest/bite-block/side guide assembly for the Planmeca Digital ProMax Pan-Ceph machine and portions of the cephalometric assembly. Name or identify the numbered parts.

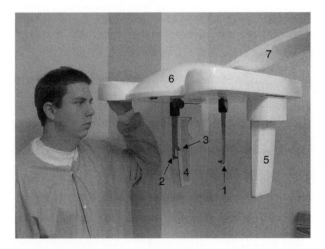

FIGURE **6-3** Name or identify the numbered parts of this ProMax machine.

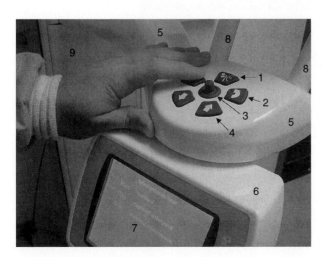

FIGURE **6-4** Name or identify the numbered parts of this ProMax machine.

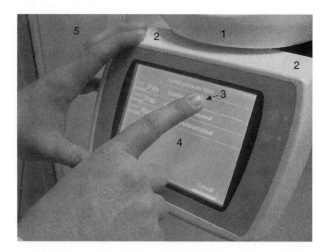

FIGURE **6-5** Name or identify the numbered parts of this ProMax machine.

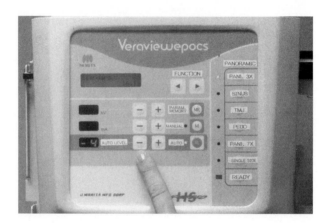

FIGURE **6-6** This is the control panel for a Veraviewepocs.
1. On the right side of the panel, the little round dots illuminate for each program group selected. How many basic program groups is this machine capable of?
2. Which program group has been activated?
3. What will the exposure time be?
4. To what adjustment is the operator pointing?
5. Do you know how fast this machine can expose a panoramic film?

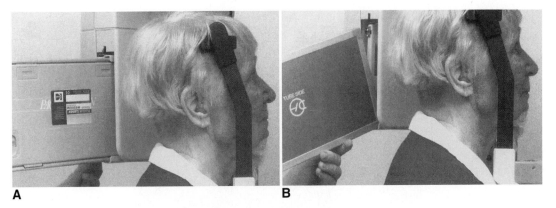

A   **B**

FIGURE **6-7** In images *A* and *B* you can see the film cassette being loaded into the Veraviewepocs panoramic machine.
1. In image *A*, what error has occurred?
2. In image *B*, how does the operator know that this is the correct way to load the cassette into the machine?

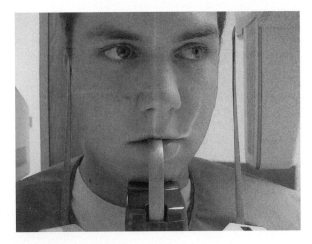

FIGURE **6-8** Only one technique error has occurred or is the most obvious in this figure. Name the error, and state how the error can be corrected.

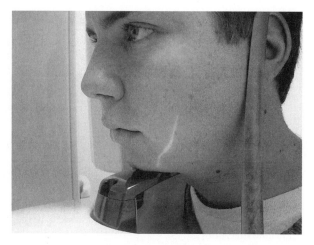

FIGURE **6-9** Only one technique error has occurred or is the most obvious in this figure. Name the error, and state how the error can be corrected.

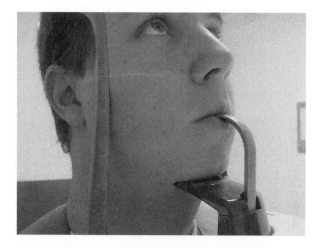

FIGURE **6-10** Only one technique error has occurred or is the most obvious in this figure. Name the error, and state how the error can be corrected.

FIGURE **6-11** Only one technique error has occurred or is the most obvious in this figure. Name the error, and state how the error can be corrected.

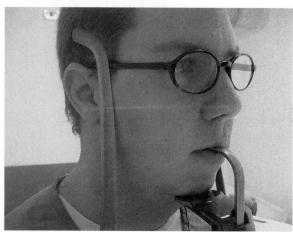

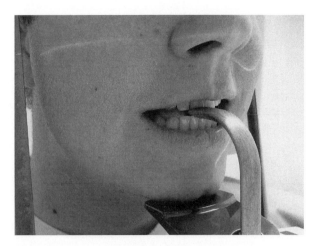

FIGURE **6-12** Only one technique error has occurred or is the most obvious in this figure. Name the error, and state how the error can be corrected.

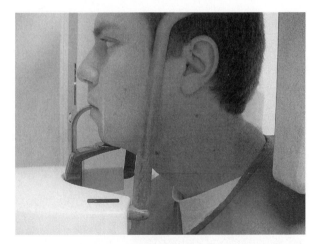

FIGURE **6-13** Only one technique error has occurred or is the most obvious in this figure. Name the error, and state how the error can be corrected.

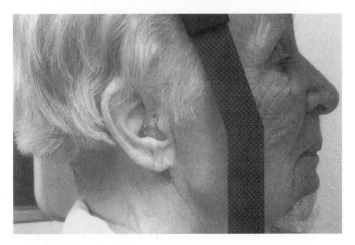

FIGURE **6-14** Only one technique error has occurred or is the most obvious in this figure. Name the error, and state how the error can be corrected.

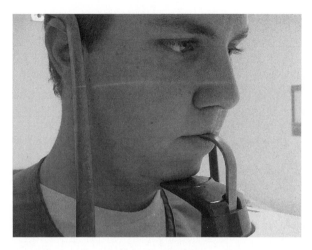

FIGURE **6-15** Only one technique error has occurred or is the most obvious in this figure. Name the error, and state how the error can be corrected.

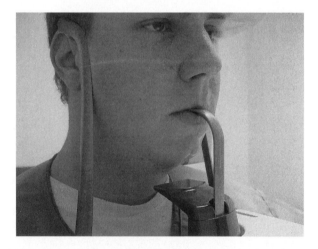

FIGURE **6-16** Only one technique error has occurred or is the most obvious in this figure. Name the error, and state how the error can be corrected.

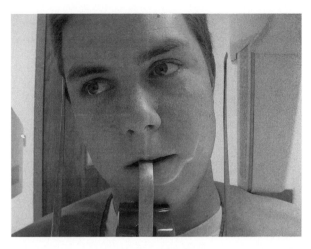

FIGURE **6-17** Only one technique error has occurred or is the most obvious in this figure. Name the error, and state how the error can be corrected.

NOTE TO STUDENTS: Remember the following steps in the generic panoramic technique:
1. Remove extraoral and intraoral items such as jewelry and prostheses.
2. Bite in the groove in the bite-block.
3. Set chin on chin rest with patient standing upright.
4. Close side guides.
5. Instruct patient to swallow and hold still; then expose to preselected machine settings.

The next two patients are father and son. In fact, both of the young patients in this section are the author's sons.

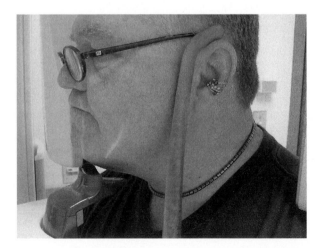

FIGURE **6-18** First the dad, who is an edentulous older patient. (Father and son like to dress alike—one as bad as the other, but the dad seems to be in some sort of identity crisis!) Study the picture carefully and see how many errors you can find.

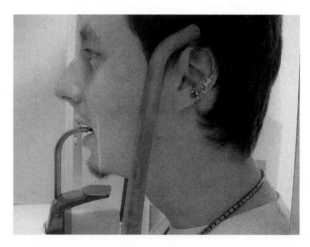

FIGURE **6-19** This is the son. See how many errors you can find here?

Chapter 7

Panoramic Radiography: Errors Seen in Radiographs

Goal

To know how to recognize and correct errors seen in panoramic radiographs

Learning Objectives

1. Identify errors in taking the panoramic radiograph
2. Know how to correct errors in taking the panoramic radiograph
3. Identify film handling and processing errors
4. Know how to correct film handling and processing errors
5. Recognize multiple errors in the same radiograph

BASIC CONCEPTS

The panoramic errors are viewed by students to be more difficult to learn than the intraoral ones. So we will limit the questions to one type of error at a time. Also to help, a preliminary explanation is provided as background information to help identify the errors. The panoramic technique is much easier to learn than the intraoral technique, and it is much less trouble with regard to clean up and infection control. However, patient positioning must be very exact, because noticeable errors develop with very small mistakes.

THE NORMAL PANORAMIC RADIOGRAPH

Mind's Eye View of the Panoramic Radiograph (Diagram 7-1)
Notice the panoramic image is divided into 9 areas that make up the 6 zones that you must learn to

picture each panoramic radiograph or image in your mind's eye. These zones are as follows:

Zone 1: The dentition. Here the occlusal plane should be mildly curved upward to make a smile-like line. The roots of the anterior teeth are in the image, and the posterior teeth are the same size on each side with no more overlapping of the contacts on one side than the other.

Zone 2: The nose-sinus. The turbinates should remain in the nose, and the hard palate shadows should cross the sinus above the apices of the posterior maxillary teeth.

Zone 3: The mandible. Here the inferior cortex should be a smooth curve and the hyoid bone and ghost image of the spine should not be superimposed.

Zone 4: The TMJs. This is a bilateral zone. Both condyles should be in about the center of the

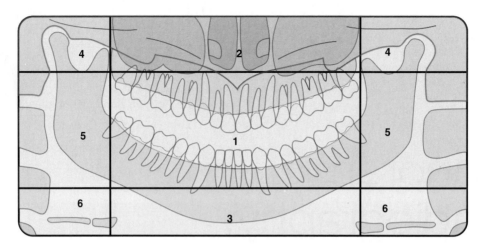

DIAGRAM **7-1**

zone. Neither condyle should be higher or bigger than the other. The condyles should not go off the top or sides of the image.

Zone 5: The spine-ramus. In many panoramic machines the double real images of the spine are not seen at the edges. If they are seen, the spine should not be superimposed on the ramus and should be at an equal distance from the ramus on both sides. The spine images should be vertical and not sloped. The ramus should be the same width on each side with no ghost images of the ramus on either side.

Zone 6: The hyoid. Here the double real images of body and greater horn(s) of the hyoid can be seen on both sides. They should be the mirror image of each other with neither of them bigger, higher, or more spread out than the other. The hyoid should not be spread out across the mandible. The distance from the body of the hyoid to the mandible should be equal on both sides.

Normal Panoramic Image (Diagram 7-2) Notice that structures have been left out. This is to emphasize that not many structures need to be identified to properly troubleshoot the image for technique errors. In this diagram, the nose and sinus as well as the maxilla are left out because nothing goes wrong here in the perfect image. There is no distinct image of the lips, nose, or ears, nor is there any undesirable air. The teeth, mandible body, ramus, TMJs, and spine are nicely imaged as just described.

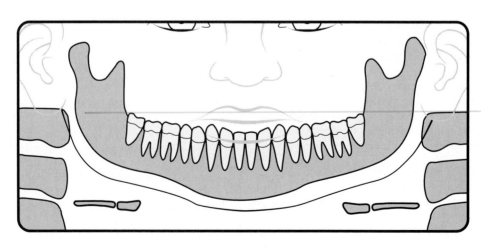

DIAGRAM **7-2**

STEPS IN TAKING A PANORAMIC RADIOGRAPH

Step 1
Assess the patient:
  Remove extraoral and intraoral items.
Load cassette into machine.
Adjust machine settings:
  kVp
Step 1 Errors
Items left in or on the patient
Cassette problems
Improper kVp setting selected:
  Image too dark
  Image too light

Step 2
Bite in the groove in the bite-block.
Check canine positioning light: should be aligned in middle of lower canine (varies a little with different machines).

Step 2 Errors
Patient positioned too far forward (Diagram 7–3)
Patient positioned too far back (Diagram 7–4)

Step 3
Position chin on chin rest, and adjust height of chin rest.
Make sure patient is standing upright with neck and back straight.
Tilt chin downward about 5 degrees.
Check Frankfort plane (ala of nose to tragus of ear) positioning light.
Check canine light to ensure it is still okay.

Step 3 Errors
Chin not on chin rest (Diagram 7–5)
Patient slumped or stooped (Diagram 7–6)
Chin tipped too low (Diagram 7–7)
Chin tipped too high (Diagram 7–8)

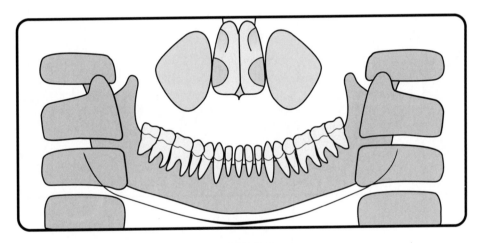

DIAGRAM **7-3**

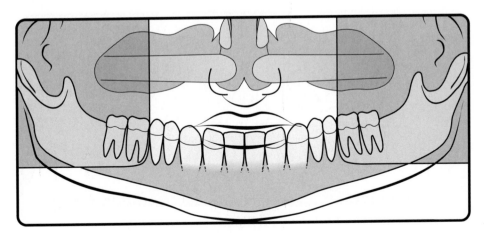

DIAGRAM **7-4**

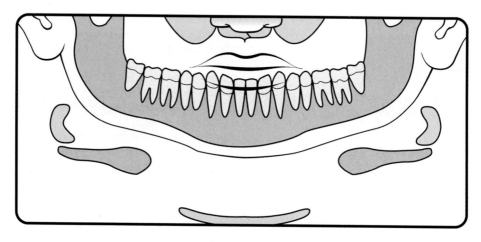

DIAGRAM **7-5**

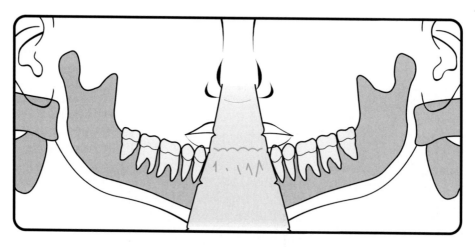

DIAGRAM **7-6**

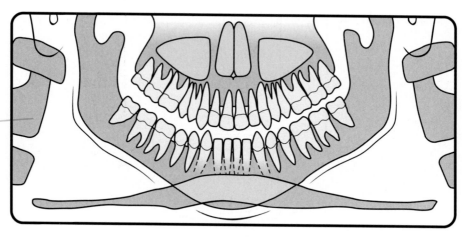

DIAGRAM **7-7**

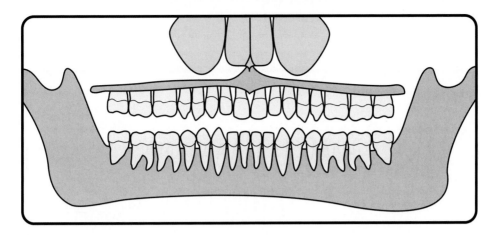

DIAGRAM **7-8**

Step 4
Close the side guides.
Check midsagittal plane positioning light
 (midface, middle of forehead, nose, and chin).
Check Frankfort plane light to ensure it is still
 okay.
Check canine light to ensure it is still okay.
Step 4 Errors
Patient shifted to one side of midline (not shown)
Patient's head twisted or turned (Diagram 7–9)
Patient's head tilted (Diagram 7–10)

Step 5
Give final instructions to patient:
 Close lips.
 Place tongue against palate.
 Hold still.
Initiate the exposure.
Step 5 Errors
Lips open; tongue not against palate (Diagram
 7–11)
Patient movement (Diagram 7–12)

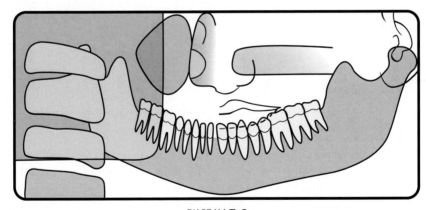

DIAGRAM **7-9**

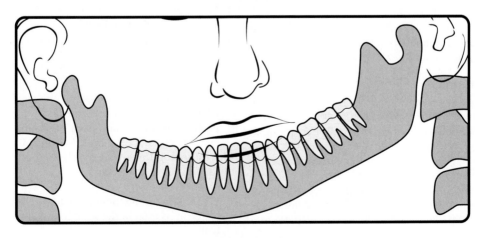

DIAGRAM **7-10**

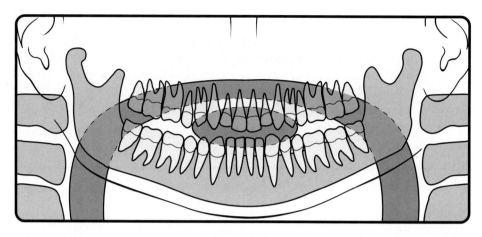

DIAGRAM **7-11**

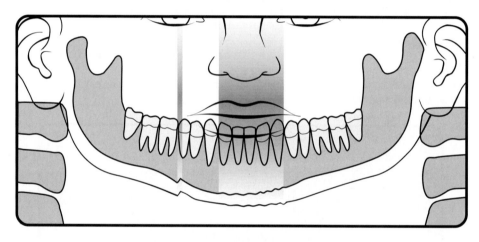

DIAGRAM **7-12**

ERRORS IN TAKING THE PANORAMIC RADIOGRAPH

Refer to Table 7-1 (*Panoramic Patient Positioning Errors*) in the Answer Key and correlate this information with Diagrams 7-1 through 7-12 as you analyze the following cases for errors. Notice that information on how to correct the errors is given in the table as well.

Instructions

For this section only, look for errors in taking the panoramic radiograph as just described in the 5 steps. There is only one radiograph per question; however, several errors may be identifiable in the same image. For each question, the number of errors being sought will be indicated.

Remember, some patients are edentulous or partially edentulous so you must identify the errors from the distorted anatomic features and not by the teeth.

The following is how teeth should look in a good panoramic image:
1. The occlusal plane should be slightly curved upwards.
2. The upper and lower teeth should be separated by the bite-block.
3. The root tips of the anterior teeth should not be cut off.
4. The anterior teeth should not be obscured by a radiopaque shadow.
5. Each posterior tooth should be the same size as its counterpart on the other side.
6. Posterior teeth should not be overlapped on one side and not overlapped on the other side.

The following three-part question applies to all of the figures in this section:
1. Name the error(s).
2. When possible, list one characteristic feature of the error as seen in the teeth and one anatomic feature.
3. Explain how to correct each error.

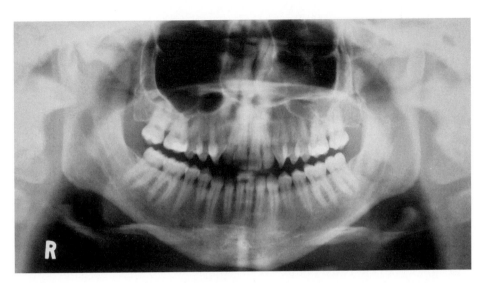

FIGURE **7-1** One error.

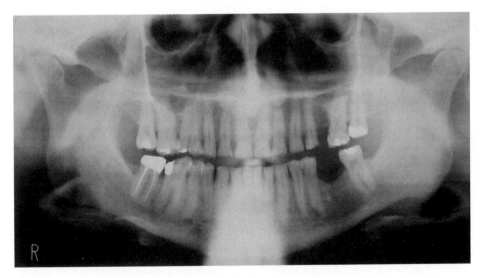

FIGURE **7-2** One error.

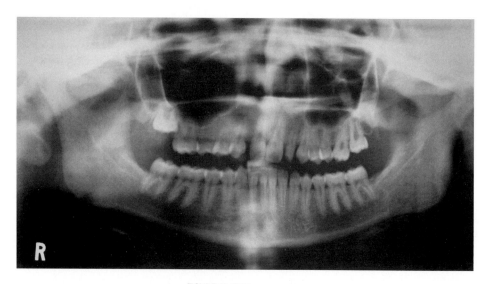

FIGURE **7-3** Two errors.

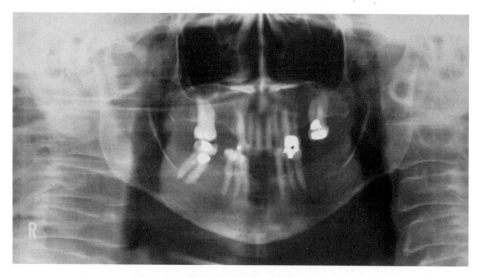

FIGURE **7-4** Two errors.

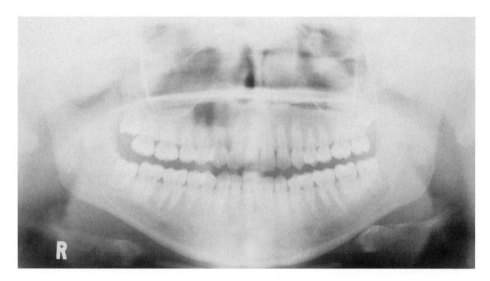

FIGURE **7-5** One error.

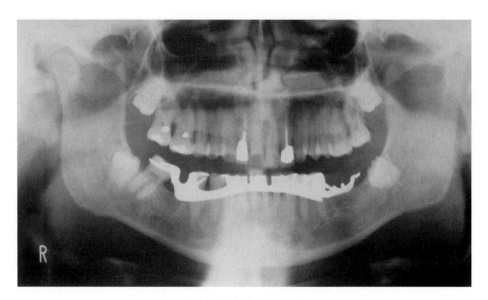

FIGURE **7-6** Two errors.

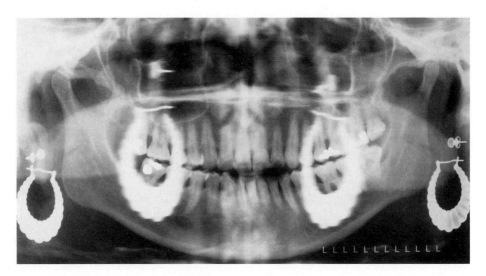

FIGURE **7-7** One error.

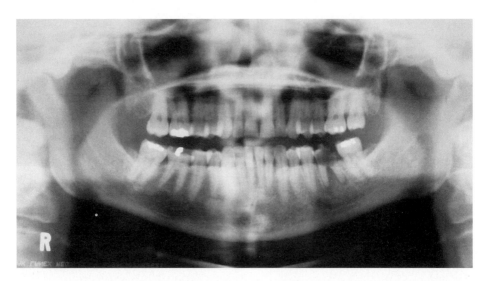

FIGURE **7-8** Two errors.

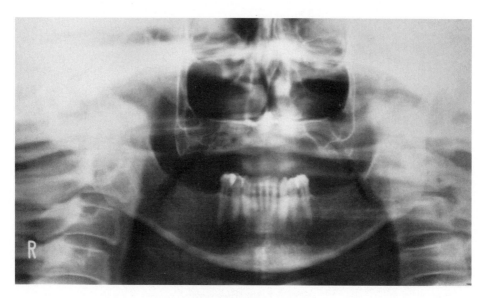

FIGURE **7-9** One error.

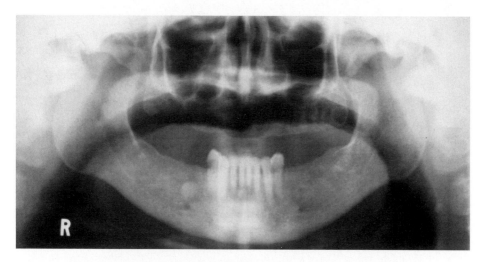

FIGURE **7-10** One error.

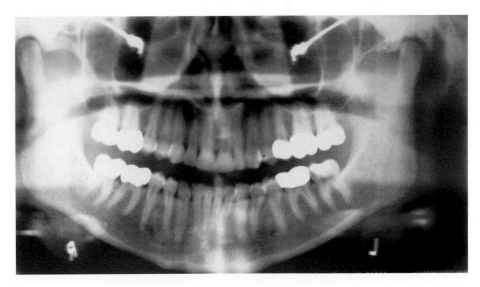

FIGURE **7-11** Three errors.

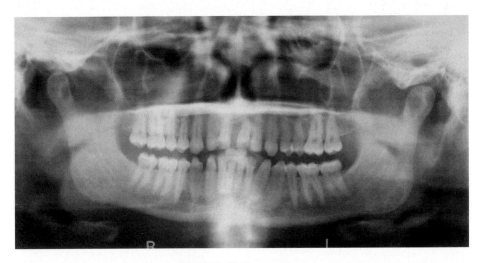

FIGURE **7-12** Four errors.

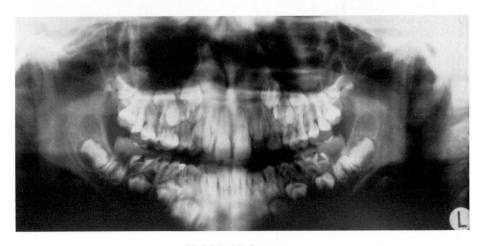

FIGURE **7-13** One error.

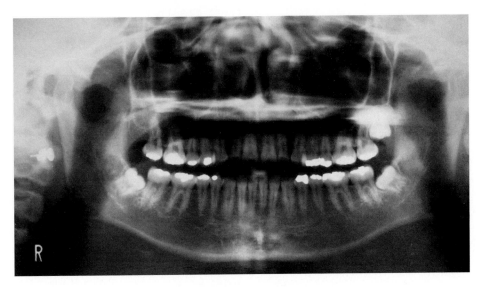

FIGURE **7-21** Four errors.

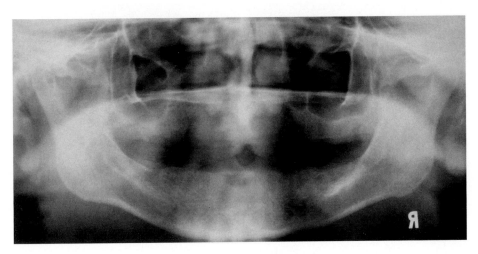

FIGURE **7-22** One error.

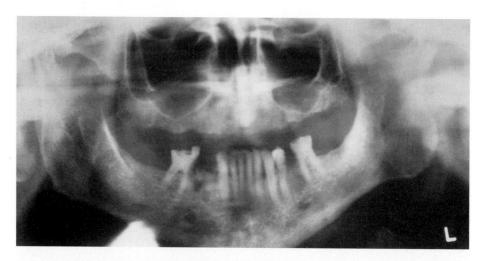

FIGURE **7-19** Two errors.

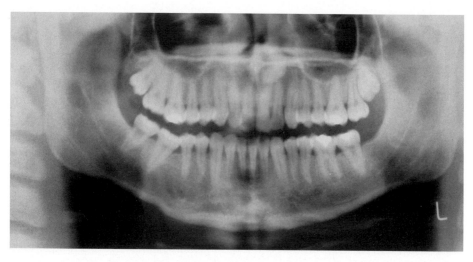

FIGURE **7-20** One error.

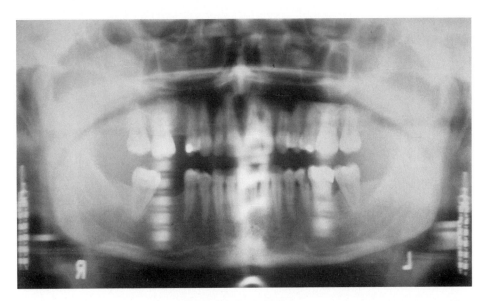

FIGURE **7-17** Five errors.

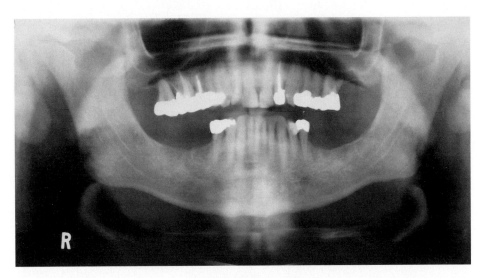

FIGURE **7-18** Two errors.

FIGURE **7-14** One error.

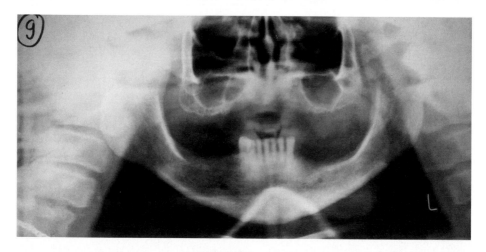

FIGURE **7-15** Two errors.

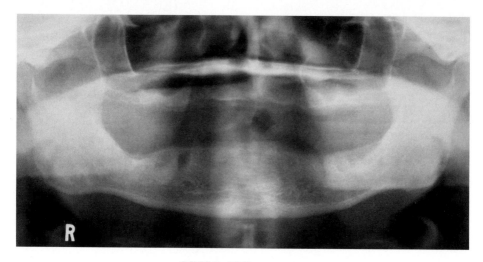

FIGURE **7-16** Two errors.

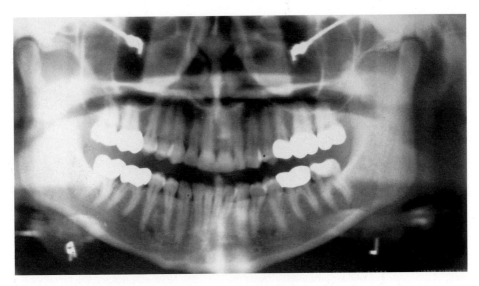

FIGURE **7-11** Three errors.

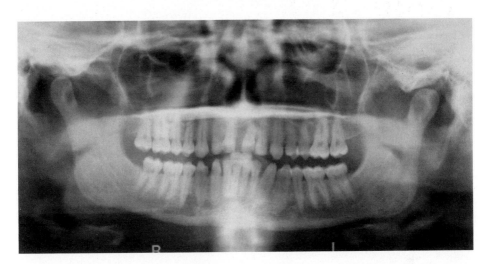

FIGURE **7-12** Four errors.

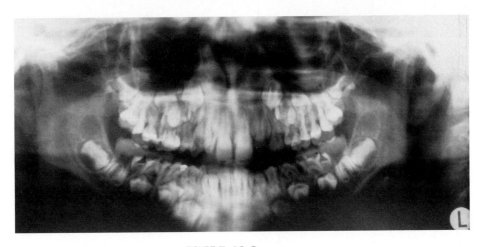

FIGURE **7-13** One error.

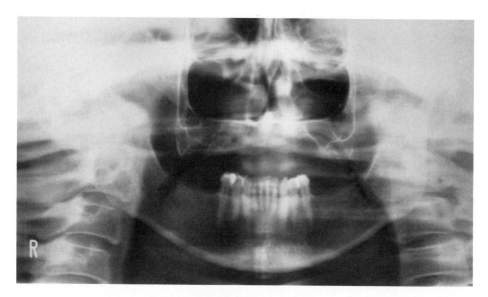

FIGURE **7-9** One error.

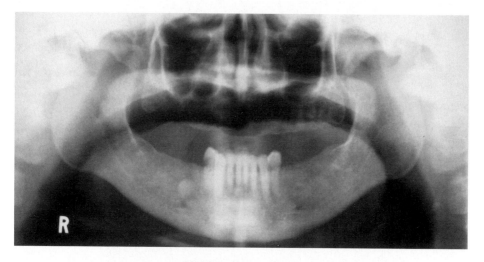

FIGURE **7-10** One error.

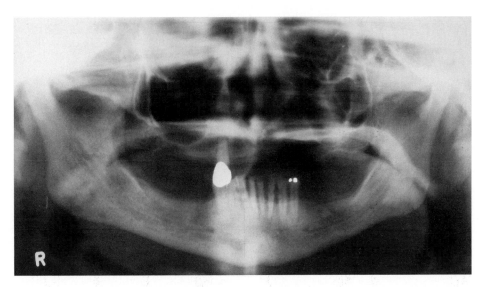

FIGURE **7-23** One error.

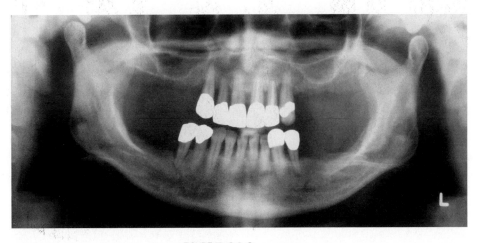

FIGURE **7-24** One error.

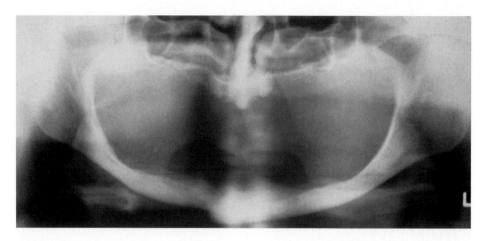

FIGURE **7-25** Three errors.

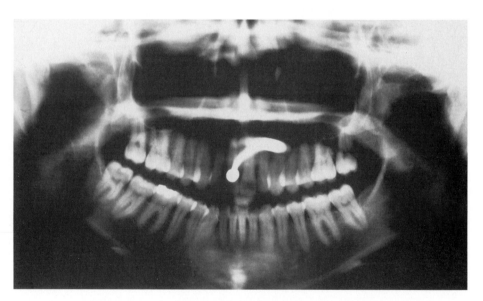

FIGURE **7-26** Three errors.

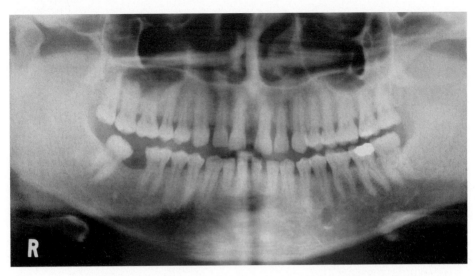

FIGURE **7-27** One error (figure is not cropped; this is the full image).

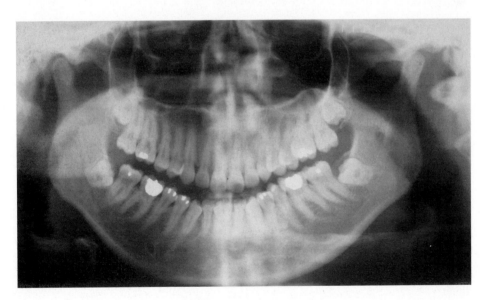

FIGURE **7-28** Two errors.

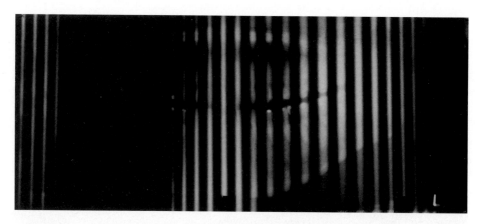

FIGURE **7-29** One error.

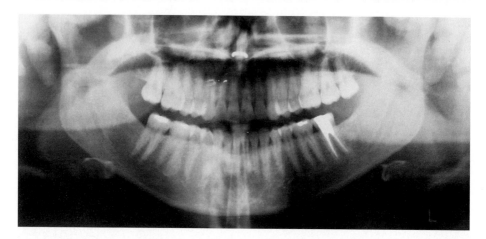

FIGURE **7-30** Four errors.

FILM HANDLING AND PROCESSING ERRORS

Instructions

Look at Table 7-2 (*Panoramic Film Handling and Processing Errors*) in the Answer Key as a guide in helping you figure out the problems and their correction.

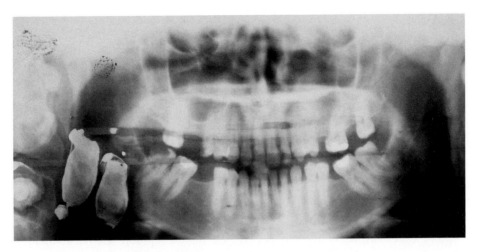

FIGURE **7-31** This film is marred by chemical stains.
1. State what chemical(s) has (have) affected this image.

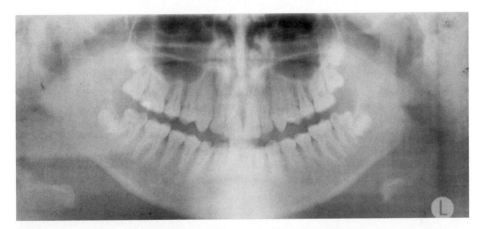

FIGURE **7-32** Though it is hard to see here, this film has an overall grayish look to it.
1. State what problem caused this.

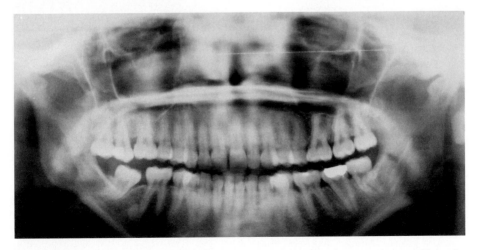

FIGURE **7-33** This film has an undesirable horizontal white line on it, and every film taken with the same cassette had the same mark.
1. State what the problem is.

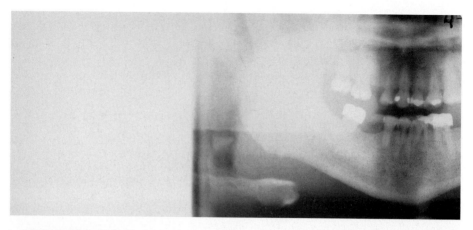

FIGURE **7-34** Only half of this film was exposed, but the exposure was not aborted.
1. What happened here?

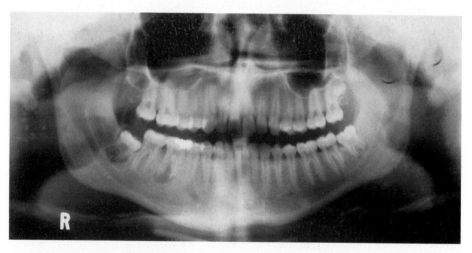

FIGURE **7-35** There are two different problems here:
1. What are the black, crescent-shaped marks from?
2. What are the little whitish spots at the right- and left-hand edges of the film?

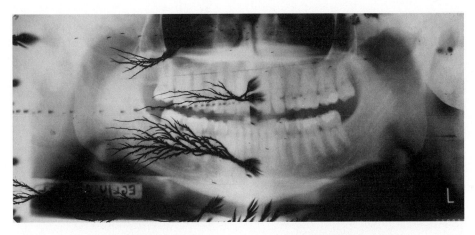

FIGURE **7-36** Observe the black spots and lightning-like marks.
1. What happened here?
2. How can this be prevented?

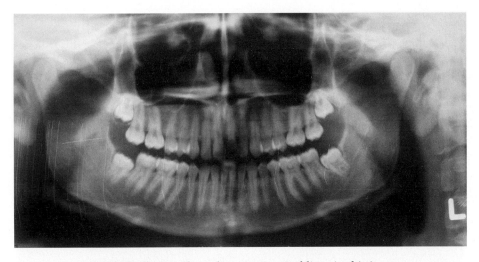

FIGURE **7-37** Observe the radiopaque vertical lines in this image.
1. What could these be?

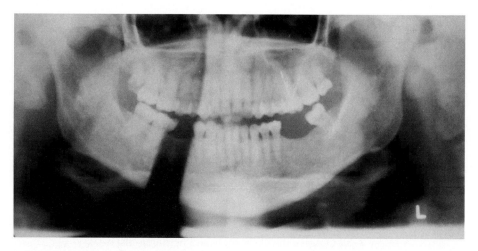

FIGURE **7-38** Here's a clue regarding the nature of this problem. The cassette is an old plastic one that is wrapped around a drum.

1. What is the undesirable black mark on the film?

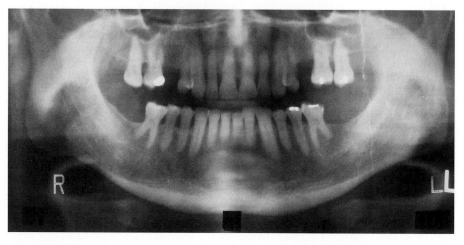

FIGURE **7-39** Look at the squiggly, thin, white vertical line on the patient's left. Every film taken with this cassette had this mark.

1. What is the problem?

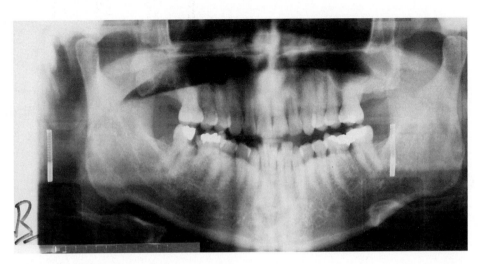

FIGURE **7-40** Notice the "Ls" at the bottom left of the figure and an "R" written in. There's also a couple of springs and darker square or rectangular areas.

1. Can you state what happened?
2. Would you keep this film?

Chapter 8

Panoramic Digital Imaging

Goal

To understand concepts and clinical techniques for panoramic digital imaging

Learning Objectives

1. Learn the differences between direct and indirect digital imaging systems
2. Learn the use of PSPs in panoramic radiology

BASIC CONCEPTS

In general, digital panoramic techniques are the same as for film-based machines. Additional skills are necessary, however, because the computer will be needed to control some machine functions like turning it on, readying a new patient file into which the image will be stored, activating the scanner if applicable, and, of course, the entirely new function of processing the image after it is captured. As with intraoral digital imaging, little information is in the textbooks except the newest editions, and panoramic digital imaging is not always included. Students should expect to see more and more of this information as the subject material begins to appear on school, state, and national tests for the various types of required certification of dentists, assistants, and hygienists.

PANORAMIC DIGITAL IMAGING

1. **Indirect Digital Imaging:** In digital imaging there are several formats. The two most basic ones are referred to as *indirect digital imaging* and *direct digital imaging*. When an existing dental office converts to a paperless electronic chart, most likely the retention and storage of film will be considered undesirable. At that time the doctor will want to convert old charts and radiographs to an electronic medium. To do this, a scanner is used. This is called

indirect digital imaging. Radiographs cannot be scanned with an ordinary scanner; a transparency adapter is needed. A home scanner with a transparency adapter is capable of scanning slides or film negatives. A full-size 8.5 × 11–inch transparency adapter will be needed for panoramic radiographs. In 2004, the price of this is $1200. An alternate method is to digitize the radiographs with a digital camera.

2. **Direct Digital Imaging:** In this instance the image is captured as a digital image right from the get-go. This is unquestionably the case when using the wired type of sensor. Remember, these are the CCD (charge-coupled device) sensor and the CMOS (complementary metal oxide sensor). Wireless CMOSs are available for intraoral radiography. Currently only CCD sensors are used in panoramic radiology. The other type of sensor is called the *PSP* (photostimulable phosphor plate). Because the plate must be scanned between exposing the plate and seeing the image in the computer, some purists have referred to the PSP system as a form of indirect digital imaging. Perhaps the PSP could be referred to as *indirect direct digital imaging.*

3. **Converting Existing Machines to Digital:** There are several considerations:

- *Step 1: Software.* Believe it or not, the first consideration is software. No matter what the brand, it absolutely must meet the international DICOM (Digital Imaging and Communication in Medicine) standard. As long as all the digital imaging software is DICOM-compliant, your intraoral, panoramic, and cephalometric images can be easily accessed. Otherwise, bridging software is needed and each type of image has to be kept in different electronic folders and the compatible software opened separately for each image type. This is a deplorable situation and non-DICOM-compliant products should be avoided without exception.
- *Step 2: Choosing a Sensor.* A decision is needed whether to select a CCD or PSP system. Both are available. If a PSP system such as DenOptix is already in use for the intraoral imaging, then going to the same brand panoramic PSP makes sense because the software and scanner will already be in place. If the office has selected a CCD or CMOS intraoral system, then converting the panoramic unit to CCD digital should be attempted. Some existing panoramic machines with soft, curved cassettes cannot be converted to CCD-type digital; instead, PSPs must be used. The best digital conversion kit is the one offered by the manufacturer; otherwise a universal converter such as the Trex Trophy system can be installed in some machines.
- *Step 3: Image Transmission.* Here we are referring to image transmission both in and out of the facility. The office must be networked. This can be with wires or wireless. The image capture computer is not where the images will be stored. They must be exported from this computer and imported into the patient's electronic chart. They can also be sent via e-mail to third parties such as insurance companies, another practitioner, or a representative of the legal system. Anytime an image is exported out of the office, the recipient must be registered with you as a HIPAA business associate or be HIPAA-exempt. One way to ensure the patient's privacy is to use bar codes, which are now readily available to dental offices.
- *Step 4: Mainframe Computer and Server.* Most likely, the computer in the front office will no longer serve as the main computer because memory for the digital images will be inadequate. Each panoramic or a 20-film, full-mouth intraoral survey requires 1 megabyte (MB) of hard disk memory. There are 1000 MB in a gigabyte (GB) so even a 100

GB hard drive will not suffice for long, especially if the doctor also has a digital video camera or even a still digital camera. So a mainframe computer is needed that is connected to a server that is in turn connected to stacks of hard drive storage disks. Essentially, the mainframe computer retrieves all of the digital information for the patient, including the accounting, HIPAA documents, chart, and images. All of the other computers communicate with the mainframe computer to add data or to call up stored data.
- *Step 5: Backup and Archiving.* Backup and archiving of the images are needed. Archiving refers to transferring the data to the storage disks via the mainframe computer and the server. These electronic records are subject to loss from flooding, fire, earthquakes, and the like, including viruses. A backup system is one in which the images or other data are transferred to another medium such as a CD or DVD disks and continuously updated each time the patient is seen; the disks are stored in a secure place such as a fireproof/waterproof safe.

4. **The Nature of PSP:** PSP is a type of fluorescent screen that does not immediately fluoresce when exposed to x-rays. The phosphor is barium europium fluorohalide. The equivalent of a latent image is in the PSP after exposure to the x-rays. Then the PSP is scanned by a laser beam, which causes the PSP to fluoresce. The fluorescing image is read by a photodiode, which reads and transmits the image information to the computer. The computer will need an internal SCSI (small computer system interface) to display the image. The SCSI will need to be installed in the full-size computer because it is not readily available for laptops although external adaptors are available.

5. **How a Panoramic System Exposes Film and the PSP.** It is important to realize that the panoramic beam is collimated to a narrow slit of radiation that is about 6 inches high and a few millimeters wide at the film. As the machine rotates around the back and sides of the patient, the cassette moves in an opposite direction such that the image is painted on the film in tall, narrow increments continually until the exposure is over. The digital sensor is a thin, narrow column of CCDs that continuously captures thin, vertical increments of the image and paints them on the screen throughout the rotation. It is for this reason that the use of a cassette with a rare earth gadolinium oxyphosphate

screen will not be able to fluoresce for long enough to totally erase the image on the PSP. Such images will, however, be light and not sharp.

Instructions

Please study the pictures and answer the questions.

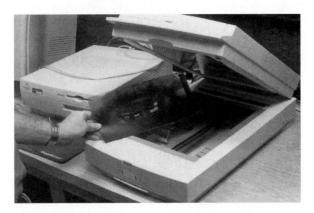

FIGURE **8-1** In the foreground of this figure we see a machine and a panoramic radiograph. What is the purpose of this device?

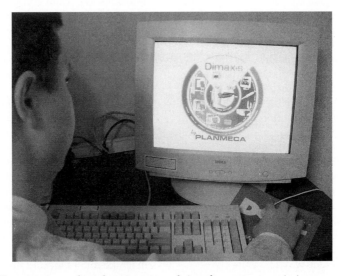

FIGURE **8-2** Here we see a dental assistant readying for a panoramic image capture. What type of system is this? Reveal as much as you know about it.

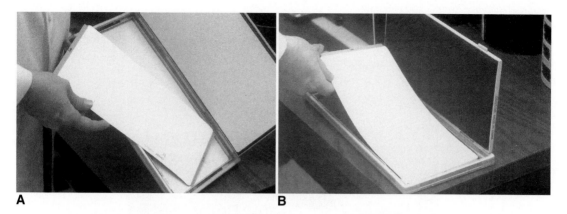

A   B

FIGURE **8-3** Here you can see a panoramic PSP being loaded into a cassette. Study *A* and *B* and answer the following questions:
1. What type of cassettes do we see here?
2. Can you see one small difference between this DenOptix PSP and a panoramic film?
3. One of the cassettes is for use with film; which one is it, and what is the difference between the two cassettes?
4. Is there an error in loading the PSP in the cassette?
5. If you used the film cassette, what would happen?

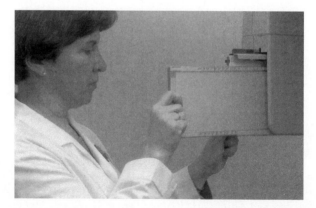

FIGURE **8-4** In this figure you can see the PSP cassette being loaded into a film-based panoramic machine.
1. Do you see anything odd in this picture?
2. Explain what is happening here.

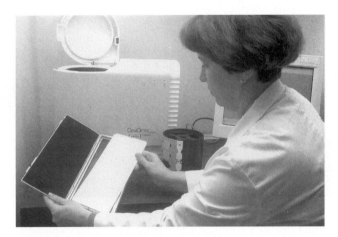

FIGURE **8-5** Now the PSP cassette is being unloaded.

1. What error has occurred with the use of this PSP?
2. What is the object to the right of the operator's right hand?
3. What is the device in the background with the open top?
4. Should this step be carried out in a darkened area because of the susceptibility of PSPs to light?

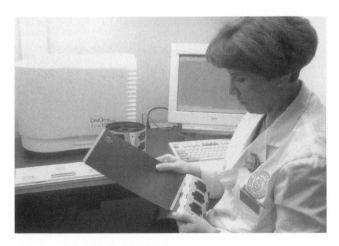

FIGURE **8-6** Here you can see the next step.

1. What is happening here?
2. Are there any errors?

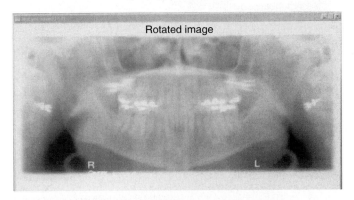

FIGURE **8-13** This screen now shows the rotated image that was done in the last step. Study this image and answer the following questions.

1. Does the overall image look okay to you? If not, can you figure out the problem?
2. What other error can you see here?

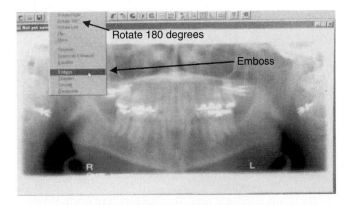

FIGURE **8-14** What are we going to try now?

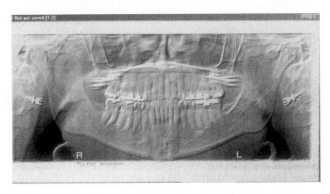

FIGURE **8-15** What do we see here?

NOTE TO STUDENTS: This completes the demonstration of the steps in acquiring, scanning, and digitally processing a panoramic image using a conventional machine and a PSP.

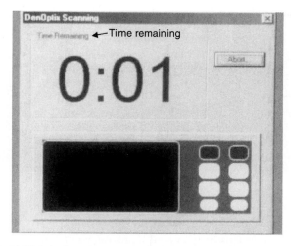

FIGURE **8-11** This is the same screen that appears at the end of the scan.
1. Describe what information is displayed on this screen.

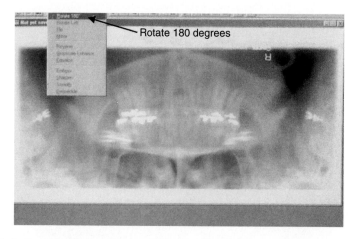

FIGURE **8-12** Only when scanning is complete can the image be displayed as we see here. This is the actual image that popped up for the pan you just saw being loaded. The screen was cropped to include only the panoramic image.
1. Is the upside-down image an error?
2. What did the operator do as seen in this screen?

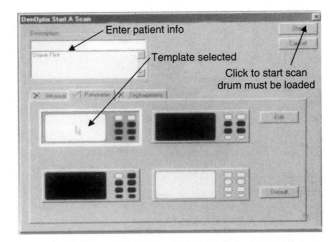

FIGURE **8-9** We are now ready to begin the scan. To do this you must go to the computer and open the DenOptix program by clicking on the icon on the computer screen (the computer screen is also known as the *desktop*). At the top left you see the screen is labeled *DenOptix*; start a scan. Take a look at the screen and information, and answer the questions.

1. What three things must you now do with the keyboard and mouse?
2. Would you be able to start the scanner if the drum were not loaded?

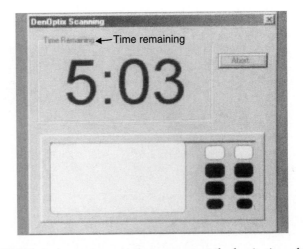

FIGURE **8-10** This is the next screen that appears at the beginning of the scan.
1. Describe what information is displayed on this screen.

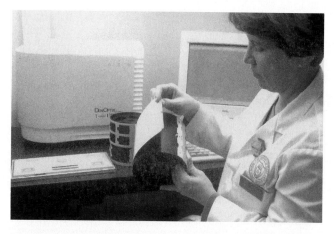

FIGURE **8-7** Here you can see a continuation of the last step.
1. What is happening here?
2. Are there any errors?

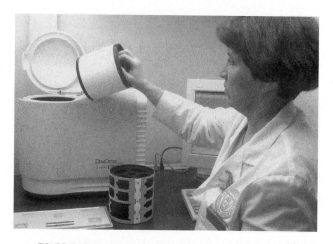

FIGURE **8-8** This is the next step in the procedure.
1. What is happening here?
2. Are there any mistakes you can see?

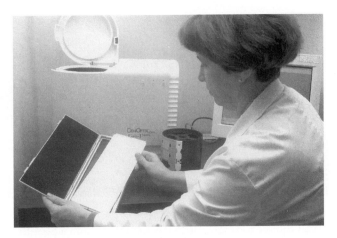

FIGURE **8-5** Now the PSP cassette is being unloaded.

1. What error has occurred with the use of this PSP?
2. What is the object to the right of the operator's right hand?
3. What is the device in the background with the open top?
4. Should this step be carried out in a darkened area because of the susceptibility of PSPs to light?

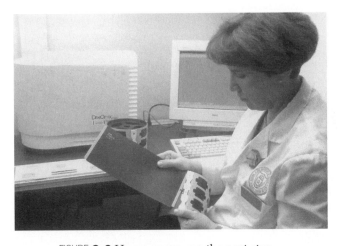

FIGURE **8-6** Here you can see the next step.

1. What is happening here?
2. Are there any errors?

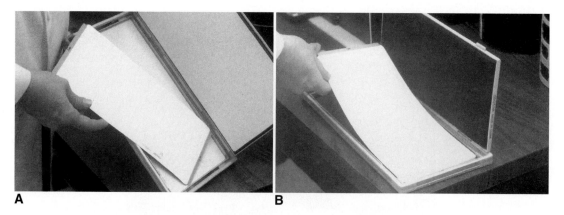

A   B

FIGURE **8-3** Here you can see a panoramic PSP being loaded into a cassette. Study *A* and *B* and answer the following questions:

1. What type of cassettes do we see here?
2. Can you see one small difference between this DenOptix PSP and a panoramic film?
3. One of the cassettes is for use with film; which one is it, and what is the difference between the two cassettes?
4. Is there an error in loading the PSP in the cassette?
5. If you used the film cassette, what would happen?

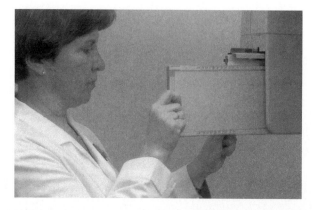

FIGURE **8-4** In this figure you can see the PSP cassette being loaded into a film-based panoramic machine.

1. Do you see anything odd in this picture?
2. Explain what is happening here.

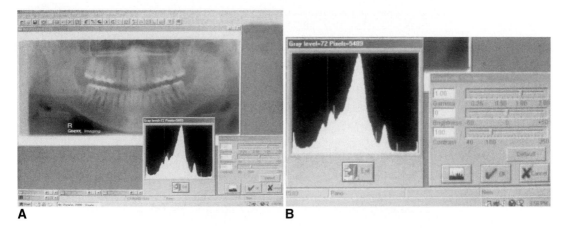

FIGURE **8-16** This is another patient. Study images *A* and *B* and then answer the questions.

1. What do we see at the bottom right of image *A* and enlarged at the left side of image *B*?
2. In image *B*, what three adjustments can we make to the image in part *A*?

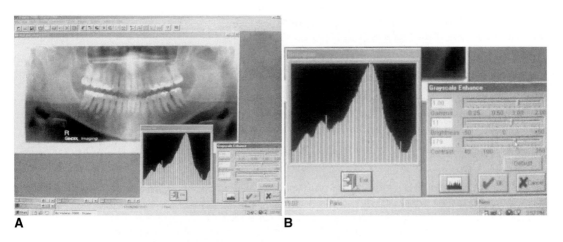

FIGURE **8-17** This is the same patient as in Figure 8-16. However some processing changes have occurred. Answer the following questions:

1. For now, look just at the image in Figure 8-17 and compare it with Figure 8-16. Describe any difference you see in Figure 8-17.
2. Look at the three controls for gamma, brightness, and contrast in Figure 8-17, *B*. What changes have been made?
3. How did the operator make the above changes?
4. Look at the histogram in Figure 8-17, *B*, and compare it with the histogram in Figure 8-16, *B*. What has happened to the histogram? What made this happen?
5. What patient positioning error occurred in taking this image?

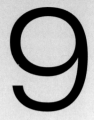

Chapter 9

Radiation Health

Goal

To know all aspects of radiation health according to current standards and practices

Learning Objectives

1. Recognize devices and supplies designed for the protection of the patient
2. Know radiologic procedures for the protection of the patient
3. Recognize infection control procedures for patient protection
4. Recognize operator radiation protection procedures
5. Identify infection control procedures for operator protection
6. Understand the use of barriers for radiation
7. Know the use of barriers for infection control

Instructions

The subject of radiation health includes the traditional concepts of patient and operator protection from biologic damage from radiation. These practices are currently under review by the Federal government, and new guidelines with significant changes are expected sometime in 2003 or 2004. In current practice, however, the subject of infection control as it applies to dental radiology must also be included as a part of radiation health or as a separate subject, since patients and operators alike must be protected from the spread of infection or communicable diseases. Infection control practices are not optional; they are mandated by the Federal OSHA regulations and by additional state laws. Offices and institutions are subject to inspections and fines for a lack of compliance. One of the limitations of our learning experience is that infection control procedures are usually learned in association with general dental practice and rarely is explicit information available for dental radiology.

NOTE TO STUDENTS: The term "cone" and "BID" (Beam Indicating Device) are used interchangeably. Another common term is "PID" (Position Indicating Device).

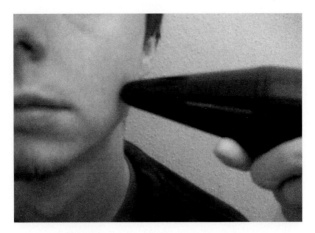

FIGURE **9-1** Here you see an older BID design.
1. What is wrong with this picture? Explain.
2. What is the usual length of these BIDs?

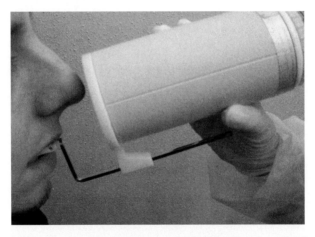

FIGURE **9-2** Here you see a short, round, open-ended BID being used with the paralleling technique. Answer the following questions:
1. What size is the diameter of the open end of the BID limited to by law?
2. What is wrong with this picture?

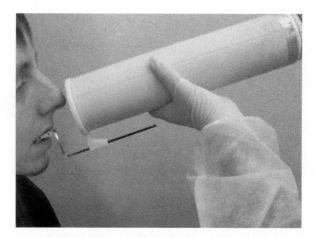

FIGURE **9-3** Here you see a long round BID being used. Answer the following questions:

1. Does the long round BID design provide the lowest amount of radiation dose to the patient?
2. The long, 16-inch, round BID is said to expose the patient to less radiation than the short, 8-inch BID. Both BIDs have a diameter of 2.75 inches at the open end. If the short BID requires exposure times 4 times shorter than the long BID (this is true), how can the long BID result in less patient exposure? Explain.

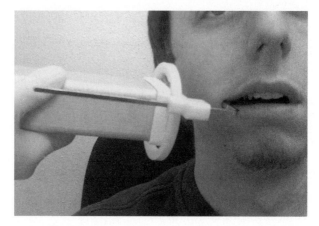

FIGURE **9-4** Here you see a long, 16-inch, rectangular BID being used. Notice the locator ring is round. Remember also, a retake doubles the dose to the patient for that exposure.

1. Why does the long rectangular BID provide less radiation exposure to the patient than the long round BID? Remember, both use the same exposure time (this is true) as long as all other factors such as machine design (AC vs. DC), kVp, mA, and film speed are the same.
2. Will a cone cut occur if a rectangular locator ring is not used?
3. In terms of BID alignment (not shape), what unique feature does the rectangular BID always have that round BIDs never have?

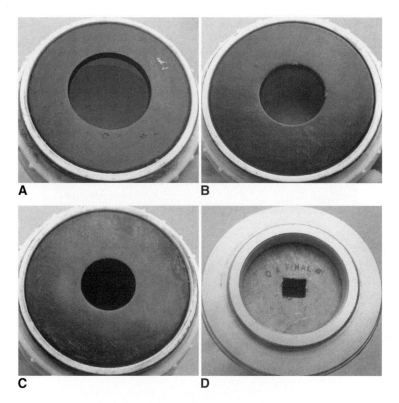

FIGURE **9-5** Here you see four current collimators labeled *A, B, C,* and *D*. Answer the following questions; be sure to answer all of the questions before going to the answer page.

1. Where in the x-ray apparatus are the collimators located?
2. What material are the collimators made from?
3. Which of these is illegal for use on new equipment?
4. Which of these delivers the least amount of radiation to the patient?
5. Collimator size is matched up to BID length. Here we have the standard short BID and two long BIDs. What is the length of the associated BIDs for *A, B, C,* and *D*?
6. Which one is a rectangular BID?
7. Which one is the pointed cone?
8. Which two have the same exposure times?

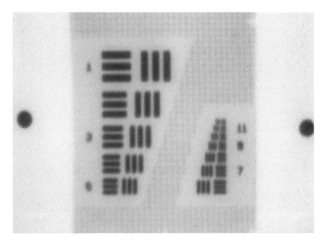

FIGURE **9-6** This is an occlusal radiograph of a test object used to check the x-ray machine.

1. What is it used for?
2. Assess this test result.

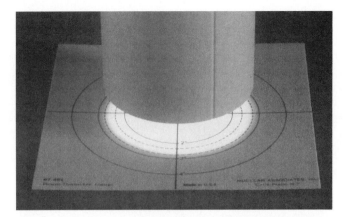

FIGURE **9-7** Here you can see the open end of a long, round cone and a piece of fluorescent screen material.
1. What part of the machine is being tested here?
2. What is the result of the test?

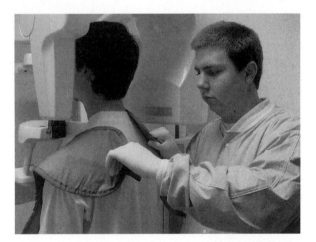

FIGURE **9-8** Here you see the patient being positioned in a digital panoramic machine.
1. What error(s) do you see in this picture?

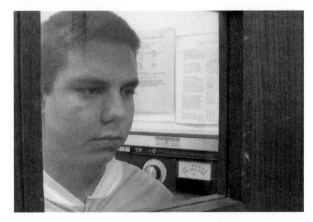

FIGURE **9-9** Here you see the operator behind a protective barrier while exposing an intraoral radiograph.
1. What material is usually incorporated in such barrier walls to protect the operator?
2. Why is the operator still protected in the area of the glass patient observation window?

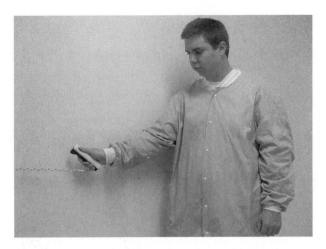

FIGURE **9-10** This student is about to take a panoramic radiograph. Appropriately, he is standing behind a protective wall.

1. What is wrong with this picture?
2. How must this be corrected?

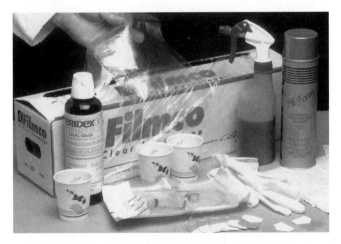

FIGURE **9-11** You are getting ready to take a set of four bitewing radiographs. These are some of the infection control products that will be needed.

1. List the needed items as seen in this picture.
2. Identify any additional items not seen in this picture.
3. What alternate radiographic procedure is available with fewer infection control requirements and reduced radiation to the patient?

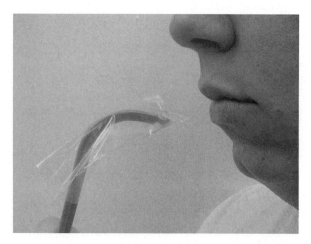

FIGURE **9-12** What do we see in this photograph?

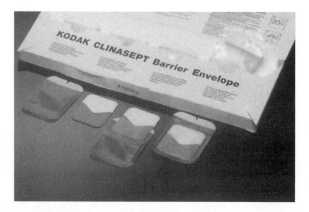

FIGURE **9-13** Discuss the utility of barrier envelopes in intraoral imaging.

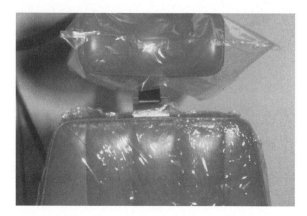

FIGURE **9-14** Here we see the headrest and upper part of the backrest of the chair wrapped for an intraoral radiographic procedure. The chair handles are also often wrapped.

1. Is this wrapping of the chair necessary, because spatter and aerosols are not created during intraoral radiographic procedures?
2. What parts of the panoramic machine should you wrap?

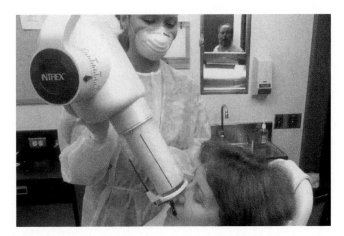

FIGURE **9-15** Here you see a radiograph being taken. This machine is of the recessed anode type and constant potential.

1. What infection control problems do you see here?
2. With the use of this machine, what dose-reduction features does it have over similar machines?
3. How many people are in the picture?

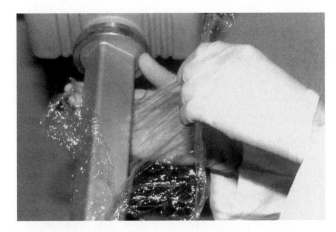

FIGURE **9-16** Here you see a machine with a long rectangular cone.

1. What infection control procedure is being carried out here?
2. What is the dose savings to the patient when the long rectangular cone is used instead of the long, round BID?
3. What will future radiation protection guidelines regarding BID shape recommend?

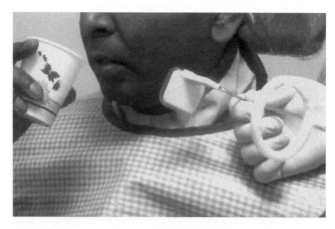

FIGURE **9-17** Here we are about to take an intraoral radiograph.

1. Identify all of the infection control measures seen in this photo.
2. Which area(s) of the mouth is the locator ring device set up for?
3. What will future radiation protection guidelines regarding patient protective aprons recommend?

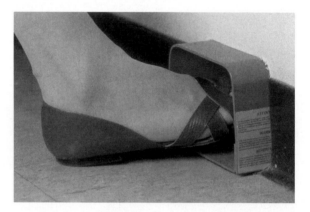

FIGURE **9-18** This is a replacement exposure switch.

1. What is the advantage of this floor-mounted design?

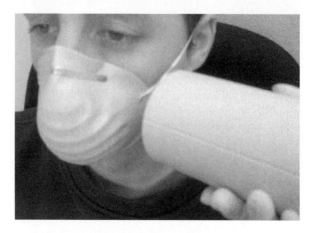

FIGURE **9-19** This patient is immune-compromised and has hepatitis B and is HIV+. He wears a mask whenever he leaves the house to protect himself from infections.

1. What infection control problem(s) do you see in this picture?

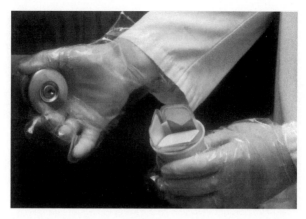

FIGURE **9-20** Here we see the contaminated film packets being transported in a clean cup to the processing area.

1. What special infection control procedure is in use as depicted in this picture?

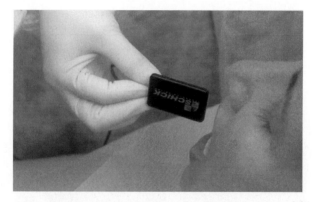

FIGURE **9-21** Here we see a CCD type digital sensor.

1. What, if any, infection control problem do we see here?

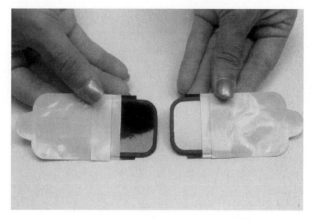

FIGURE **9-22** In this picture we see the two sides of the Digora digital sensor. Answer the following questions:

1. What type of sensor are these?
2. Which is the front or side of the sensor that must face the radiation?
3. What is the thin, dark band at the edge of the sensor as seen best on the right? What is its purpose?
4. What term is used for the wrap material for these sensors?

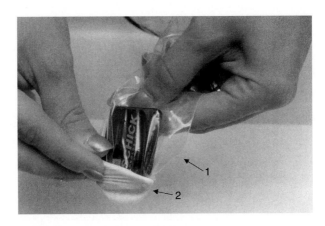

FIGURE **9-23** Here we see a wired-type CCD sensor.

1. What barrier materials (*arrows 1* and 2) are recommended and have been proven to be the most effective as reported in the literature?

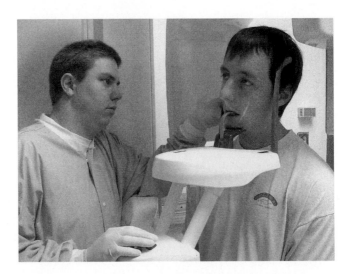

FIGURE **9-24** Here you see a patient being positioned for a panoramic radiograph.

1. What, if any, infection control problems do you see here?
2. According to current practice, what radiation protection problem do you see here?

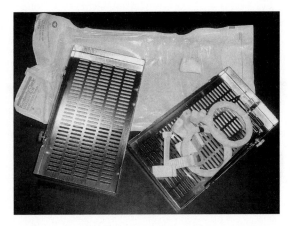

FIGURE **9-25** Here you see a complete ring positioning set being readied for sterilization in a heat sterilizer.

1. What type of sterilization container are the instruments placed in?
2. What is the other whitish colored item in the background?
3. Is heat sterilization necessary for this instrument?
4. Why don't we have the wired and/or wireless sensors in there too?

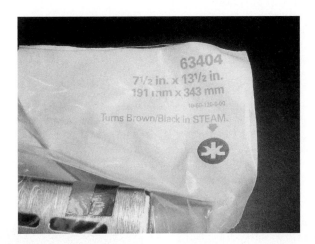

FIGURE **9-26** Notice the small arrow pointing to an icon on the sterilization packet.

1. What is the purpose of this marking?
2. Will this icon accurately indicate if used in a chemiclave or heat sterilizer?
3. Does it indicate the contents of the packet are sterile upon removal of the packet from the sterilizer? If not, how do you prove sterility?

Chapter 10

Dental Anomalies

Goal

To understand and recognize dental anomalies as seen in intraoral and panoramic images

Learning Objectives

1. Recognize variations in tooth number
2. Identify variations in tooth size
3. Identify variations in tooth shape
4. Know variations in tooth structure
5. Recognize acquired defects in teeth
6. Identify eruption problems
7. Recognize altered tooth positions
8. Classify impactions

Instructions

In this section you will find one or more examples of the conditions listed in the learning objectives. When answering the questions, try first to identify the condition from memory. Most of these conditions are common. Because they can impact on patient management, these disorders are an important group. Of course, the order in which these entities are presented here will be scrambled.
Okay, here we go!

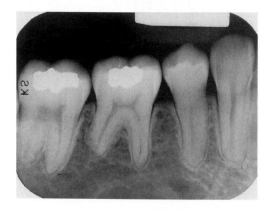

CASE **10-1** Most of this 22-year-old woman's teeth looked like this.
1. What iatrogenic treatment did she receive?
2. What condition is present?

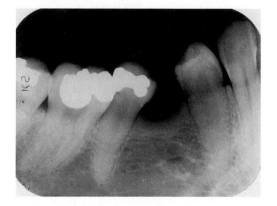

CASE **10-2** This 23-year-old man lost his 1st molar at a young age.
1. What term best describes the abnormal position of the 2nd premolar?

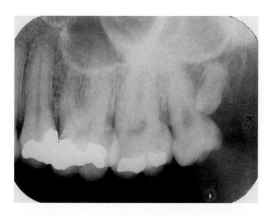

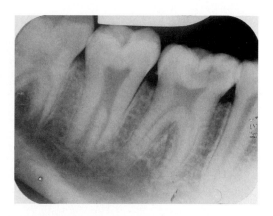

CASE **10-3** Look carefully at this posterior quadrant and notice the tiny tooth.
1. What two terms used together best describe this anomaly?

CASE **10-4** Take a look at the lower 2nd molar.
1. What term best describes its shape?
2. Is there anything characteristic about the pulp or root canal spaces?
3. Is this usually a solitary finding, or is it associated with other problems?
4. Can this condition affect the primary dentition?

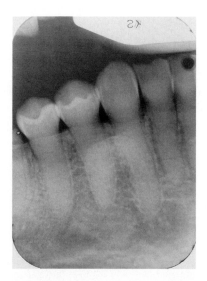

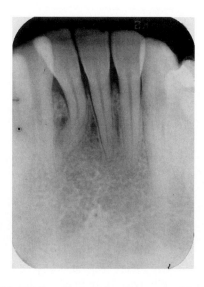

CASE **10-5** This 22-year-old man complains that several of his front teeth have begun to chip.
1. What condition is present?
2. List the characteristic radiographic features seen here and several others not seen here.
3. With what condition of bones is this dental finding sometimes associated?

CASE **10-6** Take a look at the right central incisor.
1. What term describes the altered root shape?
2. How did it get this way?

CASE-BASED **QUESTIONS**

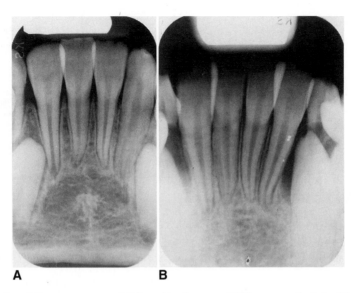

A   **B**

CASE **10-7** *A* and *B* represent two children (Andrew and Billy, respectively) of the same age. One of them is going to have a crowding problem with regard to the eruption of the permanent teeth.
1. Which one is going to have the crowding problem?
2. How did you figure that out?
3. What would you do about it?

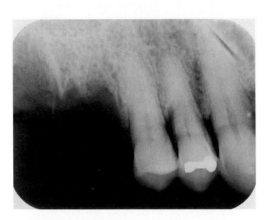

CASE **10-8** Study these teeth carefully. Notice that all three teeth have a radiolucent line in the cervical area. Clinically, the areas appeared V-shaped and were partially subgingival.
1. What is the differential diagnosis?
2. What condition do you think is present?
3. What is the cause, and how is it managed?

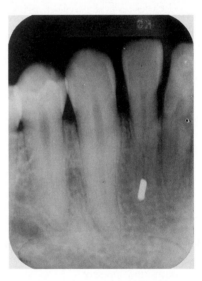

CASE **10-9** The lower right lateral incisor of this hockey player was avulsed last year during practice. The tooth was cleaned and sealed with a retrograde amalgam and then reimplanted and splinted with 009 wire and composite for several months.
1. What has happened to the root of this tooth?
2. What is the prognosis for the tooth?
3. How would you manage this case?

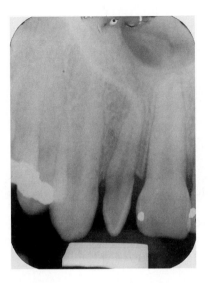

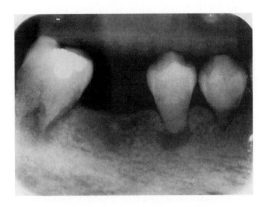

CASE **10-10** Take a look at the lateral incisor.
1. What term(s) best describe(s) this tooth's morphology?
2. How would you manage this?

CASE **10-11** Several permanent teeth of this 23-year-old man "exfoliated" spontaneously. All of his remaining teeth look like this. Notice the relative lack of root formation, the pulp is completely obliterated, and the apical radiolucencies may develop as a result of periodontal inflammation.
1. Exactly what condition is present?
2. How would you manage this?

CASE-BASED **QUESTIONS**

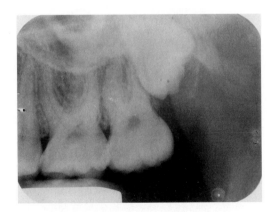

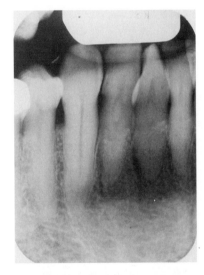

CASE **10-12** This patient complained of mild pain associated with the erupting 3rd molar.
1. See if you can identify the problem.
2. What would you do about it?

CASE **10-13** Note the pulp spaces in the central and lateral incisors. The teeth are vital.
1. What are these pulpal radiopacities called?
2. With what developmental dental problem can they be associated?
3. Does this developmental problem exist here?
4. What (if any) is the significance of this finding?

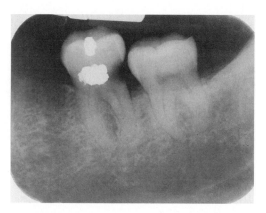

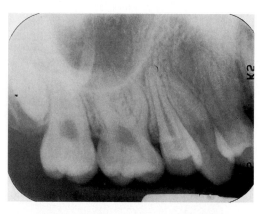

CASE **10-14** This middle-aged man has a habit that causes a factitial injury to one of his teeth. Clinically the area on the distal of the 1st molar was hard and shiny and has been a definite "meat catch" for many years.
1. Comment on the whole situation concerning the 1st molar.
2. What is the meaning of *factitial*?

CASE **10-15** Study this radiograph carefully.
1. What eruption problem has occurred here?
2. How can this be managed?

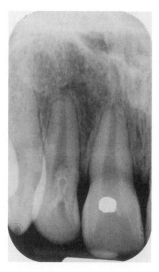

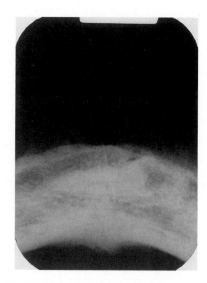

CASE **10-16** This patient is a healthy, attractive 15-year-old female. Examine her teeth carefully. Look again before going to the answer.
1. Report what you see. Be complete.

CASE **10-17** This older patient wears upper and lower dentures.
1. Exactly what do you see here (if anything)? Be specific.

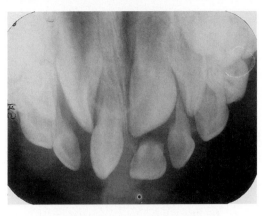

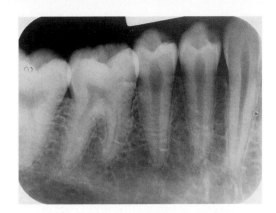

CASE **10-18** Gina is the youngest sibling among three others. Mom was a dental assistant before she married the boss (don't laugh, Denyse was my dental assistant!). The appearance of this tiny spiked tooth provoked Mom to take the brood to the dental office to get a radiograph taken.
1. What anomaly did we all discover?
2. What (if anything) should be done about it?

CASE **10-19** This patient is a healthy teenager.
1. Comment on the pulps of these teeth. Once again, look closely.

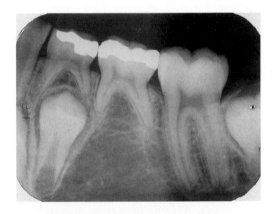

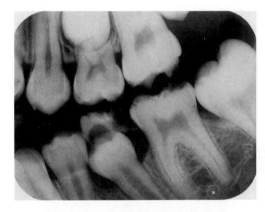

CASE **10-20** This patient is a 6-year-old girl.
1. What problem is seen here?
2. What would you report to her parents regarding the present and future management of this problem?
3. What other developmental anomaly would you suspect in this patient?

CASE **10-21** This 11-year-old boy was sick with high fevers earlier in his life. Now he is normal and healthy.
1. What condition affects the permanent 1st molars?
2. At what time in this boy's life did this occur?

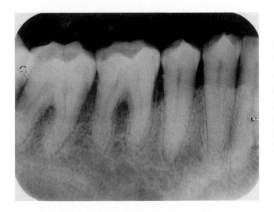

CASE **10-22** Believe it or not, this gentleman was 80 years old and had never been to the dentist. He was currently having a little discomfort because of the class 1 furcal involvement and a "meat catch" in the area. He would probably have ignored this but his favorite granddaughter was now a hygienist and insisted upon his dental visit.
1. What anomaly do we see in association with these teeth?

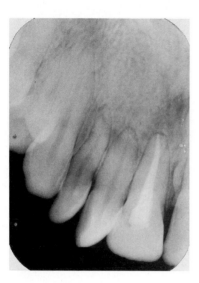

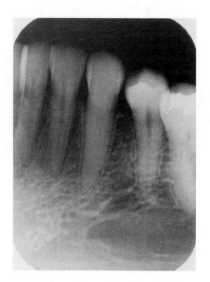

CASE **10-23** This patient is being considered for esthetic veneers in the anterior 1 X 6 of her dentition.
1. What anomaly (anomalies) can you see here?

CASE **10-24** This patient is in his late 30s. He is asymptomatic.
1. Can you pick out the non-vital tooth?
2. What are the radiographic signs of this non-vitality?
3. How would you treat this?

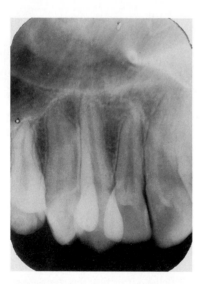

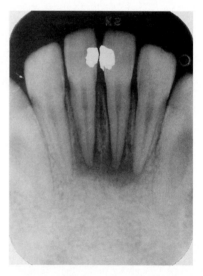

CASE **10-25** This patient's nickname in high school was "fang." Now in her mid-20s and a burgeoning chartered public accountant, she has decided to go ahead with the orthodontics.
1. What term best describes the malposition of the canine?
2. What other preventive procedure would you initiate for this patient ASAP? State your reason.

CASE **10-26** This 26-year-old man has a couple of unesthetic lower anterior restorations. Note the periapical radiolucencies in the area and the shape of the pulp chambers of the incisors. Right there you have the unique features of this anomaly. (That's a lot of clues!)
1. What anomaly is present? Be specific.
2. What material are the centrals restored with?

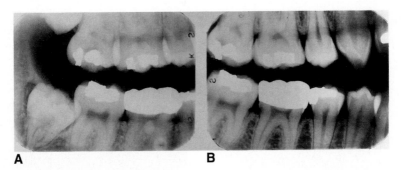

A　　　　　　**B**

CASE **10-38** Here's an interesting phenomenon. Follow these instructions carefully: Look at the posterior bitewing (*A*) and note the round, radiopaque structure (lower 1st molar). Before looking anywhere else, think about what this might be. Now look at the anterior bitewing (*B*) taken the same day. Presto! The thing you thought you saw has disappeared!
1. What entity did you think the little round radiopacity represented?
2. What is this phenomenon called, and what is the cause?
3. What is the significance of recognizing this phenomenon?

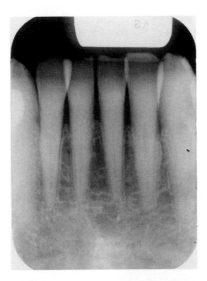

CASE **10-39** This patient is a 68-year-old woman. She takes very good care of her teeth these days. The teeth have obliterated pulps in the pulp chamber and upper root canal space.
1. What is the cause of this observation?

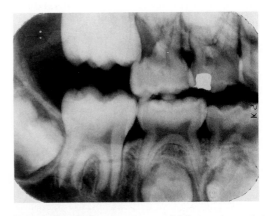

CASE **10-40** This is a 6-year-old boy whose 1st molars are just erupting. In the newly erupted molar, the root length is about the same length as the crown length. Remember, when an unerupted tooth has a root length longer than the crown length, something is delaying the eruption. In this case, there is a different eruption problem.
1. Can you identify the problem?
2. What is the significance of this finding?

CASE **10-41** This patient is a 32-year-old woman with a behavioral and psychological problem that she has not yet admitted to. The defect is maximal on the lingual aspect of the maxillary anterior teeth.
1. What dental anomaly do you think is present?
2. What is the most accurate technical term for this pattern?
3. How would you manage this case?

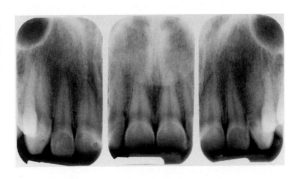

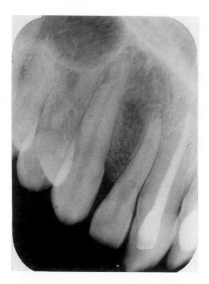

CASE **10-35** While doing endodontic therapy on an adjacent tooth, it was discovered the lateral incisor looked different.
1. What condition affects the lateral incisor?
2. How would you manage this case?

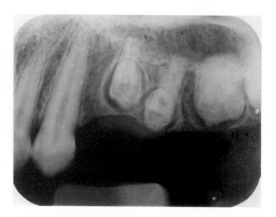

CASE **10-36** This patient received radiation therapy. The radiation was collimated to include the posterior maxilla and exclude the anterior jaws.
1. What term(s) best describe(s) the teeth in this area?
2. Will they erupt?
3. How would you manage this case?

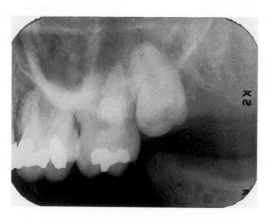

CASE **10-37** This patient has an anomaly that is hard to see in the photographic print.
1. Look carefully at these molars and see if you can identify it.

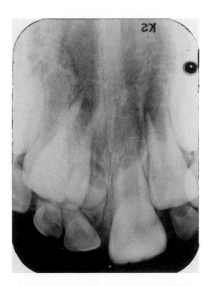

CASE **10-31** Just after the big Thanksgiving turkey meal, the mother of 6-year-old Julie noticed that Julie had not lost her 2nd front baby tooth. The tooth was not even loose at this point. "All she wants for Christmas is her two front teeth" quoted Julie's mom to her hygienist several days later.
1. Can you state what the problem is?
2. What would you do?
3. What about the two front teeth for Christmas?

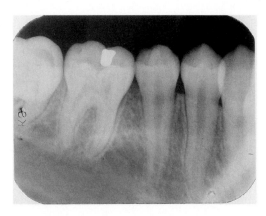

CASE **10-32** Lee Ong is a 12-year-old female of Asian extraction. Upon looking at this radiograph and subsequently examining the patient, the hygienist reported an unusual finding to the dentist.
1. What unusual finding was reported?
2. What is the significance of this discovery?

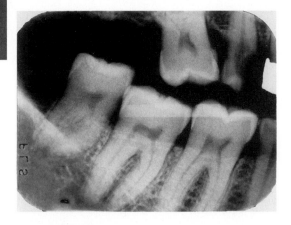

CASE **10-33** This patient is a 58-year-old man.
1. What term best describes the position of the lower 3rd molar with respect to the other teeth.
2. What generalized change in the teeth can we see here?

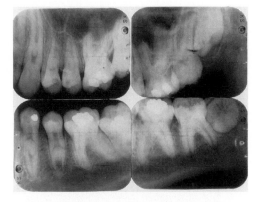

CASE **10-34** This patient is a 12-year-old male.
1. What condition affects these teeth?

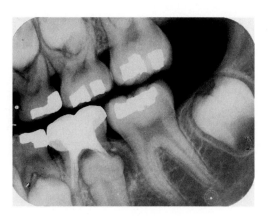

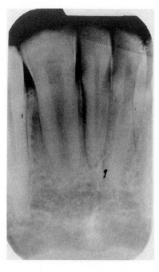

CASE **10-27** This 7-year-old boy is in for a check up.
1. What treatment has the primary 2nd molar received?
2. What condition affects the developing 2nd premolar?
3. Is there any connection between questions 1 and 2? (That's a hint!)

CASE **10-28** This is a 20-year-old man. He complains he does not like the looks of one of his bottom front teeth. He has never had an extraction. Starting at the patient's posterior right side (left side of the figure) we see the canine, a very wide incisor, the left central and lateral incisors, and the left canine.
1. Identify the anomaly present in the large incisor.
2. What clinical term best describes the large tooth?
3. Define the term you have selected.

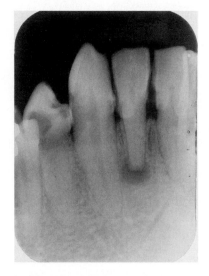

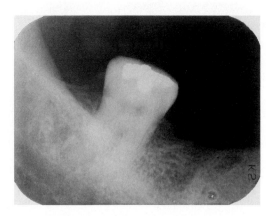

CASE **10-29** This middle-aged white man has periodontal disease. The 1st premolar is restored with an older radiolucent composite for esthetics. The right lateral incisor is a dark yellowish brown color, and he wants something done about it.
1. What condition affects the apical region of the right lateral incisor? Be complete.
2. How would you manage this case?

CASE **10-30** This patient came in with a broken lower partial denture. He wears a complete upper denture, which he was very satisfied with. Because of this, he was wondering if he should get a complete lower denture. If so, this tooth would need to be extracted.
1. What factor would you consider regarding the removal of this tooth?
2. Of what use (if any) would percussion be in the clinical evaluation of this tooth?

CASE-BASED **QUESTIONS**

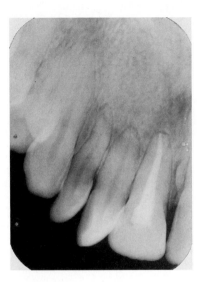

CASE **10-23** This patient is being considered for esthetic veneers in the anterior 1 X 6 of her dentition.
1. What anomaly (anomalies) can you see here?

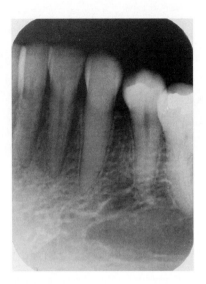

CASE **10-24** This patient is in his late 30s. He is asymptomatic.
1. Can you pick out the non-vital tooth?
2. What are the radiographic signs of this non-vitality?
3. How would you treat this?

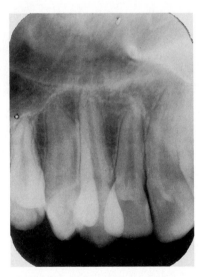

CASE **10-25** This patient's nickname in high school was "fang." Now in her mid-20s and a burgeoning chartered public accountant, she has decided to go ahead with the orthodontics.
1. What term best describes the malposition of the canine?
2. What other preventive procedure would you initiate for this patient ASAP? State your reason.

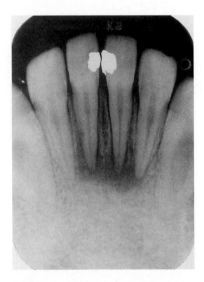

CASE **10-26** This 26-year-old man has a couple of unesthetic lower anterior restorations. Note the periapical radiolucencies in the area and the shape of the pulp chambers of the incisors. Right there you have the unique features of this anomaly. (That's a lot of clues!)
1. What anomaly is present? Be specific.
2. What material are the centrals restored with?

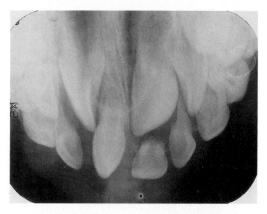

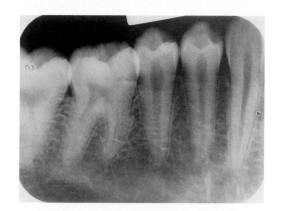

CASE **10-18** Gina is the youngest sibling among three others. Mom was a dental assistant before she married the boss (don't laugh, Denyse was my dental assistant!). The appearance of this tiny spiked tooth provoked Mom to take the brood to the dental office to get a radiograph taken.
1. What anomaly did we all discover?
2. What (if anything) should be done about it?

CASE **10-19** This patient is a healthy teenager.
1. Comment on the pulps of these teeth. Once again, look closely.

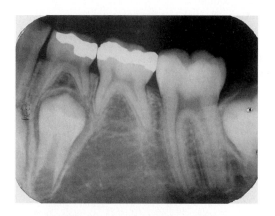

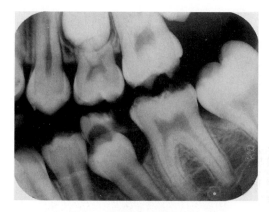

CASE **10-20** This patient is a 6-year-old girl.
1. What problem is seen here?
2. What would you report to her parents regarding the present and future management of this problem?
3. What other developmental anomaly would you suspect in this patient?

CASE **10-21** This 11-year-old boy was sick with high fevers earlier in his life. Now he is normal and healthy.
1. What condition affects the permanent 1st molars?
2. At what time in this boy's life did this occur?

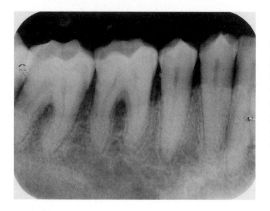

CASE **10-22** Believe it or not, this gentleman was 80 years old and had never been to the dentist. He was currently having a little discomfort because of the class 1 furcal involvement and a "meat catch" in the area. He would probably have ignored this but his favorite granddaughter was now a hygienist and insisted upon his dental visit.
1. What anomaly do we see in association with these teeth?

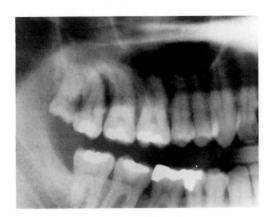

CASE **10-42** This patient has an anomalous problem.
1. Identify the problem.

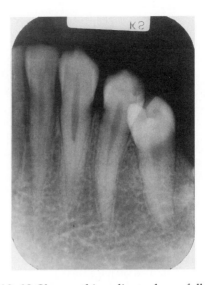

CASE **10-43** Observe this radiograph carefully.
1. What endodontically significant finding do these teeth demonstrate? These teeth do not require endodontic therapy.

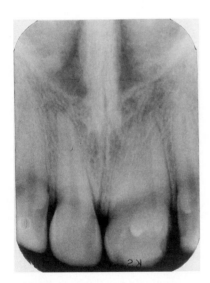

CASE **10-44** Here's a 23-year-old man who says his left front tooth is just too big. Here we see his two central and lateral incisors.
1. What general term can be used to describe the big tooth?
2. What specific problem affects this tooth?
3. Define the term you have selected for your previous answer.

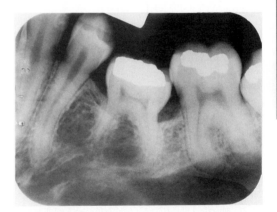

CASE **10-45** This patient is an adult in his 20s, and something needs to be done about this situation.
1. What terms can we use to describe the primary 2nd molar?
2. Can you see any problem developing as a result of this situation?
3. What treatment would you recommend?

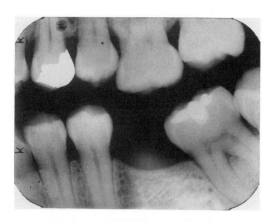

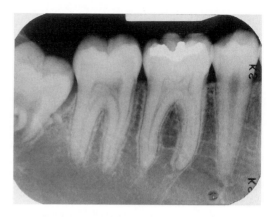

CASE **10-46** This situation is common. The lower 1st molar has been missing for a long time.
1. What do you see here?
2. How would you manage this?

CASE **10-47** Okay. Here's an easy one. Study this radiograph.
1. How old is this patient?
2. Comment on the pulp chambers of the 1st and 2nd molars.
3. What is the significance of this observation?

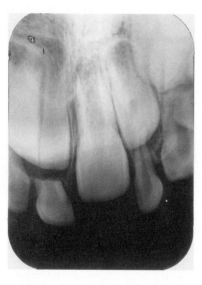

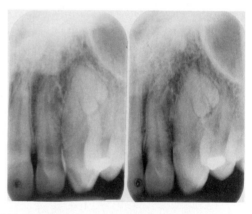

CASE **10-49** This patient is a 28-year-old man. He is asymptomatic. A radiopacity was noted in the apical region of the canine.
1. What anomaly do you think is present clinically?

CASE **10-48** This is a 5½-year-old girl. There is an indication she may have crowding of her permanent dentition. To avoid misleading you, note the film was bent and caused distortion in the left central incisor that is not associated with the sign being sought.
1. What sign indicates probable crowding in the permanent dentition?

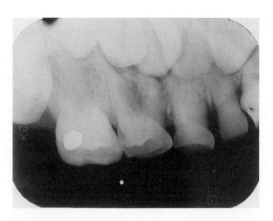

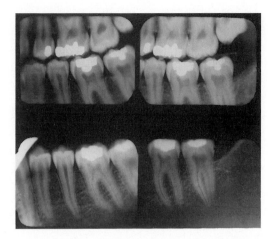

CASE **10-50** This patient is in his late teens with delayed eruption of all his permanent teeth. He has an underdeveloped set of bones in his upper torso, frontal bossing, and hypertelorism.
1. What condition do you think he has?
2. Which bone is underdeveloped?
3. What is hypertelorism, and exactly how do you determine this is present?

CASE **10-51** This patient is in his late 20s. He has a metabolic problem and takes huge amounts of vitamin D with a poor response. He is small in stature, especially in the lower body. The sign associated with his problem affects most of his teeth.
1. Describe the abnormal dental findings you need to look at carefully.
2. What condition do you think is present?

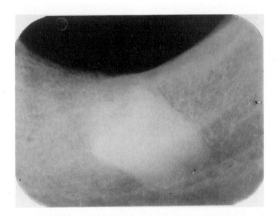

CASE **10-52** This edentulous patient has a radiopaque area in his left jaw.
1. Precisely what is this radiopaque entity?
2. How would you manage this?

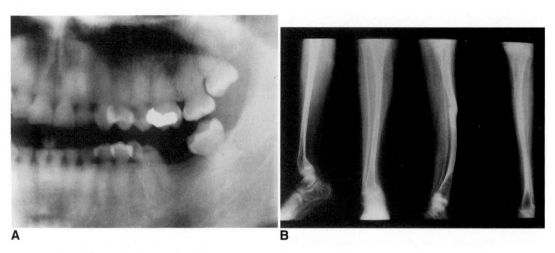

A   B

CASE **10-53** This patient is an 18-year-old white female. She has a problem with her teeth (*A*) and with her bones (*B*), and her eyes have a very visible anomaly.
1. What condition affects the teeth?
2. What is the overall systemic condition called?
3. What do you think can be seen in the eyes?

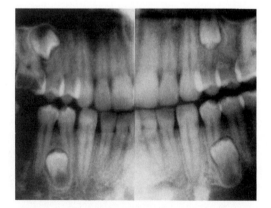

CASE **10-54** Here is a patient with a very apparent finding.
1. What anomaly is present?
2. How would you treat this?
3. What is the most common site of this anomaly?

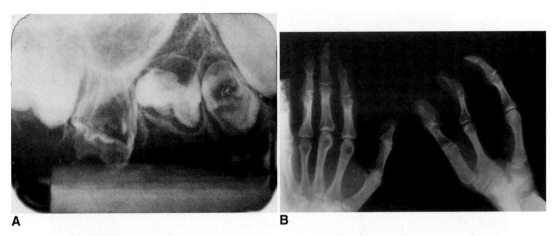

A   B

CASE **10-55** This patient has a syndrome named after the same folks who first reported the jaw cyst basal cell nevus syndrome. (Big clue!) The patient is a young man in his early 20s and had some abnormal looking teeth (*A*). Among other stigmata, he has a claw-like hand because of missing fingers (*B*), hypoplasia of the dermis in patches, and skin lesions.
1. What term best characterizes the appearance of these teeth?
2. What syndrome does this patient have?

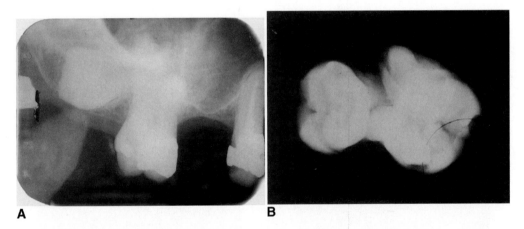

A   B

CASE **10-56** This simulated case demonstrates an impacted 3rd molar (*A*) whose roots are in proximity to each other. When the 3rd molar was elevated (during extraction), the erupted 2nd molar moved with it. As a result, both teeth were removed (*B*).
1. What condition affects these teeth?
2. Define the term you have chosen for the above answer.

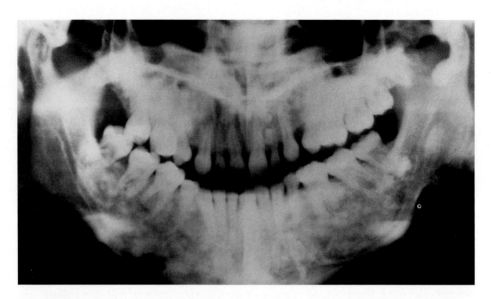

CASE **10-57** This patient is a 27-year-old man who had a large radiopaque mass removed from the left angle area of the mandible.
1. What dental anomaly involving numbers of teeth can you find?
2. What are the radiopaque lesions?
3. What syndrome does this patient have?
4. What important feature of the syndrome would you discuss with this patient?

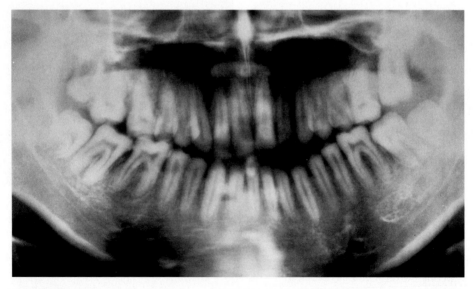

CASE **10-58** Study this radiograph carefully. This patient has a generalized condition affecting all of his teeth. A sibling is also affected the same way.
1. What condition of the teeth is present here?

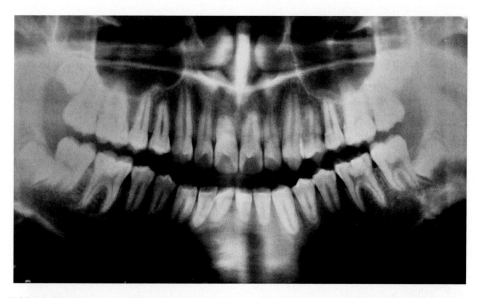

CASE **10-59** Henry is a 12-year-old Hispanic boy. He has never had orthodontic treatment.
1. Name at least two dental anomalies seen in this case.
2. What syndrome is present?
3. What other features are sometimes seen?

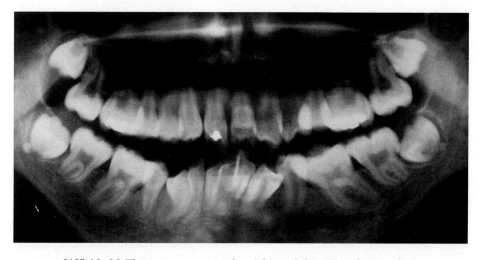

CASE **10-60** This teenage patient has "the real thing!" and in spades!
1. Can you name the anomaly (anomalies) present in this case?
2. Can you quantify your finding?
3. What other anomalies do you see?

CASE-BASED **QUESTIONS**

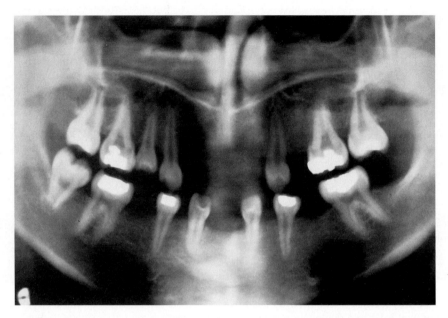

CASE **10-61** This patient has fine, sparse, blond hair; he has no eyebrows; and his nails don't grow out because they crumble once they get beyond the nail bed. His complexion is a ruddy, dry, reddish color. He has one other affected sibling. He has never had any teeth extracted.

1. What condition affects this patient?

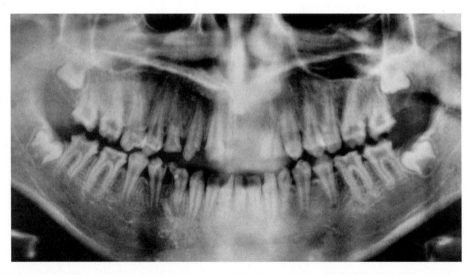

CASE **10-62** This patient is a 12-year-old female who rarely smiles with an open mouth or otherwise shows her teeth.

1. What condition affects her teeth?

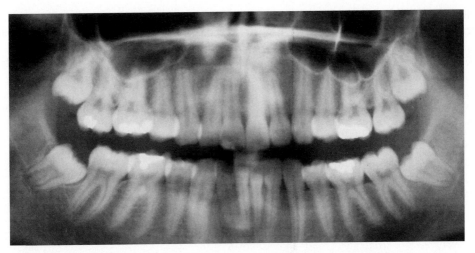

CASE **10-63** This patient is a 19-year-old male. He has just completed a full course of orthodontic therapy with extraction of all four 1st premolars.
1. Should we consider the developing 3rd molars as impacted and extract them or leave them alone because they are still erupting?
2. Do you think the erupting 3rd molars can cause a regression of the original crowding?

SPECIAL SECTION ON THIRD MOLAR IMPACTIONS

Study Figure 10-1, *A* to *F*, (pp. 158-159) which demonstrates classification for impacted 3rd molars. Having a classification is important in medico-legal record keeping and confirms that the dentist has thoroughly evaluated the tooth's position in relation to the adjacent tooth, to the potential space available, and to structures like the maxillary sinus. The relationship to the inferior alveolar canal will be considered separately. This classification is based on the work of Pell and Gregory and Winter and Archer.

Mandibular Impactions (Figure 10-1, A to C)

FACTOR I: Space (distance) between the distal of 2nd molar and ramus:

Class 1: Equal to or greater than m-d diameter of 3rd molar crown.

Class 2: Less than m-d diameter of 3rd molar crown.

Class 3: All or most of 3rd molar is in ramus.

FACTOR II: Depth of 3rd molar in bone:

Position A: Most superior aspect of 3rd molar level with or above occlusal plane of 2nd molar.

Position B: Most superior aspect of 3rd molar below occlusal plane but above cervical line of 2nd molar.

Position C: Most superior aspect of 3rd molar below cervical line of 2nd molar.

FACTOR III: Position of long axis of 3rd molar relative to long axis of 2nd molar:

Vertical	Mesioangular
Horizontal	Distoangular
Inverted	Buccoangular
Rotated	Linguoangular

CLASS 1

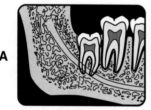 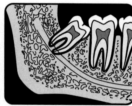 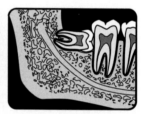

VERTICAL	**MESIOANGULAR**	**HORIZONTAL**
Position C	Position A	Position B

CLASS 2

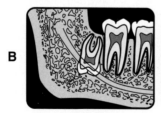 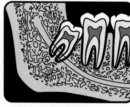 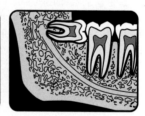

INVERTED	**MESIOANGULAR**	**HORIZONTAL**
Position C	Position B	Position A

CLASS 3

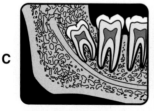 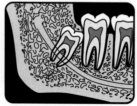 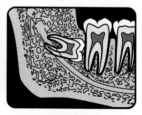

DISTOANGULAR	**MESIOANGULAR**	**HORIZONTAL**
Position B	Position C	Position C

FIGURE **10-1,** A to C

Maxillary Impactions (Figure 10-1, D to F)

FACTOR I: Depth of 3rd molar in bone:

Class A: Most inferior aspect of 3rd molar crown is on level with or below occlusal plane of 2nd molar.

Class B: Most inferior aspect of 3rd molar crown is between occlusal plane and cervical line of 2nd molar.

Class C: Most inferior aspect of 3rd molar crown is at or above cervical line of 2nd molar.

FACTOR II: Position of long axis of 3rd molar relative to long axis of 2nd molar:

Vertical	Mesioangular
Horizontal	Distoangular
Inverted	Buccoangular
Rotated	Linguoangular

FACTOR III: Relationship of 3rd molar to maxillary sinus:

Sinus approximation (SA)

No sinus approximation (NSA)

CLASS A

D

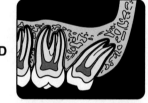
MESIOANGULAR NSA

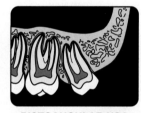
DISTOANGULAR NSA

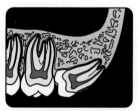
HORIZONTAL NSA

CLASS B

E

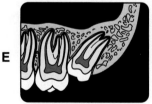
MESIOANGULAR NSA

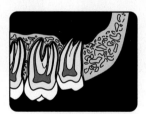
VERTICAL SA

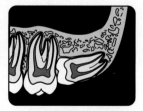
HORIZONTAL NSA

CLASS C

F

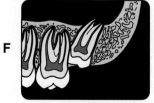
MESIOANGULAR SA

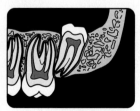
INVERTED SA

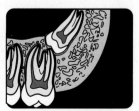
DISTOANGULAR SA

FIGURE **10-1,** D to F

All of these patients have impacted 3rd molars. Classify the impacted 3rd molars for each case.

Some cases include upper and lower 3rd molar impactions.

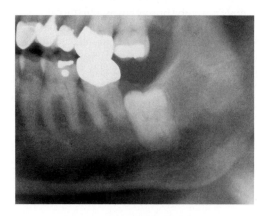

CASE **10-63.1**

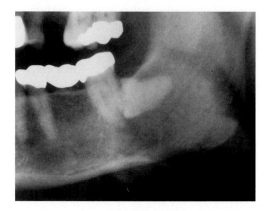

CASE **10-63.2**

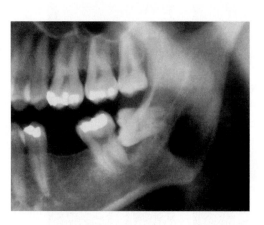

CASE **10-63.3**

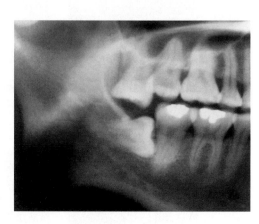

CASE **10-63.4**

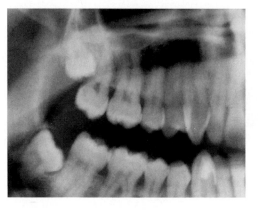

CASE **10-63.5**

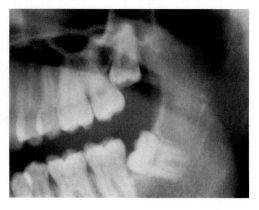

CASE **10-63.6**

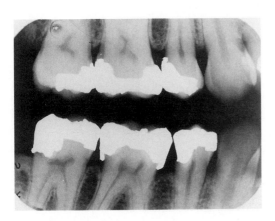

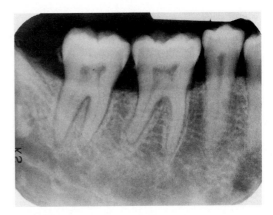

CASE **10-73** Here we have a lot of periodontally significant defective restorations.
1. Identify the defective restorations, describe the defect, and suggest how each should be managed.

CASE **10-74** Look at the two molars and the 2nd premolar.
1. What periodontally significant findings can you see?

SPECIAL SECTION ON CARIES AND CARIES SEQUELAE

Caries can be classified and/or described in many ways. It can be described by the classic classification: class I is occlusal; class II is interproximal, usually involving the contact point(s) of adjacent posterior teeth and sometimes including the distal of the canines; class III is anterior interproximal caries involving the contact points; class IV involves the incisal edge of an anterior tooth; class V is usually located on the buccal or lingual surface of any tooth; class VI involves a cusp tip only.

Caries may also be referred to as *incipient* when the caries is less than halfway through the enamel, *enamel caries* involving half or more of the depth into enamel but not into dentin, *dentinal caries*, and *pulpal caries*. Caries can be acute or chronic.

Here are some further descriptive terms.
- *Bottle caries* is seen in young children who are bottle-fed fluids with high sugar content.
- *Rampant caries* is often seen in teenagers and is associated with dietary, hygiene, and hormonal factors. Caries affects many teeth and advances at a rapid rate.
- *Xerostomia caries* is a form of rampant caries associated with xerostomia secondary to factors such as drugs and age; it often affects the roots of teeth.
- *Radiation caries* is similar to xerostomia caries, but the etiology is different and multifactorial, involving radiation effects on the oral ecology, immune factors, quantity of saliva, and dietary factors in post-irradiation patients. It ultimately results in a rubbery circumferential caries and eventual fracture of the tooth.

- *Recurrent caries* is seen at the margin or under a restoration.
- *Arrested caries* is when the caries process has ceased and the affected area becomes hard remineralize and often stained a brownish or blackish color and the caries advancement may be anywhere from incipient to very advanced.
- *Root caries* is seen on any surface of the root; when on the interproximal, it must be distinguished from class II caries by its location below the cemento-enamel junction. A special form of root caries is associated with overdentures.

Caries sequelae include space loss; periapical conditions of pulpal origin such as abscess, radicular cyst, periapical granuloma, and the rare cholesteatoma; also a lateral periodontal cyst can develop from a lateral canal in the root of a non-vital tooth; pulp polyp and residual cyst that remains upon extraction of the tooth, and Turner's enamel hypoplasia is a sequela of caries or trauma to a developing permanent tooth.

Radiographically, other conditions may resemble caries such as:
- Abfraction
- Toothbrush abrasion
- Abrasion from a partial denture clasp
- Adumbration, or cervical burnout, especially seen at the cervical of anterior teeth, the distal of canines, and upper 1st and 2nd molars
- Mach band effect seen in the dentin immediately beneath enamel and disappears when the enamel is covered with an opaque material like the paper wrap from a film packet

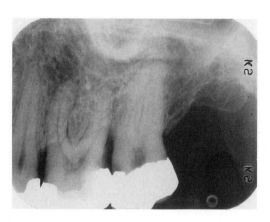

CASE **10-69** This radiograph is part of the patient's routine radiographic examination.
1. Report your findings in association with the 1st molar.
2. Report your findings in association with the 2nd molar.

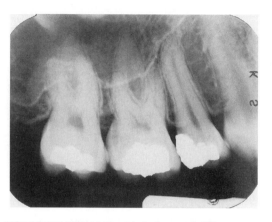

CASE **10-70** This patient is in her early 30s.
1. List one periodontally significant finding associated with each of the three most posterior teeth seen here.

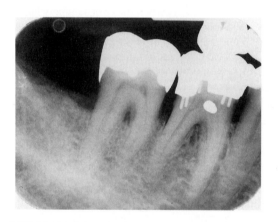

CASE **10-71** Take a look at these two molars.
1. What would you report?

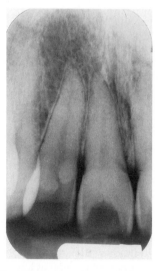

CASE **10-72** Look at this radiograph closely and the shovel-shaped incisors. (Prominent marginal ridges, deep lingual pit, and tendency for class III caries.) There is some horizontal bone loss. The lamina dura is much more prominent for the lateral than for the central incisor.
1. In this area and especially in this case, what further additional periodontally significant finding would you look for in this radiograph? Explain.

SPECIAL SECTION ON PERIODONTAL ASSESSMENT

The following cases are presented in no particular order. All of the selected cases demonstrate some radiographic finding(s) that may be associated with periodontal disease.

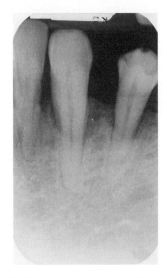

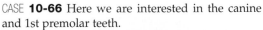

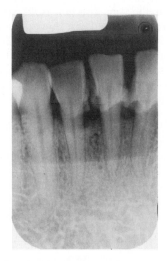

CASE **10-66** Here we are interested in the canine and 1st premolar teeth.
1. Describe your findings associated with the canine.
2. Describe your findings in association with the premolar?

CASE **10-67** This is the lower anterior region of a periodontal patient.
1. What term is used to classify this calculus regarding its location above the gingiva?
2. What term describes such copious amounts of calculus?
3. What periodontally significant factor can such copious amounts of calculus mask?
4. Classify the type of bone loss in association with these teeth.
5. What periodontal disease do you think is present?
6. What is the horizontal radiopaque line at the apical region of all these teeth?

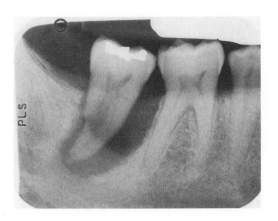

CASE **10-68** Note this patient's molars.
1. What term describes the periodontal status of the 2nd molar?
2. In this circumstance, what other disease(s) must be ruled out?
3. Describe the periodontal defect associated with the 2nd molar.
4. What finding suggests this tooth has been mobile for a long time?
5. Is there anything that may suggest the cause of this mobility?
6. What do we see in the furcal area of the 1st molar?

SPECIAL SECTION ON LOCALIZATION

There are three "rules" for the localization of objects toward the buccal or lingual within the jaws using two periapical radiographs taken at different angles.

- First described by C. Clark in 1909, this rule requires a fixed vertical angulation and a different horizontal angle of the beam for the two radiographs. If the object in question moves in the same direction as the horizontal shift of the tube head, it is toward the lingual; if the object moves in the opposite direction, it is on the buccal. This is where the *SLOB rule* comes from: **S**ame on **L**ingual; **O**pposite on **B**uccal. The problem for many is that it is hard to figure out which way the tube head moved in the two comparison radiographs.
- The *buccal object rule* was first described by Richards in 1952. Here the buccal object will move with the angulation change of the BID (cone), including up, down, mesial, or distal when the two radiographs are compared. This rule is easier because students can recognize the effects of vertical and horizontal changes in the BID.
- The *known object rule* was first popularized by Langlais in the early 1980s. In this instance

there is no need to figure out which way the tube head or BID has moved. The only requirements are the two comparison radiographs taken at different vertical or horizontal angles and a known object you can identify as buccal or lingual. The known object will have moved either up or down or mesially or distally in the two comparison radiographs. Some known objects are the buccal cusps, the buccal malar process of the maxilla, the lingual mandibular and palatal tori and the incisive foramen, the buccal mental foramen and external oblique ridge, the lingual genial tubercles and internal oblique ridge, etc. Now look at the unknown object and compare its movement to the movement of the known object. If the unknown object moves in the same way as the known object, it is located in the same place (either buccal or lingual); if it moves in the opposite direction as the known object, it is opposite in location. If it does not move, it is in the middle of the jaw in question. If the movement is in the same direction as the known object but not as much, it is not as far out on the side (buccal or lingual) of the known object.

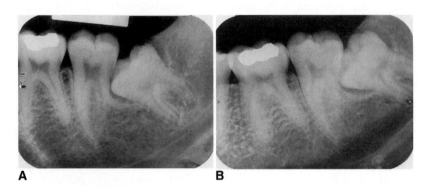

A   **B**

CASE **10-64** Notice the impacted 3rd molar.
1. On which side of the mandible is the impacted 3rd molar located?

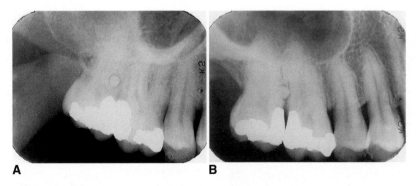

A   **B**

CASE **10-65** Notice the enamel pearl on the maxillary 2nd molar.
1. Because you suspect an associated periodontal defect, toward which side (the buccal or lingual) will you probe for the enamel pearl?

All of these patients have impacted 3rd molars. Classify the impacted 3rd molars for each case.

Some cases include upper and lower 3rd molar impactions.

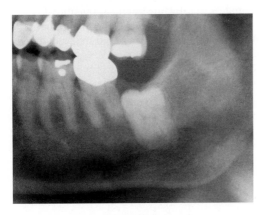

CASE **10-63.1**

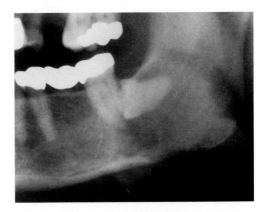

CASE **10-63.2**

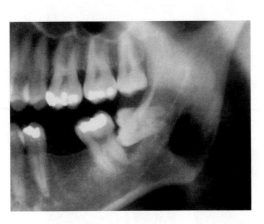

CASE **10-63.3**

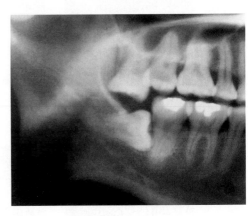

CASE **10-63.4**

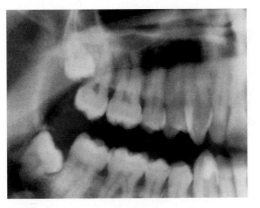

CASE **10-63.5**

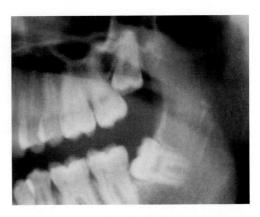

CASE **10-63.6**

Maxillary Impactions (Figure 10-1, D to F)

FACTOR I: Depth of 3rd molar in bone:

Class A: Most inferior aspect of 3rd molar crown is on level with or below occlusal plane of 2nd molar.

Class B: Most inferior aspect of 3rd molar crown is between occlusal plane and cervical line of 2nd molar.

Class C: Most inferior aspect of 3rd molar crown is at or above cervical line of 2nd molar.

FACTOR II: Position of long axis of 3rd molar relative to long axis of 2nd molar:

Vertical	Mesioangular
Horizontal	Distoangular
Inverted	Buccoangular
Rotated	Linguoangular

FACTOR III: Relationship of 3rd molar to maxillary sinus:

Sinus approximation (SA)

No sinus approximation (NSA)

CLASS A

D

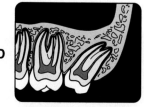
MESIOANGULAR NSA

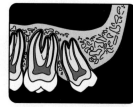
DISTOANGULAR NSA

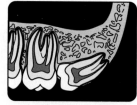
HORIZONTAL NSA

CLASS B

E

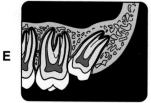
MESIOANGULAR NSA

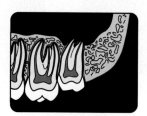
VERTICAL SA

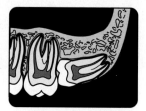
HORIZONTAL NSA

CLASS C

F

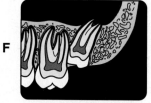
MESIOANGULAR SA

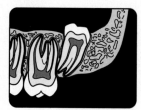
INVERTED SA

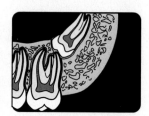
DISTOANGULAR SA

FIGURE **10-1,** D to F

CASE-BASED **QUESTIONS**

- Some forms of erosion
- Older, radiolucent, tooth-colored filling materials, radiolucent cements, and pulp capping materials
- Developmental defects such as the various presentations of enamel hypoplasia

- The so-called controversial pre-eruptive caries, whereby a tooth becomes "carious" before eruption, when not exposed to the oral environment by, for example, a periodontal defect; such cases most likely represent external or internal resorption

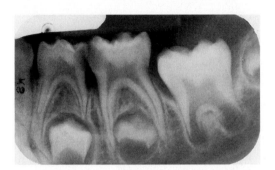

CASE **10-75** This patient is a 6-year-old boy with an erupting 1st permanent molar. Note how root formation does not exceed crown length when the tooth first emerges into the mouth; the apical half of the root will develop from first emergence until the tooth is in occlusion. This is important in the early identification of delayed eruption.
1. Classify the caries in the two primary molars
2. What caries sequela must we avoid in this situation?
3. When will these teeth be shed?
4. How would these teeth be treated?

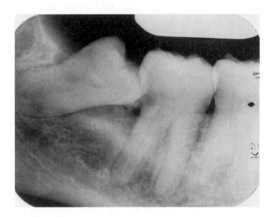

CASE **10-76** This is a patient with a toothache. It is relieved by a cold drink. He is now in his 40s and has never needed to go to the dentist. The tooth is sensitive to percussion. This is a common situation in people with a partially erupted 3rd molar that was not extracted.
1. What periodontally significant factor(s) can you see in association with the 3rd molar?
2. Is there any problem with the 2nd molar? Explain.

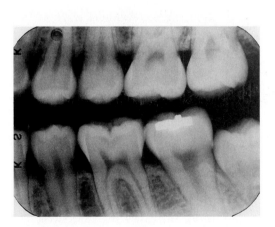

CASE **10-77** This is a patient under consideration for preventive treatment.
1. Which one surface would you not seal as the only treatment? Why?
2. On which one tooth can cervical burnout be most clearly seen?

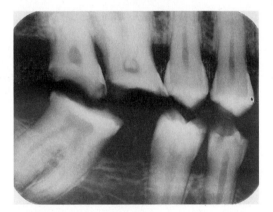

CASE **10-78** This patient's molars are rock-hard on the occlusal surface, which is dark brown in color, smooth, and shiny.
1. What type of caries has affected the molars?
2. What is the radiolucent area on the distal of the mandibular 1st premolar?
3. Do you see any occlusal caries anywhere?
4. Classify the caries on the mesial of the lower 2nd premolar.

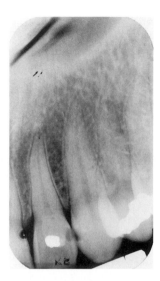

CASE **10-79** Here we are interested in the lesions on the lateral and canine.
1. Classify the caries on these two teeth.
2. What would you conclude if no caries could be found upon clinical examination?
3. With what material is the lingual pit restored?

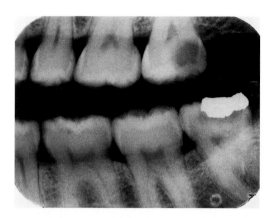

CASE **10-80** This patient has a number of carious lesions.
1. Classify the caries in the following teeth:
   Maxilla:
   - 1st premolar
   - 2nd premolar
   - 2nd molar
   Mandible:
   - 1st molar
   - 2nd molar
   - 3rd molar
2. On which one surface is the most obvious cervical burnout?

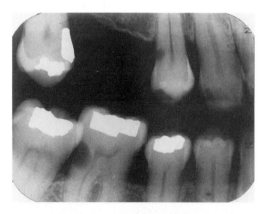

CASE **10-81** This patient has two very obvious carious lesions of interest to us here.
1. Classify the lesions on the upper 1st premolar and on the lower 1st molar.
2. Comment on the etiology (cause).

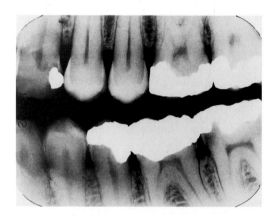

CASE **10-82** This case is short and sweet.
1. Where is the recurrent caries?

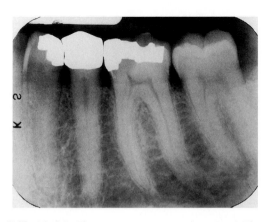

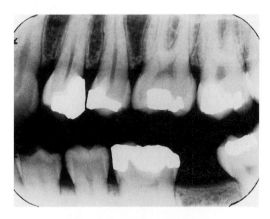

CASE **10-83** This is a common situation. This patient does not have any clinically detectable caries though the problem was easily seen during the clinical examination.
1. What problem do you think affects the lower 1st molar?
2. What treatment would you recommend?

CASE **10-84** This is an important and somewhat frequent situation. This patient complains of a slight twinge or sensitivity in one of his teeth on this side, which he just cannot seem to localize. This sensation comes and goes, never stays for long, and is absent for long periods. He also complains of a "meat catch" in the upper premolar area but is not certain the pain he is speaking of comes from there. The problem is actually obvious if you know what to look for.
1. Which one tooth would you suspect as the source of the problem? Explain.

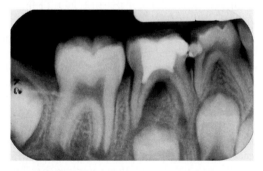

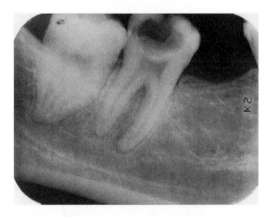

CASE **10-85** Here we see an important set of circumstances that must be recognized. The pulpotomy was done 6 months ago at the last dental visit. A gum boil still comes and goes. Note that the root formation is only about two-thirds complete; thus eruption of the 1st molar is still in progress. Remember, the occlusal plane of the permanent dentition is higher than that of the primary dentition.
1. What problem relative to the mandibular 2nd premolar do we need to prevent?
2. What treatment would you suggest?

CASE **10-86**
1. Comment on the mandibular 2nd molar vitality status.
2. How would this case be restored?

CASE-BASED **QUESTIONS**

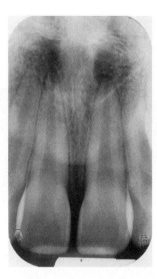

CASE **10-87** This 8-year-old boy fell off his skateboard and traumatized his upper lip. The teeth did not appear fractured clinically; however, this radiograph was taken to make sure.
1. What problem(s) (if any) do you see?

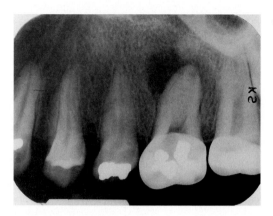

CASE **10-88** Here we are interested primarily in the maxillary 1st molar.
1. Comment on the vitality status of this tooth.
2. What condition is present at the apex?
3. What type of crown is on the 1st molar?
4. What condition affects the 2nd molar?

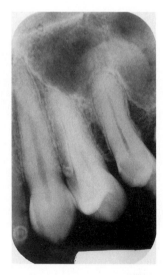

CASE **10-89** This is an unusual periapical radiograph of the premolars. It is actually a botched canine radiograph. The tooth in question is the 2nd premolar.
1. Classify the caries in the 2nd premolar.
2. Comment on the root shape of this tooth.
3. What periapical reaction (if any) do we see here?
4. How would this tooth be managed? Comment on extraction.

SPECIAL SECTION ON THIRD MOLAR RELATIONSHIP TO THE MANDIBULAR CANAL

Depicted are some of the most important means of determining a very close relationship of the 3rd molar root to the inferior alveolar canal. The suspicion of this intimate relationship is important to incorporate into the treatment plan because neurogenic symptoms such as a numb or burning lower lip or vascular problems such as severe bleeding can occur if the structures within the canal are damaged during the procedure. More recently, the validity of these findings has been questioned. However, it is certainly desirable to be cautious whenever these findings are seen. In Case 10-90, *A*, note that one or both walls of the canal are not apparent in the region of the roots; here the roots may have resorbed or thinned the canal wall. In *B*, a radiolucent band is on one or more roots where the canal crosses the roots; here there may be a groove in the roots, making this area more radiolucent and caused by the proximity of the canal during root development. In *C*, the canal is narrowed where it crosses the roots; here we may actually have the canal going right between the roots or being completely or partially enveloped by the roots. Also, any two or three combinations are an even stronger suggestion that the 3rd molar roots are close to the canal.

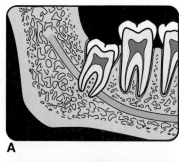

A

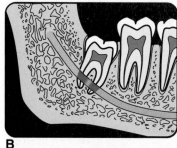

B

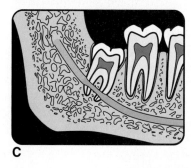

C

CASE **10-90**

1. Having studied the above diagrams, can a close relationship of the 3rd molars and the mandibular canal be suspected?

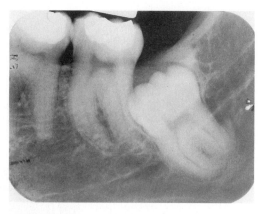

CASE **10-91**

1. What feature(s) cause(s) you to suspect a close relationship between the 3rd molar and the inferior alveolar canal?

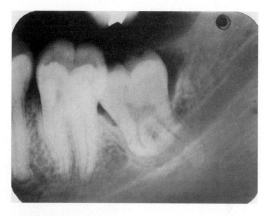

CASE **10-92**

1. What feature(s) cause(s) you to suspect a close relationship between the 3rd molar and the inferior alveolar canal?

SPECIAL SECTION ON SINUS PNEUMATIZATION

In Case 10-93 you can see the stages (*A* to *C*) by which pneumatization of the maxillary sinus develops. This concept is more important than ever as implant therapy is common.

The pneumatization process seems to vary over time and from one person to another. It may be most prominent in persons with chronic sinus problems such as allergy or sinusitis. In any case, the available alveolar bone for an implant in this area may alter over time and the patient should be informed.

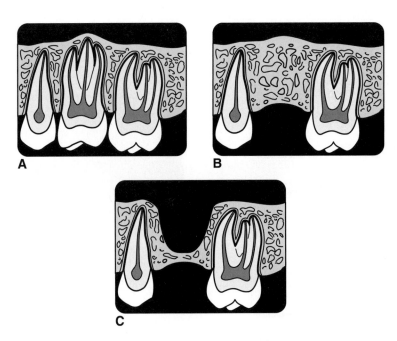

CASE **10-93**
1. Based on the diagrams, can pneumatization be seen in periapical radiographs?

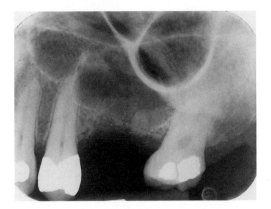

CASE **10-94** This patient wishes to have the edentulous space replaced with several implants. This radiograph was taken as part of the initial assessment.
1. How do things look for one or more implants here? (Good, not bad, or bad)
2. What pathology do you see in the edentulous area?
3. What condition affects the sinus?
4. Is there anything that can be done if the patient insists on exhausting every possibility in order to have implants?

Assessment/ Interpretation of Pathology of the Jaws

Goal

To know how to assess and/or interpret radiographic images for the presence of disease

Learning Objectives

1. Recognize abnormal features in the jaws
2. Recognize cysts of the jaws
3. Know the features of tumors of the jaws
4. Recognize developmental or genetically related disorders
5. Identify fibro-osseous conditions
6. Recognize inflammatory disorders and infections
7. Review the most common pathologic abnormalities affecting the jaws

Instructions

The questions are short and to the point. They do contain clues such as the age and sex of the patient, laboratory values, and even in the patient's name! So watch for the clues.

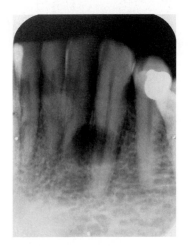

CASE **11-1** Bill is an asymptomatic 47-year-old who presented for routine dental treatment. This radiograph was taken as part of the full mouth survey.

1. On what side of the mandible (buccal or lingual) is the radiolucent lesion in the canine area located?
2. What developmental anomaly do you think this finding represents?
3. What treatment (if any) would you recommend?

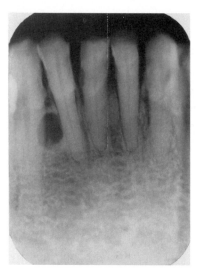

CASE **11-2** Mary is a 67-year-old who was referred to the periodontist. As part of the radiographic examination, this small radiolucent lesion was detected. The teeth were vital.

1. Give a differential diagnosis for this lesion. Include three conditions, stating your most likely choice first and least likely last.
2. Considering the patient's age and the location, size, and clinical findings, what is your diagnostic impression?
3. What treatment would you recommend? Why?

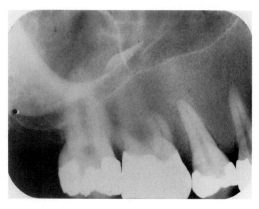

CASE **11-3** This is a 35-year-old asymptomatic woman who has slight buccal and palatal enlargement of the alveolar bone in this area. Other studies indicated portions of the zygoma were involved. This condition was first detected at age 19 years and is slowly progressive. Her alkaline phosphatase was normal to high-normal, and the serum calcium was normal.

1. Describe the significant radiographic findings.
2. Give a differential diagnosis consisting of three conditions, with your best choice first.
3. What is your diagnostic impression?
4. What treatment (if any) would you recommend?

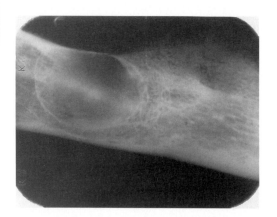

CASE **11-4** This 72-year-old woman presented with loose 20-year-old dentures and slight intermittent pain under the lower denture. She stated she had her teeth extracted because of severe untreated caries and abscessed teeth. The radiolucent lesion was detected on a radiograph of the painful area.

1. Describe the lesion.
2. What is your diagnostic impression?
3. Name several other lesions that could look like this.
4. What treatment would you recommend?

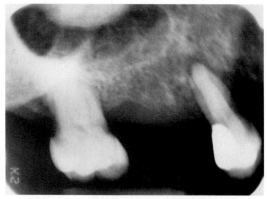

CASE **11-5** Mary is a 55-year-old who is about to have dentures made.

1. Study this radiograph and determine what significant factor might affect the treatment plan.

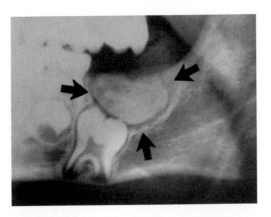

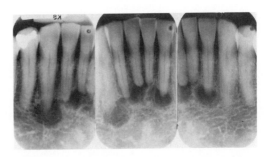

CASE **11-6** This 6-year-old boy presented with intermittent pain in the left posterior mandible. A clinically missing lower left 1st molar was noted, and the other three 1st molars were erupted. No bony expansion was in this area (*arrows*); however, the tissue at the crest of the ridge was slightly reddish and swollen.
1. What is the cause of the patient's pain?
2. Describe the lesion causing the delayed eruption.
3. Give a differential diagnosis of four conditions.
4. What is the most probable diagnosis?
5. Upon removal of the mass, will the 1st molar erupt?

CASE **11-7** This asymptomatic patient is a 45-year-old woman. Her routine radiographs indicated several periapical radiolucencies in the lower anterior region.
1. What is the probable race of this patient?
2. What condition is present?
3. In all likelihood, are the teeth vital?
4. If applicable, what stage(s) is (are) present?
5. What treatment (if any) would you recommend?

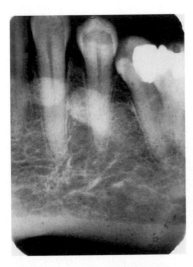

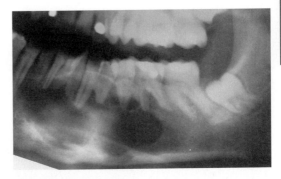

CASE **11-8** This patient is missing all of his lower molars bilaterally, and a removable partial denture is being planned.
1. What (if any) treatment plan modification(s) would you consider after studying this radiograph? Comment on the prognosis of your treatment plan.

CASE **11-9** This is a 16-year-old female with a lesion in the left mandible. All of the teeth are vital.
1. Describe the lesion.
2. Give a differential diagnosis of five conditions in a descending order of certainty.
3. State your diagnostic impression.
4. Discuss the certainty and prognosis of your diagnostic impression.

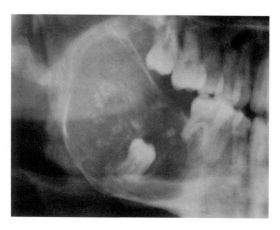

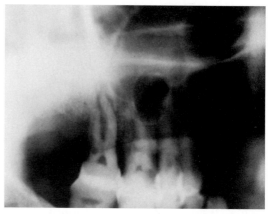

CASE **11-10** Terry is a 12-year-old boy with intermittent pain and swelling in the right posterior mandible.
1. Describe the lesion.
2. Give a differential diagnosis.
3. State your diagnostic impression.
4. What is the treatment, and state the prognosis?

CASE **11-11** Clara is a 72-year-old who reports pain and slight facial swelling in the right maxilla. Clinically, you could see swelling at the mucobuccal fold between the 1st molar and 2nd premolar. Her history revealed she had a Caldwell-Luc procedure performed on the right maxillary sinus some 20 years ago.
1. Based on this history and radiographic findings, what lesion is present?
2. Briefly describe the three variations in location with which this lesion presents.

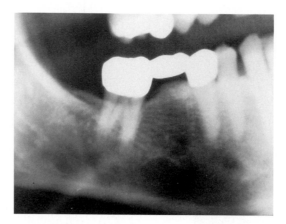

CASE **11-12** George is a 41-year-old with slight discomfort in the area of this 15-year-old bridge. Clinically, the gingiva beneath the pontic was red and swollen.
1. What condition do you think is present?
2. What is the treatment and prognosis?

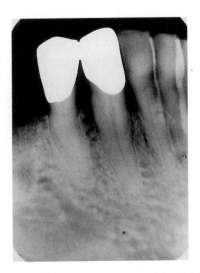

CASE **11-13** Ollie is 64 years old. He has a removable partial denture with bilateral free end bases, which he has worn for years. Look at the most distal tooth in the lower right quadrant; it was the only tooth affected.
1. What condition affects the root of this tooth?
2. What is the characteristic radiographic appearance?
3. With what systemic disease is this associated, and do you think this case applies?
4. Comment on how this may have developed.
5. Has the dilacerated root developed in association with this condition or its history?

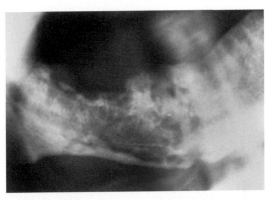

CASE **11-14** Mr. X is a 59-year-old homeless person. He recently had his remaining mandibular teeth extracted for tenderness, redness, swelling, and intraoral and submandibular fistula formation in the right quadrant. However, the pain has not regressed. Now paresthesia has developed in the lower right lip. The radiograph revealed a possible partially healed fracture of the mandible in the right canine region, the cause of which the patient could neither affirm nor deny.
1. Describe the radiographic findings.
2. State your diagnostic impression.
3. In normal extraction socket healing, how long does it take for the lamina dura to disappear?
4. How would you treat this?

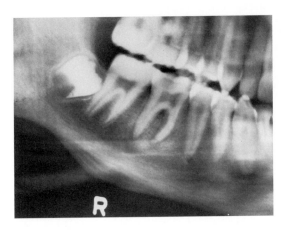

CASE **11-15** Denis is a 13-year-old boy with a slightly swollen face on the right side. Clinically, a non-tender, bony, hard swelling was in the mucobuccal fold adjacent to the 1st molar. There was a history of past toothache, but it went away.
1. Describe the significant radiographic findings.
2. State your diagnostic impression.
3. How would you treat this?
4. With successful treatment, how long would you expect it to take for the swelling to go away?
5. Describe the radiographic evidence of resolution.

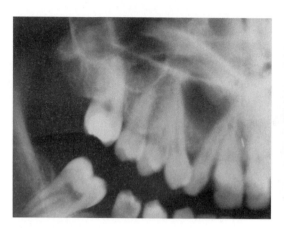 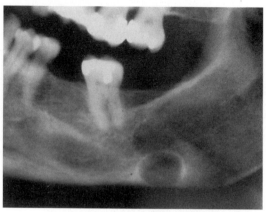

CASE **11-16** Denise is a 27-year-old who complained her "front tooth" seemed to be getting "crooked." The radiolucency in the right maxilla was a serendipitous finding.

1. Regarding the lesion, what diagnostic test would you perform?
2. What is your diagnostic impression?
3. How would you manage this case? Remember the chief complaint!

CASE **11-17** This 52-year-old man gave us the okay for a fixed prosthesis to replace the lower left molar. Everybody was surprised to find the radiolucent lesion at the inferior border of the mandible.

1. What is your diagnostic impression?
2. How would you manage this lesion?
3. About the bridge, can the angular relationship of teeth (such as abutment tooth parallelism) be assessed accurately from a panoramic radiograph?

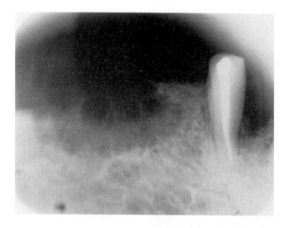

CASE **11-18** Mrs. Sally S. is 42 years old. She complained that her overdenture no longer fit well and chewing was painful. Clinically, a reddish, slightly swollen area was at the crest of the edentulous ridge in the right posterior mandible.

1. Describe the lesion.
2. What is your diagnostic impression?
3. How would you manage this case?

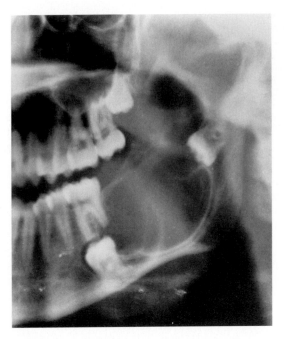

CASE **11-19** This patient is a 16-year-old male. He complained of pain on chewing, and his mother noticed the left side of his face seemed a bit swollen. He had never been to the dentist. At surgery, some straw-colored fluid could be aspirated.
1. Describe the lesion.
2. Give a differential diagnosis of five lesions.
3. State your diagnostic impression.
4. How would you manage this case?

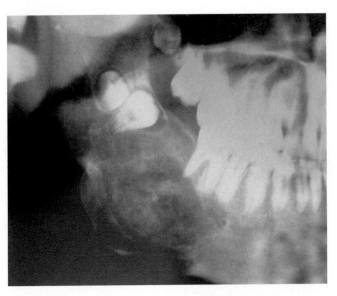

CASE **11-20** Normie is an 11-year-old boy who presented with a slowly progressive facial swelling over the past 6 to 8 months and mild pain on chewing.
1. Describe the lesion.
2. Give a differential diagnosis.
3. State your diagnostic impression.
4. How would you manage this case?

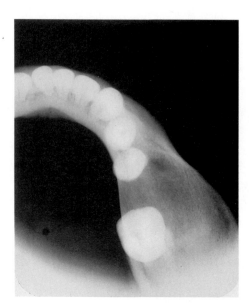

CASE **11-21** While working up this patient for a bridge, this lesion was noted. There is a radiographic feature here that almost certainly suggests the diagnosis.
1. Describe the "pathognomonic" (almost certain) feature.
2. What is the diagnosis?

NOTE TO STUDENTS: Okay, are you ready for the next one? Take a break, come back, and let's see what you can do.

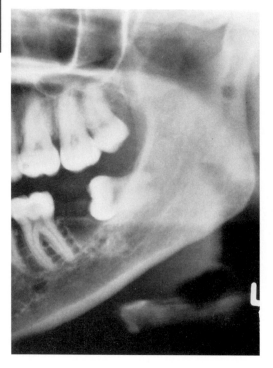

CASE **11-22** This patient has not seen a dentist in 10 years. There are two radiologically distinct conditions affecting the mandible.
1. Name the two conditions.
2. What is the significance of these two findings (if any)?
3. What is the probable sex of this patient?

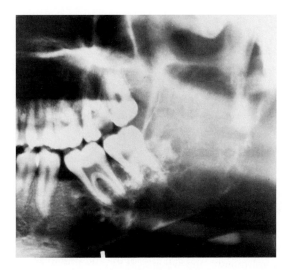

CASE **11-23** Okay, this is a hard one... but this general group of lesions is really important to recognize in x-rays. As with all of the histories given with the cases, watch for the clues! Sang is a 20-year-old woman who reports a rather recent development of swelling and pain in the left side of her face. There was a deep carious lesion in the upper left 2nd molar, but the tooth proved to be non-vital. The lower 2nd molar displayed +2 mobility. There was a "welling up" of blood when the lesion was incised at surgery.
1. What basic radiologic pattern does this lesion display?
2. What radiographic features can you see that, when correlated with the history, suggest a diagnosis?
3. State your diagnostic impression.

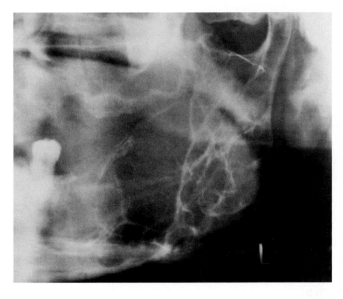

CASE **11-24** This patient is a 32-year-old man. The maxilla is edentulous, but he does not wear a denture. At surgery, the lesional tissue was an amber, gelatinous, gooey material.
1. What is the overall radiographic pattern of the lesion in the left posterior mandible?
2. Clinically, what does this pattern suggest regarding the nature and behavior of this lesion?
3. Describe the lesion.
4. Give a differential diagnosis.
5. What is your diagnostic impression?
6. Comment on the 2nd premolar.

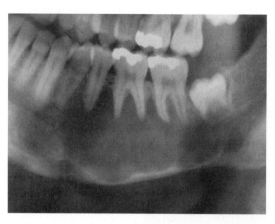

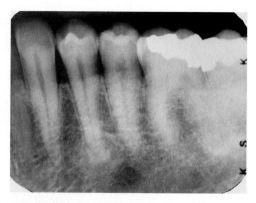

CASE **11-25** Solitaire is a 14-year-old member of the all-girl softball team. She remembers the ball slamming into her jaw several months ago when the sun got into her eyes and she missed a pop fly.
1. What is the radiographic pattern of this lesion?
2. Describe this lesion.
3. State your diagnostic impression.

CASE **11-26** Jenny A. is a 38-year-old asymptomatic white woman. There is a radiopacity at the apex of the 1st premolar and a radiolucency at the root end of the 2nd premolar.
1. Are these findings part and parcel of the same condition (yes or no)?
Answer either question #2 or #3:
2. If yes, state the condition and explain your choice.
3. If no, identify the two conditions.

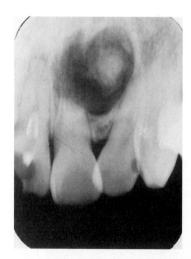

CASE **11-27** Monsieur Phantome is a 45-year-old Frenchman who noticed his front tooth has been getting crooked. Clinically, a slight bony swelling was at the mucobuccal fold and on the palate. The associated left central and lateral incisors were vital.
1. Give a differential diagnosis for this lesion.
2. Notice the root resorption; what, in general, does this indicate regarding the nature of the lesion?
3. Can you take a guess as to the diagnosis?

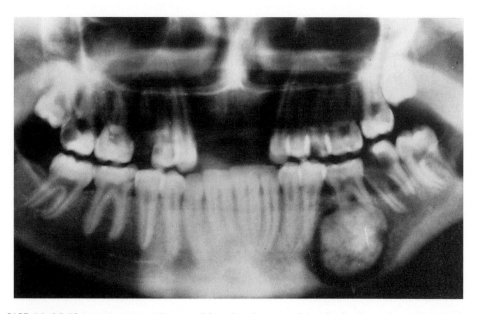

CASE **11-28** This patient is a 17-year-old male who complained of pain and swelling in the left side of his jaw.
1. Describe the lesion at the apex of the left 1st molar.
2. What is your diagnostic impression of the lesion?
3. What do you see regarding the mandibular left 2nd molar? (*Hint*: you've seen this before.)
4. Why are the roots of the maxillary teeth obscured?

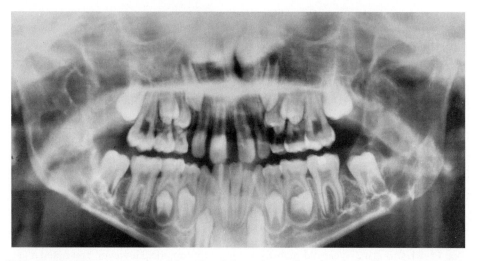

CASE **11-29** Jill is an 11-year-old with a bilateral, painless facial swelling that has been present since about age 5 years. When looking straight ahead, her eyes appeared "turned upward to heaven."
1. What condition is present?
2. What is the cause of the eye problem?
3. How would you manage this case?

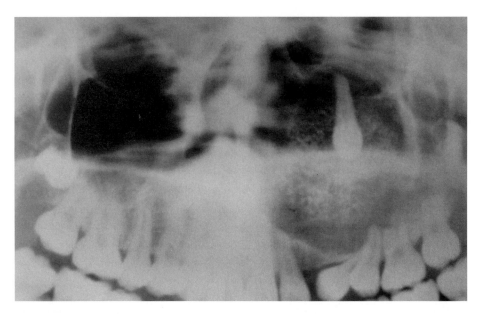

CASE **11-30** This patient is a 13-year-old girl. She had surprisingly little swelling but complained of a space between her teeth on the left side and several crooked teeth.
1. What condition is present?
2. How should this be managed, and what is the prognosis?

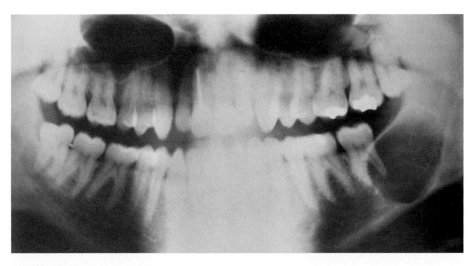

CASE **11-31** This is a 27-year-old man who was asymptomatic. However, you noted a very slight buccal swelling on the left side. Study this entire radiograph carefully.
1. What is your diagnostic impression?
2. Histologically, what would you expect the pathologic diagnosis to be?
3. How would you manage this case?

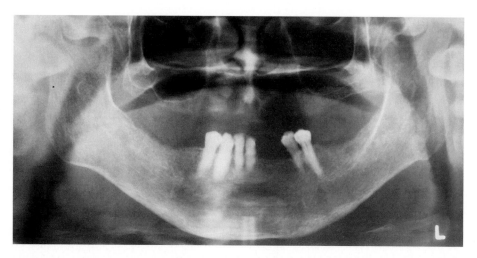

CASE **11-32** Take a good look at this entire radiograph of a 63-year-old woman of British descent.
1. In this case the radiologic diagnosis being sought is a systemic problem.
2. What features did you observe to come to this conclusion...or did you just guess?

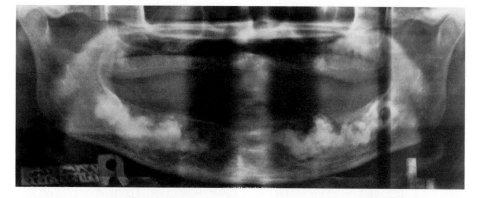

CASE **11-33** This edentulous 65-year-old black woman came in complaining of pain beneath her lower denture. The tissue in the mandibular premolar area appeared red and ulcerated with a bony spicule clinically visible at the base of the ulcer.
1. What condition affects her jaws?
2. What specific complication of this condition has occurred?

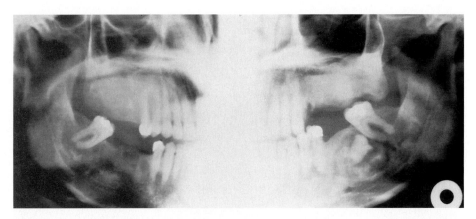

CASE **11-34** Elizabeth J-L, age 37 years, has kept both her maiden and married names. On her torso she has several café au lait spots whose outline resembles the coast of Maine. Her problem was first discovered when she complained of pain in her hip after a long day of shopping. Her alkaline phosphatase is a little bit elevated.
1. What does "café au lait" mean anyway?
2. What condition do you think is present?
3. Comment on the lesions in the jaws.
4. What is the radiopaque area in the middle of the radiograph?

CASE-BASED **QUESTIONS**

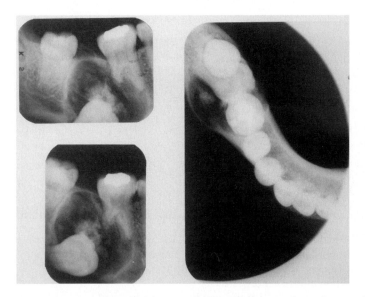

CASE **11-35** This patient is a 27-year-old woman with swelling in the right mandible.
1. What radiographic pattern characterizes this lesion?
2. Give a differential diagnosis for this lesion.
3. State your diagnostic impression.

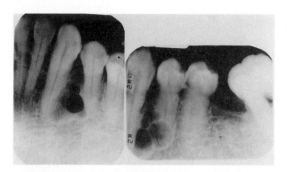

CASE **11-36** This patient is a 50-year-old man. Clinically, a slight swelling was between the left canine and 1st premolar.
1. Classify the radiographic appearance of this lesion.
2. Give a differential diagnosis.
3. State your diagnostic impression
4. How would you manage this case?

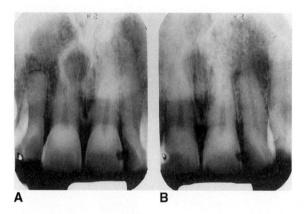

A   B

CASE **11-37** This patient is a 37-year-old woman. She reported a vague, slight discomfort in the maxillary anterior area and a more definite, transient salty taste. The lesion in question is in the maxillary midline.
1. What is your diagnostic impression?
2. Can you make any comment(s) on the radiographic appearance of this case?
3. With what anatomic structure might this pathologic entity be confused?
4. What previous dental treatment has this patient had?
5. What type of radiograph do we see in part *B,* and what does it show?

NOTE TO STUDENTS: Study Cases 11-38 and 11-39 together. It is very important to be able to distinguish these two conditions because one requires treatment and the other does not.

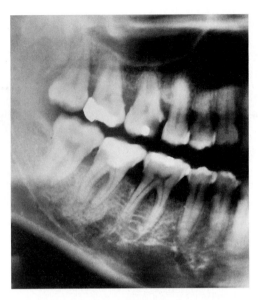

CASE **11-38** This 40-year-old man has restorations, active small and large caries, periodontal disease with horizontal bone loss with calculus, and erupted 3rd molars. The asymptomatic mandibular right 2nd molar is the main focus of this case: note the large and apparently deep restoration and the radiopaque area at the apex.
1. What is your diagnostic impression of the condition affecting the mandibular right 2nd molar? What important clinical test would you perform to confirm your diagnosis?
2. What treatment (if any) is needed? Does this condition regress?
3. *In passing:* Do you see any caries in association with the lower 3rd molar? Explain.

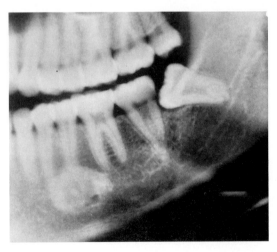

CASE **11-39** This 42-year-old man has had little need for dental treatment for either caries or periodontal disease. The asymptomatic mandibular left 2nd premolar is the main focus of this case. Note the lack of caries or restorations and the radiopaque area at the apex.
1. What is your diagnostic impression of the condition affecting the mandibular left 2nd premolar? What important clinical test would you perform to confirm your diagnosis? In this case, why do any test at all?
2. What treatment (if any) is needed? Does this condition regress?
3. *In passing:* Do you see any caries in association with the lower 3rd molar? Explain. Can you classify the 3rd molar impaction?

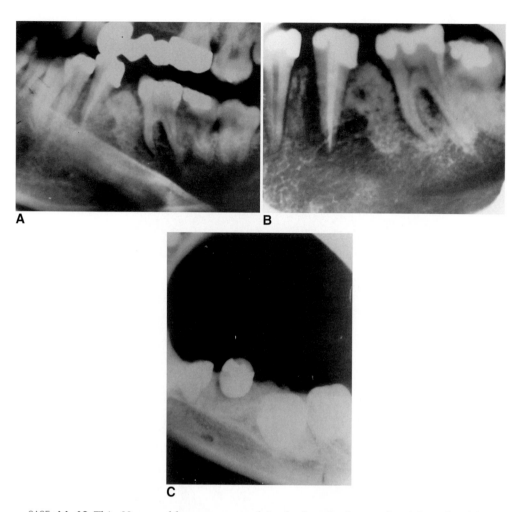

A

B

C

CASE **11-40** This 32-year-old woman complained of toothache on the right side of her mandible. A panoramic radiograph (*A*) was taken, and the radiopaque area was discovered on the other (left) side. Upon consultation, there was disagreement as to whether this lesion was idiopathic osteosclerosis (can be seen in non-apical areas) or if it represented something else. As a result, the additional intraoral periapical (*B*) and occlusal (*C*) radiographs were taken. Clinically, the upper fixed prosthesis appeared to have been constructed to occlude with the lingually displaced 2nd premolar about 12 months ago by a dentist in Germany.

1. Looking at all three radiographs, what is your diagnostic impression? Explain.
2. Look at the 2nd premolar: in the panoramic radiograph it appears to be supra-erupted, whereas in the periapical view it is on the same occlusal plane as the adjacent teeth. Explain this apparent contradiction.

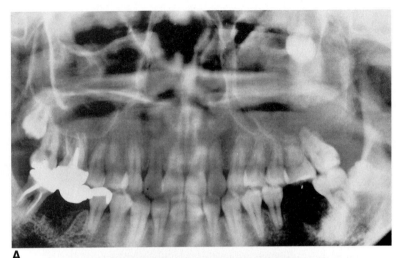

A

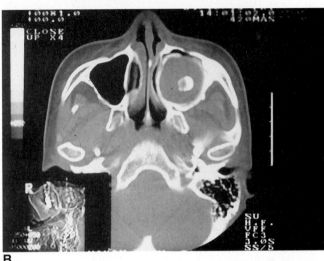

B

CASE **11-41** This is a 20-year-old man who has had a lot of work done for his age. Note that the maxillary right 3rd molar appears to be still erupting as the apex is open. The problem is with the upper left 3rd molar.

1. Study the images and give your diagnostic impression.
2. Why does the left 3rd molar appear to be in the orbit (above the infraorbital margin) on the panoramic radiograph and well below the orbit in the CT image?

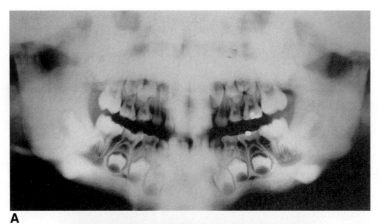

A

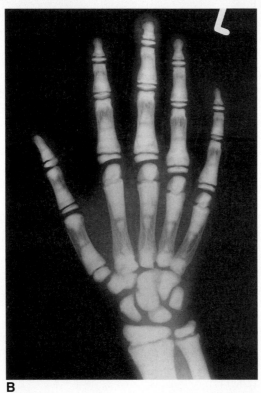

B

CASE **11-42** Peter is a 6-year-old boy with a problem that made it difficult for us to get a good panoramic radiograph. The hand film demonstrates the "bone within a bone" feature, especially in the metacarpals and in some phalanges.
1. What condition affects this patient?
2. How would you manage this case?

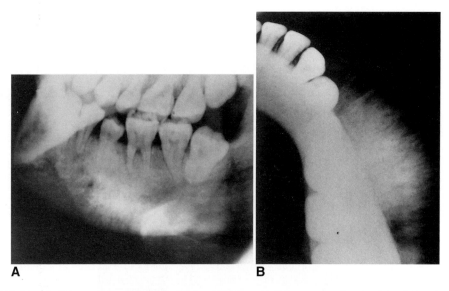

A   B

CASE **11-43** This patient, a 28-year-old man, had never been to the dentist. The left side of his face has become noticeably swollen lately. Now he is experiencing deep bone pain in his jaw, paresthesia in the lower left lip, and a loosening of his lower 1st molar.
1. Describe the radiographic findings.
2. What is your diagnostic impression?

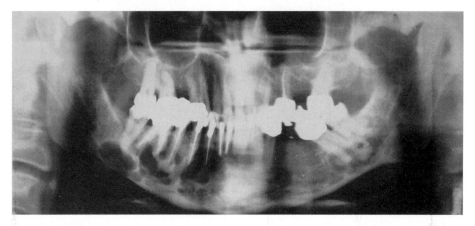

CASE **11-44** This patient is a 42-year-old black woman. She has continuing mild to moderate pain in the right mandible. She has had one surgery on the radiolucent lesion in the right canine area and endodontic treatment of the adjacent teeth. The area did not heal but actually enlarged after the surgery. Meanwhile, several other radiolucent lesions developed in the same quadrant.
1. Believe it or not, this history and radiograph are typical of this condition. See if you can state your diagnostic impression.
2. How would you manage this case?

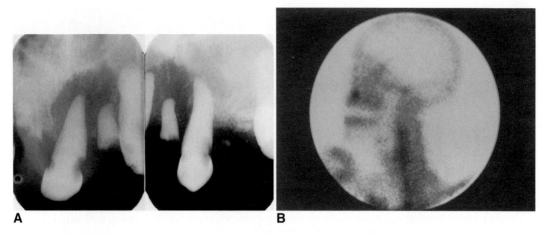

A   B

CASE **11-45** This is a person who has neglected himself. He is an alcoholic, smokes 2 to 3 packs of cigarettes a day, and has poor oral hygiene. Though he had difficulty breathing, especially on exertion, he had no known lung disease. The technetium scan you see in *B* was taken before biopsy and in association with a nuclear scan of the lungs.
1. What radiographic pattern can we ascribe to this lesion?
2. Describe the lesion.
3. State your diagnostic impression.

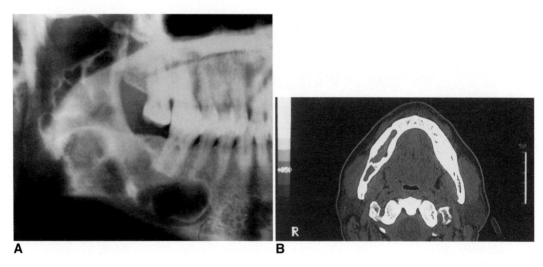

A   B

CASE **11-46** This patient is a 52-year-old man with no clinically visible swelling. However, he had pain because his extruding maxillary 2nd molar was traumatizing the opposing mandibular edentulous ridge. If you have been getting discouraged with these hard cases, this one is classic if you know your stuff!
1. What radiologic pattern do we see here?
2. Correlate the findings between the panoramic and CT images.
3. Give a differential diagnosis.
4. State your diagnostic impression.

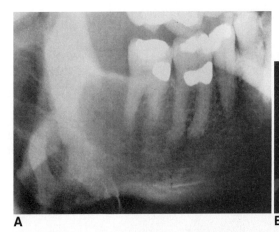 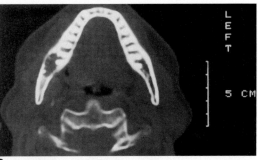

A   B

CASE **11-47** This is a 57-year-old woman who complained of pain in her right jaw and paresthesia in the right lower lip. Clinically, she had ever-so-slight right facial swelling that she noticed but that was hard to see by the clinicians who saw her. The radiograph and CT image were taken at the time of presentation to the oral and maxillofacial radiology clinic.
1. Describe the radiographic findings.
2. Do you have any idea as to what is going on here? If so, state your diagnostic impression.

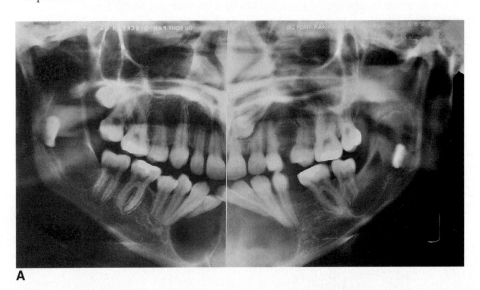

A

CASE **11-48** This is a 14-year-old teenager. She has several anomalous ribs, although you can see the clavicles are present (*B*). She has no facial swelling although she does have several small skin lesions.

Jaw lesions: (*A*)
1. What is your diagnostic impression?
2. The lesion in the left mandible appears to contain some radiopaque material. Can you state what that is?
3. How would you manage these lesions?

Skin lesions:
4. What skin lesions do you suppose she has?

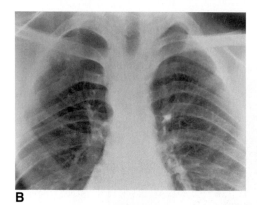

B

CASE **11-48, cont'd**

Ribs: (B)

5. Name three rib deformities on the right (*left side of photo*) side of her chest.

Diagnostic impression:

6. State the diagnosis. By now bells should be ringing loud and clear!

Bonus questions:

Forget about the details of this case for a moment. What if in another patient the finding was hypoplastic or missing clavicles:

7. What condition would you suspect?

8. What would you look for in the jaws?

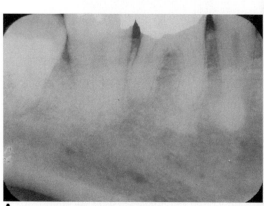

A

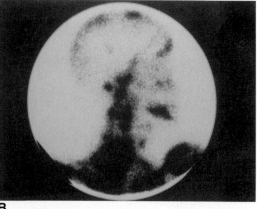

B

CASE **11-49** This is a 75-year-old man on medication for frequent nocturia. He has pain in his right mandible and subsequently had the technetium scan done.

1. Describe the radiographic findings in *A*.
2. What is your diagnostic impression without considering *B*?
3. What do you see in *B*?
4. Considering the history and the findings in *A* and *B*, what is your diagnostic impression?

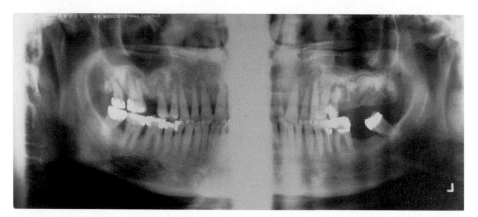

CASE **11-50** This 56-year-old white man from England now lives in the United States. He takes medication to lower his alkaline phosphatase levels and to curb progression of his disease. He has one family member back in England with the same condition.

1. Describe the radiographic findings.
2. What is your diagnostic impression?
3. What anomaly affecting the roots of the teeth might we watch for in this patient?
4. If we make a removable maxillary partial denture, would we warn the patient about it getting loose over time?
5. On long-term follow-up, what else would we look for (if anything) in his jawbones?

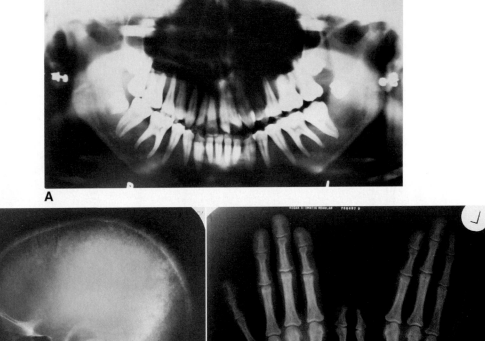

A

B

C

CASE **11-51** Rene P. is a 13-year-old female with a systemic disease characterized by glandular and organ components. She has a high serum calcium and high urinary calcium when placed on a low-calcium diet. The radiographs were all overexposed (too dark) on the normal settings. Her desire was to have orthodontic treatment.

1. Radiographically, what do you see in the panoramic radiograph (*A*)? Focus on the mandibular posterior areas only. (No, this is not a trick; the rest is not readable.)
2. Radiographically, what do you see in the skull (*B*)?
3. Radiographically, what do you see in the hands (*C*)?
4. State your diagnostic impression.
5. Can you state the tetrad of features that characterize this disease?
6. How would you manage this case? Don't forget the ortho!

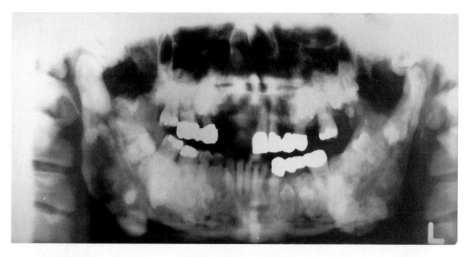

CASE **11-52** Getting tired of hard cases? This one should be easy, but it is important. Mary Quitecontrary is 35 years old. She is aware of her diagnosis.
1. Describe the radiographic findings.
2. What is your diagnostic impression?
3. Relative to her diagnosis, what serious counsel would you offer?

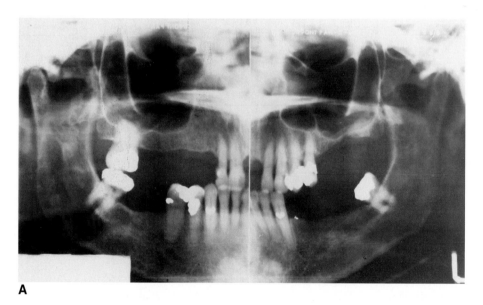

A

CASE **11-53** This is a 62-year-old man with a disease that affects the jaws, skull, and other bones in the skeleton. His primary complaint is back pain caused by involvement of the vertebral column. Bence Jones protein was found in the urine, and the serum calcium and alkaline phosphatase were elevated.
1. What findings can you see in the panoramic radiograph? (Findings are subtle.)

Continued

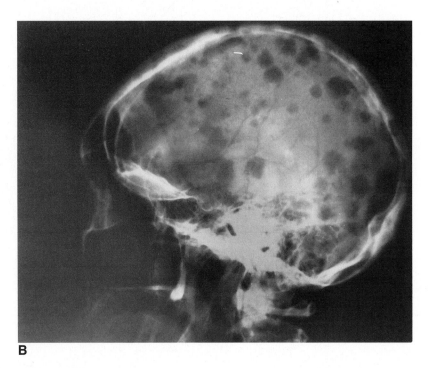

B

CASE **11-53 cont'd**
2. What findings can you see in the skull?
3. What is your diagnostic impression?

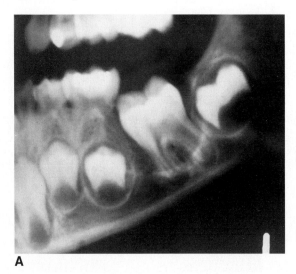

A

CASE **11-54** This patient is a 6½-year-old boy from Toronto, Canada, where they told his mom he needed some treatment. He had pain in the area and slight facial swelling that was relieved following an initial course of antibiotic treatment. The family was transferred to the United States where the problem was not immediately recognized. Ultimately the radiologist saw him; this is what was found.
1. Panoramic radiograph (A): describe what you see.
2. What is the eruptive potential of the mandibular 1st molar?

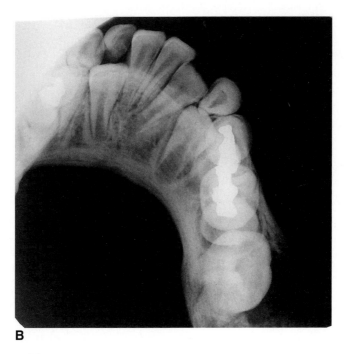

B

CASE **11-54 cont'd**

3. Occlusal radiograph (*B*): describe what you see.
4. Give a differential diagnosis.
5. State your diagnostic impression.
6. What treatment would you recommend?

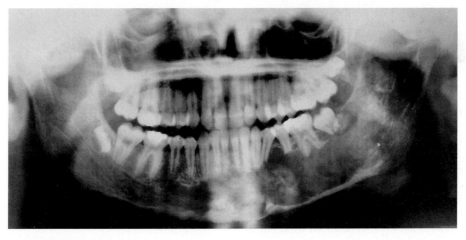

CASE **11-55** This patient is a 12-year-old girl who presented with a slight swelling in her left submandibular area and in the midline mental region. There was no pain or systemic disease.

1. Describe the radiographic findings.
2. What is your diagnostic impression?

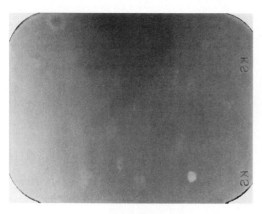

CASE **11-56** This patient is a 38-year-old woman who has had acne since age 12. This is a radiograph of her buccal mucosa.
1. State your diagnostic impression.

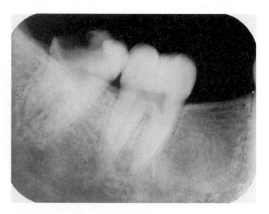

CASE **11-57** This patient is a 45-year-old Hispanic man.
1. State your diagnostic impression regarding the target-like lesion mesial to the molar.

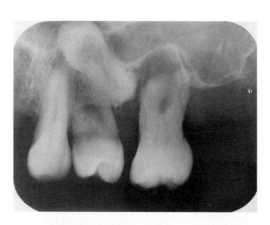

CASE **11-58** This patient is a 60-year-old man with a history of having teeth extracted as they become bothersome. This molar has now become loose, it hurts, and he wants it extracted. Interestingly, he is taking an antibiotic for an aching sinus on this side. The medical doctor did not examine his teeth.
1. First, what pattern of bone loss do you see in association with the molar?
2. What is the etiology of this molar problem?
3. Report as much as possible about what you can see regarding the unerupted tooth.
4. How would you manage this case?

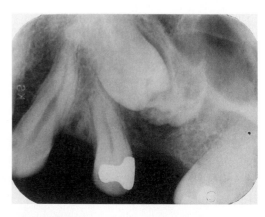

CASE **11-59** This case involves "what do you see" sorts of questions. The patient complains of sensitivity to hot and cold in this area.
1. Describe what you see in association with the 1st premolar.
2. How about the 2nd premolar?
3. Do you see anything in the sinus?

PART Two

School, State, and National Board Examination Review

Section 1: Principles of Radiation Physics, Health, and Biology

Section 2: Radiographic Assessment and Interpretation

SECTION 1: PRINCIPLES OF RADIATION PHYSICS, HEALTH, AND BIOLOGY

Instructions

Read the questions carefully. In some questions the answer being sought is related to an "is not" phrasing of the question. The answer choices are based on the statement(s) in the question that, with rare exceptions, are factual. On the other hand, the answer sections contain inaccurate or irrelevant, but seemingly plausible, selections and the goal is for the reader to recognize the one most correct answer. This may require the selection of the "all of the above" choice or the "none of the above" choice as the correct answer. Also, the reader should be wary of selecting the longest answer or the "C" choice. On the other hand, some of the correct answers are the longest or "C" choice. Also, the correct answer, such as the "B" choice, may occur several or more times in a row.

MULTIPLE CHOICE QUESTIONS

1. An atom is said to be neutral when:

A. It is ionized
B. There are more electrons than protons
C. The number of positive charges in the nucleus equals the number of negative charges of the orbital electrons
D. It has a positive charge

2. X-rays interact with matter to produce:

A. Ionization and desiccation
B. Ionization and excitation
C. Desiccation and excitation
D. Ionization and replication

3. Which electron is bound most tightly to the nucleus?

A. J-shell electron
B. K-shell electron
C. L-shell electron
D. Q-shell electron

4. Electromagnetic radiation wavelengths are measured in:

A. Kilometers
B. Meters
C. Angstrom units
D. All of the above

5. Which of the following statements is true?

A. X-rays have wavelengths, frequencies, and velocities.
B. X-rays can be reflected like light.
C. X-rays have mass and carry a positive electric charge.
D. X-rays do not travel in straight lines.

6. Which of the following most adequately describes the radiation produced by high kilovoltages?

A. Short wavelengths of low frequency
B. Long wavelengths of high frequency
C. Short wavelengths of high frequency
D. High penetrating waves of low frequency

7. Secondary radiation is:

A. Less when kVp is increased
B. Most detrimental to the patient
C. Less deeply penetrating than primary radiation
D. Proportional to the square of the distance the operator stands from the patient

8. Pocket dosimetry is an example of:

A. Chemical dosimetry
B. Photographic dosimetry
C. Luminescent dosimetry
D. Biologic dosimetry
E. Air-ionization dosimetry

9. Which of the following is not applicable to thermoluminescent dosimetry?

A. Ultraviolet light
B. Heat
C. Trapping centers
D. Lithium fluoride
E. Measurement of light

10. The long BID (cone) is recommended when using the paralleling technique because we can:

A. Use the shorter time intervals allowable with an electronic timer
B. Use a longer focal spot-film distance to compensate for a greater object-film distance to reduce magnification and distortion
C. Hold the film closer to the tooth so there is less magnification and a better image
D. Use a lower kVp
E. B and C

11. The paralleling technique is recommended over the bisecting-angle technique because:

A. Positioning the film is easier
B. It uses slower film
C. It gives a less-distorted picture of root length
D. It shortens developing time
E. A, B, and C

12. What is the main cause of foreshortening in the bisecting-angle technique?

A. Improper placement of the film
B. Improper horizontal angulation of the BID
C. Vertical angulation of the BID is excessive
D. Vertical angulation of the BID is insufficient

13. Which statement is the most correct?

A. The long BID is used with the paralleling or the bisecting-angle technique.
B. The long BID is used with the paralleling technique only.
C. The short BID is used with either the paralleling or the bisecting-angle technique.
D. Film holders are not necessary with the paralleling technique.

14. The intensity of x-radiation at any given distance from the source of radiation varies:

A. Inversely with the square of the distance
B. Directly with the square of the distance
C. Inversely with the distance
D. Directly with the distance

15. When an 8-inch target-film distance is changed to a 16-inch target-film distance (kVp and mA kept constant), the exposure time should be:

A. Doubled
B. Decreased by half
C. Increased by half
D. Quadrupled

16. In hand processing, if you place the film in the fixer first, this results in:

A. A black film
B. A clear film
C. A mottled film
D. No change

17. A tire track or other pattern throughout the image results from:

A. Developer and fixer with different temperatures
B. Bending the film
C. Reversing the film to the beam
D. Fluoride

18. Fluoride contamination of a film from the operator's fingers results in:

A. White marks
B. Black marks
C. Generally increased density
D. No change

19. The optimum time and temperature for hand development of film is:

A. 3 to 4 minutes at 70 degrees F
B. 4.5 to 5 minutes at 83 degrees F
C. 4.5 to 5 minutes at 65 degrees F
D. 4.5 to 5 minutes at 68 to 70 degrees F

20. To test for chemically fogged or age-fogged film:

A. Develop the film without exposing it
B. Develop the film after exposing it
C. Hold the film up to a bright safelight
D. Fix the film only
E. C and D

21. In manual processing, the fixing time for films is usually:

A. 5 minutes
B. 10 minutes
C. 15 minutes
D. 20 minutes
E. Dependent on the temperature

22. A radiographic film is underexposed. In manual processing, which of the following manipulations will produce diagnostically acceptable radiographs?

A. Overdevelopment
B. Sight-development
C. Treatment with Farmer's reducer
D. None of the above

23. Which of the following are the components of Farmer's reducer that can be used to decrease the radiographic density (too dark) in a processed film?

A. Sodium sulfite and hyposulfite
B. Sodium sulfite and potassium ferricyanide
C. Potassium bromide and potassium ferricyanide
D. Sodium thiosulfate and potassium ferricyanide
E. X-rays and duplicating film

24. Which is the hardening agent in film processing?

A. Acetic acid
B. Potassium bromide
C. Potassium alum
D. Potassium hydroxide

25. Which of the following tissues is most susceptible to radiation?

A. Nerve tissue
B. Muscle tissue
C. Brain tissue
D. Blood-forming tissue

26. Which of the following is the most
radiosensitive?

A. Young bone
B. Nerve
C. Muscle
D. Reproductive organs

27. Which of the following is not a critical factor
in the radiation response of cells?

A. Cellular differentiation
B. Size of cells
C. Metabolic activity
D. Mitotic rate

28. Which of the following effects can be
associated with low-dose, whole body
radiation?

A. Shock
B. Epistaxis
C. Epilation
D. Leukemia

29. Relative to radiation biology, the latent
period is that period between:

A. Exposure of the film and development of the
images
B. Exposure to radiation and the appearance of
clinical symptoms
C. The states of cell rest and cell mitosis
D. Subsequent doses of x-radiation

30. Which of the following effects is not
considered to be dependent on dose rate?

A. Death of the organism
B. Local somatic effects
C. Genetic effects
D. Fetal somatic effects

31. Which of the following is the earliest clinical
symptom for an individual exposed to a
mid-lethal radiation dose sufficient to cause
acute radiation syndrome?

A. Nausea and vomiting
B. Diarrhea
C. Loss of hair
D. General discomfort
E. Fever

32. Which of the following is a unit of radiation
absorbed dose expressed
in joules per kilogram of irradiated
tissue?

A. Roentgen (R)
B. Curie (Cu)
C. Rem
D. Gray (Gy)

33. The doubling dose is that dose:
A. In which the LD-50 is doubled
B. In which the rads delivered are doubled
C. That causes a doubling of gene mutation
D. That causes a doubling of interactions
along the track of a high-speed
electron

34. For dental radiography, the recommended
collimation of the radiation beam
of the BID at the patient's skin
surface is:

A. 2.65 inches
B. 2.75 inches
C. 3 inches
D. 3.65 inches

35. A pregnant patient:
A. Should be advised of her legal rights before
being irradiated
B. Should be warned about a possible
miscarriage
C. Should never be irradiated for dental
radiographs
D. May be irradiated for dental radiographs by
taking the proper precautions

36. Which of the following reduces the radiation
dose to the patient?

A. Gonadal shields
B. High-speed film
C. Collimator
D. Digital imaging
E. All of the above

37. Which of the following is the most
effective in reducing patient radiation dose?

A. Fast films
B. Proper collimation
C. Higher kilovoltage
D. Digital imaging

38. The electrons that revolve around the
nucleus:

A. Have a positive charge
B. Have no charge; either positive or
negative
C. Have a negative charge
D. Can be either positive or negative

39. Isotopes of an element have the
same:

A. Half-life
B. A number
C. Z number
D. N number

40. The transformer used to heat the filament of the x-ray tube is:

A. The autotransformer
B. The step-up transformer
C. The step-down transformer
D. The rechargeable DC battery circuit

41. At diagnostic levels, what percent of the electron energy is converted to x-radiation at the anode?

A. Less than 1%
B. 2%
C. 10%
D. About 98%

42. In a standard non-constant potential machine, about 70% of the radiation in the x-ray tube is:

A. Monochromatic
B. Bremsstrahlung
C. Characteristic
D. Asynchronous

43. The substance that is the most resistant to the passage of x-rays is:

A. Leaded glass
B. Plastic
C. Wood
D. Rubber

44. X-rays are produced when:

A. The anode is heated above 3000 degrees C
B. The filament becomes positively charged
C. Electrons strike the cathode
D. Electrons strike the anode

45. The x-ray beam of a standard non-constant potential x-ray machine consists of photons of many different wavelengths, with the shortest wavelength photons determined by:

A. Milliamperage (mA)
B. Kilovoltage peak (kVp)
C. Filtration
D. Exposure time

46. The target material (in the anode) for dental x-ray tubes is:

A. Copper
B. Tungsten
C. Lead
D. Gadolinium

47. In a standard dental x-ray unit, the quality of x-radiation produced during the exposure is controlled primarily by:

A. Exposure time
B. Kilovoltage peak (kVp)
C. Milliamperage (mA)
D. Inherent filtration

48. In a standard AC-type x-ray machine, a 0.5 (½) second exposure would produce how many impulses of x-radiation?

A. 5
B. 15
C. 30
D. None of the above

49. To reduce the amount of heat given off during x-ray production, the source of x-ray energy is surrounded by:

A. Copper
B. Water
C. Oil
D. Lead
E. Air

50. The number of electrons in a dental x-ray tube is determined by the:

A. Kilovoltage used
B. Distance between the filament and the target
C. Step-up transformer
D. Size of the focusing cup
E. Low-voltage circuit

51. The efficiency of x-ray production in an x-ray generating tube (i.e., the percentage of electron kinetic energy converted to x-rays) is directly related to the:

A. Z number of the target material
B. Operational kVp
C. Melting point of the target material
D. A and B
E. All of the above

52. Which of the following statements about radiation is true?

A. General radiation is Bremsstrahlung radiation.
B. Bremsstrahlung radiation is the same as characteristic radiation.
C. All atoms have the same characteristic radiation.
D. Characteristic radiation is produced when cathode electrons collide with electrons of the outermost shell.

53. To increase the penetrability of the x-ray rays, their wavelength should be:

A. Shortened by increasing the kVp
B. Shortened by decreasing the kVp
C. Lengthened by increasing the kVp
D. Shortened by increasing the mA
E. Lengthened by increasing the mA

54. In a constant potential (DC) x-ray machine, the x-ray beam is:

A. A continuous beam of radiation
B. A pulsating beam of radiation
C. A pulsating divergent beam of radiation
D. A continuous divergent beam

55. Which of the following statements is not correct?

A. X-rays can penetrate opaque matter.
B. X-rays are differentially absorbed by matter.
C. X-rays cannot ionize gasses.
D. X-rays affect photographic film emulsion much like light.

56. The number of oscillations or waves passing a point per second is known as the:

A. Heat capacity of an x-ray photon
B. Melting coefficient of an x-ray photon
C. The tube capacity of the x-ray machine
D. Frequency of an x-ray photon

57. The mean penetrability of an x-ray beam is not related to which of the following?

A. kVp
B. Filtration
C. Wavelength
D. Frequency
E. mA

58. X-rays are a form of ionizing radiation. Ionization is:

A. The separation of the nucleus into positive and negative ions
B. Produced by photoelectric absorption only
C. Produced by the Compton effect and Bremsstrahlung only
D. Produced by photoelectric absorption and Compton scatter

59. The interaction in which the entire photon of x-radiation is removed from the beam by atomic interaction is known as:

A. The Thompson effect
B. The photoelectric effect
C. Compton scatter
D. Excitation

60. A recoil electron is produced during which of the following reactions?

A. The photoelectric effect
B. The Compton effect
C. Pair production
D. Photonuclear disintegration

61. The predominant mechanism of x-ray interaction with matter in the dental setting is:

A. Thompson (unmodified scatter)
B. The photoelectric effect
C. Compton scatter
D. Pair production

62. X-ray filters are usually made of:

A. Copper
B. Lead
C. Aluminum
D. Stainless steel

63. Collimators are usually made of:

A. Copper
B. Lead
C. Aluminum
D. Stainless steel

64. Dental x-ray machines that use 65 kVp are required to have a half-value layer (HVL) equivalent to at least:

A. 0.5 mm aluminum
B. 1.5 mm aluminum
C. 2.0 mm aluminum
D. 2.5 mm aluminum

65. The HVL is the amount of:

A. Lead necessary to absorb all of the radiation in the beam
B. Copper in the target needed to dissipate heat
C. Absorber necessary to attenuate the x-ray beam by one-half and is used to measure beam quality
D. Opening in the lead diaphragm needed to collimate the beam to its proper size
E. All of the above

66. The radiation weighting factor is used in the determination of which of the following radiation units?

A. R
B. Sv
C. Gy
D. Rad

67. The unit of x-radiation measurement that deals with the absorbed energy per kilogram of tissue is the:

A. R
B. Sv
C. Gy
D. rem

68. A pocket dosimeter should be _____ before each use.

A. Checked for x-ray translucency
B. Sensitized with a standard radiation exposure
C. Loaded in the darkroom
D. Charged with the charging unit

69. Which of the following properties of x-rays is the basis for the rules of geometric projection?

A. X-rays travel at the speed of light.
B. X-rays travel in diverging straight lines from a point source.
C. The course of an x-ray photon can be diverted with an electromagnetic source.
D. X-rays can form a latent image on photographic film.

70. Regardless of the target-film distance, incorrect horizontal angulation will cause:

A. Elongation of the x-ray image
B. Foreshortening of the x-ray image
C. No significant change in the x-ray image
D. Overlapping of teeth in the x-ray image

71. The size of the focal spot in the x-ray tube influences radiographic:

A. Density
B. Contrast
C. Definition
D. Distortion

72. Which of the following does not control total magnification (includes penumbra) of the radiographed object?

A. Focal spot-film distance
B. Focal spot size
C. Object-film distance
D. Cathode size
E. None of the above

73. The optical density of an intraoral film indicates the:

A. Degree of darkness in an image
B. Difference between observers
C. Speed of the screens
D. Kilovoltage used
E. None of the above

74. Optical density is a function of:

A. kVp
B. mA
C. mAs
D. Exposure time
E. All of the above

75. Subject contrast is primarily a function of:

A. kVp
B. kVp and mA
C. mA
D. kVp, mA, and exposure time

76. Fog affects the contrast of an intraoral film because it:

A. Decreases film density
B. Increases film density
C. Produces white stains on the film
D. Produces dark stains on the film

77. The primary advantage of the paralleling technique over the bisecting-angle technique is:

A. The increased anatomic accuracy of the image
B. The increased object-film distance
C. The greater magnification of the image
D. The long BID is easier to handle

78. Why is the long BID considered a necessary adjunct to the paralleling technique?

A. To avoid magnification of the image
B. To avoid shape distortion of the image
C. To reduce secondary radiation
D. The long BID is easier to handle
E. To avoid superimposition of structures

79. The technique that shows the upper and lower crowns and associated alveolar bone on the same radiograph is called the:

A. Retro-coronal technique
B. Bitewing technique
C. Bisecting-angle technique if a BID indicator is not used
D. Paralleling technique if a BID indicator is used
E. C and D

80. If a satisfactory radiograph was produced using a target-film distance of 8 inches and an exposure time of 5 impulses, what would be the correct exposure time for a target-film distance of 16 inches?

A. 10 impulses
B. 20 impulses
C. ⅓ sec
D. ½ sec
E. B or C

81. In the bisecting-angle technique, the central ray of the beam is directed:

A. Perpendicular to the long axis of the object
B. Parallel to the long axis of the object
C. Perpendicular to a line bisecting the angle formed by the object and the film packet
D. Perpendicular to the film packet

82. Which of the following is a correct statement about intensifying screens?

A. Thinner phosphor layers result in faster screens.
B. Thinner phosphor layers result in more unsharpness.
C. Thicker phosphor layers result in faster screens.
D. Thicker phosphor layers result in less unsharpness.

83. BID (cone) cutting (partial image) on a radiograph is caused by:

A. Underexposure
B. Improper exposure technique
C. A damaged BID
D. Improper coverage of the film with the beam of radiation

84. A cassette:

A. Emits light
B. Is a container for films and screens
C. Is an instrument to align the BID
D. Records the patient's exposure

85. Intensifying screens are used with extraoral and panoramic films to:

A. Increase the exposure time
B. Improve image quality
C. Decrease the radiation to the patient
D. Increase the kVp

86. The efficiency with which film responds to x-ray exposure is known as *film sensitivity* or *film speed*. Which speed range is the best for reducing radiation to the patient?

A. Speed B
B. Speed D
C. Speed E+
D. Speed F

87. A film is stripped from its packet and exposed to light. After processing it will:

A. Be unaffected
B. Turn clear
C. Turn black
D. Turn white

88. Which of the following films can be used intraorally and extraorally?

A. Screen film
B. Occlusal film
C. Periapical film
D. Bitewing film

89. Which of the following will not produce film fog?

A. Unprotected films in the x-ray room or x-ray equipped operatory
B. Films stored for a long time in an unsafe place
C. Light leaks in the darkroom
D. Films stored in a refrigerator in the lab

90. Which of the following will produce film fog?

A. Light leaks in the darkroom
B. Films stored for a long time in an unsafe place
C. Unprotected films in the x-ray room or x-ray equipped operatory
D. All of the above

91. The primary purpose of the lead foil in the back of the film packet is to:

A. Eliminate penumbra
B. Absorb remnant radiation after film exposure
C. Identify film placed backwards (back to front)
D. Stiffen the x-ray packet

92. The base material used in dental films is:

A. Sodium thiosulfate
B. Metol
C. Cellulose acetate
D. Gelatin

93. Radiographic film emulsion is:

A. Cellulose acetate
B. Gelatin
C. Gadolinium oxyphosphate
D. Gelatin and silver bromide

94. Sensitization specks:

A. Are defects in the gadolinium oxyphosphate crystals
B. Are defects in the silver bromide crystals
C. Act as electron traps
D. A and C
E. B and C

95. In hand processing, films should be washed in running water for at least:

A. 10 minutes
B. 20 minutes
C. 30 minutes
D. 40 minutes

96. What is the cause of yellow or brown stains appearing on films some time after processing?

A. Aged film
B. Improper exposure technique
C. Films stored in a hot place
D. Incomplete fixing and washing

97. The latent image consists of the accumulation of:

A. Electrons in exposed silver bromide crystals
B. Atomic silver at the sensitized specs
C. Atomic silver in gelatin molecules
D. Electrons in exposed silver bromide crystals and in the gelatin molecules

98. The safety of a darkroom safelight depends on the:

A. Distance of the safelight from the workbench
B. Time the films are exposed to the safelight
C. Wattage of the bulb in the safelight
D. Speed of the film
E. All of the above

99. Differences between manual and automatic processing include which of the following?

A. Processing solution chemistry
B. Solution temperature
C. Solution concentration
D. Time to completion of processing
E. All of the above.

100. During the processing of Insight "F" speed film in the private dental office, which of the following is the most important source of film fog?

A. Secondary radiation to the dental operatory
B. Unsafe safelight
C. Developing solutions that are too cold
D. Use of an automatic processor

101. The theory that explains cellular damage by x-rays is the:

A. Direct action poison chemical theory
B. Indirect action poison chemical theory
C. Bremsstrahlung theory
D. Indirect non-ionizing theory

102. Theoretically the biologic response to a given dose of radiation would be greater (more severe) with:

A. The tissue being anoxic at the time of irradiation
B. A higher dose rate
C. A smaller area of tissue exposure
D. Lower linear energy transfer (LET)

103. Which of the following x-ray photons (x-rays) are most apt to be absorbed by the skin?

A. Central x-ray photons
B. Filtered x-ray photons
C. Long wavelength x-ray photons
D. Short wavelength x-ray photons

104. The first clinically observable reaction to radiation overexposure is:

A. Loss of hair
B. Reddening of the skin (erythema)
C. Cataract formation
D. Agenesis of blood cells

105. In intraoral periapical radiography, which of the following is currently (2004) under consideration for abolition?

A. Round, open-ended BIDs of any length
B. ANSI "D" speed film
C. The protective apron for the patient
D. None of the above
E. All of the above

106. Ionization occurs:

A. When atoms lose electrons; they become deficient in negative charges and therefore behave as positively charged atoms
B. When atoms gain electrons; they become positively charged
C. When an atom loses its nucleus
D. Only when a K-orbit electron is ejected and replaced with an L-orbit electron

107. The structure that has a nucleus containing positive protons with surrounding orbits of one or more negative electrons is called:

A. A molecule
B. A neutron
C. An atom
D. A proton

108. Neutrons have:

A. A negative charge
B. A positive charge
C. No charge
D. A positive and a negative charge

109. The step-up transformer is used to:

A. Step up the current to heat up the filament
B. Allow the operator to vary the kVp
C. Change low input voltage to high output voltage
D. None of the above

110. If you wanted to increase the penetrating quality of the x-ray beam, what machine setting(s) would you change?

A. Increase the mA
B. Increase the kVp
C. Increase the mA and the kVp
D. Increase exposure time, mA, and kVp

111. Which of the following series indicates the correct progression of energy transformation in the production of x-ray photons?

A. Kinetic energy, electrical energy, and radiation
B. Kinetic energy, radiation, and electrical energy
C. Electrical energy, kinetic energy, and radiation
D. Electrical energy, radiation, and kinetic energy

112. Which of the following most adequately describes the radiation produced by high kilovoltage?

A. Short wavelengths of low frequency
B. Long wavelengths of high frequency
C. Short wavelengths of high frequency
D. High penetrating waves of low frequency

113. A dental hygienist wishes to change his mA from 10 to 15. If the original exposure time is 1.5 seconds, what must the new exposure time be to maintain the same density?

A. 0.75 seconds
B. 1.0 second
C. 0.5 seconds
D. 2 seconds

114. Thermionic emission is found at the:

A. Positive anode
B. Negative anode
C. Positive cathode
D. Negative cathode

115. The filament circuit in a dental x-ray tube:

A. Requires a step-up transformer
B. Is observed on a voltmeter
C. Provides a cloud of electrons when the cathode is heated sufficiently
D. Regulates the speed of the electrons

116. In a step-up transformer, the:

A. Secondary coil has more wire turns than the primary coil
B. Primary coil has the same number of wire turns as the secondary coil
C. Primary coil has more wire turns than the secondary coil
D. None of the above

117. The kilovoltage in an x-ray generating system regulates:

A. The number of electrons produced
B. Thermionic emission
C. The velocity of the electrons traveling from the filament to the target
D. The velocity of the x-ray photons produced

118. To increase the penetrability of x-ray photons, their wavelengths should be:

A. Shortened by increasing the kVp
B. Lengthened by increasing the kVp
C. Shortened by increasing the mA
D. Lengthened by increasing the mA

119. Which of the following statements about radiation is true?

A. Electromagnetic radiation is the propagation of wavelike energy.
B. Light waves are electromagnetic radiation.
C. Radio waves are electromagnetic radiation.
D. A and C.
E. All of the above.

120. Select the correct statement.

A. X-rays cannot be focused to a point.
B. X-rays can be focused to a point.
C. X-rays cannot increase the electrical conductivity of a gas.
D. X-rays do not always travel in a straight line.

121. Increased quantum energy of electromagnetic radiation is associated with increased:

A. LET
B. Velocity
C. Frequency
D. Wavelength

122. Bremsstrahlung production is:

A. The primary source of x-ray photons in the dental x-ray tube
B. The process by which x-ray energy is released as electrons rearrange themselves in the inner shells of an atom
C. Important only in x-ray machines with rotating anodes
D. Not important in the kilovoltage range below 69 kVp

123. Which of the following statements describes Compton scatter?

A. The photon uses some of its energy to remove an electron from its orbit and then transfers the remaining energy to the electron in the form of kinetic energy that is capable of ionizing molecules.
B. The photon gives up some of its energy in ejecting an orbiting electron and is then deflected with a longer wavelength.
C. A high-energy photon passes close to a nucleus, releasing an electron and a positron. Some of the energy is used to give kinetic energy to the two particles.
D. None of the above.

124. Diagnostic radiology is based on which of the following interactions of x-rays with matter?

A. The Compton effect
B. Coherent scatter
C. The photoelectric effect
D. All of the above

125. Radiopaque tissues:

A. Absorb little of the x-rays
B. Absorb x-rays more fully
C. Are hollow regions
D. Are cysts, granulomas, or abscesses
E. None of the above

126. Which of the following statements is true regarding characteristic radiation?

A. It is produced by the interaction of cathode electrons with target nuclei.
B. It is produced by the interaction of cathode electrons with target electrons.
C. It comprises the major component of the x-ray beam (more than 50%).
D. A and B.
E. All of the above.

127. Collimation of the beam refers to the:

A. Selective removal of soft radiation from the beam
B. Selective removal of hard radiation from the beam
C. Reduction of the beam diameter
D. Process of reducing the beam intensity by 50%

128. Filtration is used in dental x-ray machines to remove:

A. Scatter radiation
B. High energy photons
C. Long-wavelength photons
D. Low energy electrons

129. A lead diaphragm is used in dental x-ray machines to:

A. Prevent Compton scatter
B. Limit beam size
C. Remove low energy radiation
D. Increase the photoelectric effect

130. Which of the following is true regarding the collimator?

A. It is an aluminum disk with a hole in the center.
B. It has a smaller aperture for a long BID than for a short BID.
C. It removes soft radiation.
D. A and B.
E. All of the above.

131. In the paralleling technique, an increased source-object distance:

A. Prevents enlargement of the image
B. Avoids overlapping
C. Prevents shadows
D. Causes blurring of the image outline
E. None of the above

132. Which property of x-radiation must be utilized to control magnification of the radiographic image?

A. X-rays travel in divergent paths from their source.
B. X-rays penetrate opaque objects.
C. X-rays cannot be focused.
D. X-rays cause secondary radiation when they strike the patient's face.

133. An increase of which of the following factors causes an increase in subject contrast?

A. Exposure time
B. mA
C. kVp
D. None of the above

134. Increasing kVp results in:

A. Low contrast (long scale contrast)
B. High contrast (short scale contrast)
C. Lighter film density (medium contrast)
D. None of the above

135. How do you change from a low contrast to a high contrast image and still maintain density?

A. Decrease the kVp and increase the mAs
B. Decrease the kVp and mAs
C. Increase the kVp and decrease the mAs
D. Increase the kVp and the mAs

136. The localization rule whereby the lingual object follows the movement of the radiation source (tube head) is known as:

A. Clark's rule
B. Rapier's technique
C. Miller's technique
D. Richards' technique

137. The localization rule whereby the buccal object follows the movement of the tip of the BID is known as the *buccal object rule,* first described by _____ in 1952.

A. Clark
B. Rapier
C. Miller
D. Richards

138. The *SLOB* rule usually refers to _____ rule and stands for **S**ame on **L**ingual; **O**pposite on **B**uccal.

A. Clark's
B. Rapier's
C. Miller's
D. Richards'

139. With the paralleling technique, it is important to use:

A. A short target film distance to avoid the loss of detail
B. A short BID to decrease magnification
C. A long target film distance to increase magnification
D. A long target film distance to decrease penumbra

140. In the paralleling technique, the most accurate image of a tooth is produced on the radiograph when the central ray is:

A. 30 degrees to the long axis of the tooth
B. 90 degrees to the film and the tooth
C. 90 degrees to the plane of the x-ray photon
D. 90 degrees to a plane bisecting the long axis of the tooth and the plane of the film

141. The focal spot-object distance is 8 inches, kVp is 65, mA is 10, exposure time is 12 impulses, and the resulting radiograph is acceptable. If we change the distance to 16 inches, what should the new exposure time be?

A. 3 impulses
B. 6 impulses
C. 24 impulses
D. 48 impulses

142. The "tire track" pattern appears in an image if it is:

A. Not processed properly
B. Given too much radiation
C. Not exposed to a sufficient amount of radiation
D. Placed in the oral cavity backwards

143. A latent image is:

A. An image late in its formation
B. A very light image
C. Produced after exposure but before developing
D. A very dark image

144. What is the function of the raised dot embossed on intraoral film?

A. It identifies the side of the film facing the occlusal line.
B. It identifies the side of the film facing the tongue.
C. It identifies the side of the film facing the beam of radiation.
D. It identifies the maxillary or mandibular teeth depending on how the film is placed in the mouth.

145. When the patient's lips are not kept closed during the panoramic exposure, what happens?

A. A radiolucent shadow obscures the anterior teeth.
B. A radiolucent band obscures the apices of the maxillary teeth.
C. A radiopaque band obscures the anterior teeth.
D. No appreciable change is noted in the radiograph.

146. In panoramic radiology, the collimator is:

A. A thin narrow slit oriented in the vertical plane
B. A thin narrow slit oriented in the horizontal plane
C. A small rectangular aperture of the same proportions as the panoramic film
D. Similar to the rectangular collimator used with the rectangular BID

147. On a panoramic radiograph, the soft tissue of the nose appears as:

A. Bilateral radiopaque images
B. A midline radiopaque image
C. A midline real radiopaque image and bilateral ghost images
D. Bilateral real radiopaque images and a midline ghost image

148. On most newer panoramic machines, the tube head of the machine is:

A. Angled upward 4 to 7 degrees
B. Horizontal and directs the beam perpendicular to the film
C. Angled downward to avoid thick structures at the back of the head
D. Designed to adjust automatically for patient size

149. A dark shadow that obscures the apical region of the maxillary teeth in a panoramic image is usually caused by:

A. Positioning the patient too far forward
B. Positioning the patient too far back
C. The lips not closed
D. Not having the tongue against the palate

150. In most panoramic machine designs, the one adjustment the operator can make for patient size is:

A. kVp
B. mA
C. Exposure time
D. mAs
E. Exposure cycle time

151. A single or series of dark, even, vertical radiolucent bands extending from the top to the bottom of the image is seen. This is usually caused by a:

A. Cracked screen
B. Momentary obstruction of the machine by the patient
C. Defect on the rollers of the automatic processor
D. Static electricity

152. In current panoramic machines, special lights are fitted to:

A. Illuminate the patient
B. Assess proper patient exposure parameters
C. Ensure proper film density
D. Aid with patient positioning

153. Intraoral film speed is directly related to the:

A. Size of the AgBr crystals
B. Image exposure time
C. Exposure latitude
D. None of the above

154. In the darkroom, a cassette was opened to remove an exposed film. A piece of black paper was discovered on the surface of the intensifying screen. The paper would most likely produce:

A. A white or light artifact
B. A black artifact
C. No artifact as the x-ray photons pass right through
D. Black filament-like marks as is seen in intraoral films

155. Gelatin is a good radiographic film emulsion vehicle because it:

A. Enhances contrast
B. Is soluble in water at processing temperatures
C. Is chemically inert
D. All of the above

156. With the use of an automatic processor:

A. Total darkness must be maintained in the darkroom
B. Solutions should be kept as near to room temperature as possible
C. Installation requires a properly designed darkroom
D. Frequent solution replenishment is essential

157. Though rarely seen, reticulation is said to occur when the:

A. Developer is too hot
B. Fixer is too cold
C. Developer and fixer temperatures differ too greatly
D. Automatic processor needs cleaning

158. In the automatic processor:

A. Unexposed silver salts are precipitated into the developer solution
B. The latent image is activated by the action of the rollers in the fixer section
C. Exposed silver salts are precipitated onto the film base
D. Developer solution can be used for silver recovery
E. A and D

159. In automatic processors, the daylight loader:

A. Permits the loading of cassettes in daylight
B. Can be contaminated by film wrappers
C. Eliminates the need for a darkroom
D. Requires filtration to protect film from fog
E. All of the above

160. The normal cycle time for most automatic processing units is:

A. 2 minutes
B. 4-6 minutes
C. About 10 minutes
D. Significantly different for every machine

161. The rinse cycle in the water bath of automatic processors is to:

A. Rid the film of chemicals
B. Dissolve metallic silver
C. Harden the emulsion
D. There is no water bath in automatic processors

162. In manual processing, radiographs are rinsed in clean running water to:

A. Rid the film of chemicals
B. Dissolve metallic silver
C. Shrink the emulsion
D. Remove the latent image

163. The safety of safelight illumination does not depend on which of the following?

A. Size of the darkroom
B. Wattage of the lightbulb
C. Distance of the safelight from the work surface
D. Duration of time the film is exposed to the safelight

164. When using the automatic processor, what is the most common cause of lost films?

A. Mixing film up with wrappers
B. Improper film identification
C. Feeding bent films into the processor
D. Combined use with intraoral and panoramic films

165. The perception of radiographic density varies inversely with the:

A. Radiolucency of the object
B. Quantity of silver in the radiograph
C. Quantity of x-radiation exposing the radiograph
D. Quantity of incident viewing light transmitted through the radiograph

166. When viewing a direct digital image on a monitor, the limiting factor in image perception is:

A. Modified by reflected light in a dark room
B. The quality of the original scanned radiograph
C. The software
D. The quality of the monitor

167. If resolution is measured in line pairs distinguishable by the eye within a millimeter of space (line pairs per millimeter, or lp/mm), what is considered as the outer limit of the eye?

A. 6 lp/mm
B. 10-12 lp/mm
C. 14 lp/mm
D. 22 lp/mm

168. In digital imaging exposure, dynamic range is best when using:

A. Photostimulable phosphor plates (PSPs)
B. Charge coupled device (CCD) sensors
C. Complimentary metal oxide (CMOS) sensors
D. Film and then scanning it into the computer

169. The first "wireless" sensor in digital imaging was which one of the following:

A. PSP
B. CCD
C. CMOS
D. None of the above because all are "wired"

170. In digital radiology, "image processing" means:

A. Using software to alter the original image
B. Using processed film
C. The process of capturing, storing, and archiving the image
D. The conversion of the digital image to an analogue image

171. The currently recognized official maximum permissible dose (MPD) of radiation to an occupationally exposed person is:

A. .01 mSv/week
B. 1 mSv/week
C. 10 mSv/week
D. 100 mSv/week

172. When a photon of x-radiation interacts with a molecule of water (H_2O) it results in the production of H• and OH•; radiobiologically this is referred to as:

A. Excitation
B. Electrolyte formation
C. Attenuation
D. Free radical formation

173. On average, the dose rate from natural background radiation is:

A. 0.005 mSv /year
B. 0.05 mSv/year
C. 0.6 mSv/year
D. 1.3 mSv/year

174. Sievert (Sv) is a newer unit of radiation measurement. One Sv is equivalent to:

A. 1 mrem
B. 100 mrem
C. 10 rem
D. 100 rem
E. None of the above; Sv is equivalent to rads

175. In terms of therapy, radiation is used to:

A. Destroy tissue
B. Increase mitotic activity
C. Heat tissue
D. Dehydrate tissue

176. A certain amount of radiation is needed before the clinical signs of damage to somatic cells appear. The amount of radiation after which damage can be produced is called the:

A. Latent dose
B. Threshold dose
C. Maximum permissible dose (MPD)
D. Background radiation dose
E. Scattered radiation dose

177. As a radiation worker, you should not be exposed to more than 0.05 Sv (50 mSv) per year. But when you are a patient, you can easily receive 0.15 Sv (150 mSv) from certain types of dental radiographic procedures or an oral and maxillofacial CT scan. Which of the following statements best reconciles these contradictory statements?

A. Any appropriate radiation dose may be given for diagnostic purposes.
B. A patient can be given any amount of radiation regardless of damage.
C. Documented exceptions recorded in the chart can be made.
D. Whole body radiation is different from specific region radiation.

178. The maximum permissible dose from diagnostic x-rays for a patient in 1 year is:

A. 0.05 mSv
B. 0.5 mSv
C. 5 mSv
D. 50 mSv
E. Not specified

179. A dental assistant is using a radiation monitoring badge service. The service reports the badge was exposed to 0.05 mSv in the previous month. The assistant should:

A. Stop taking x-ray films immediately
B. Report to a radiation oncologist for a blood count
C. Ignore the report because the reading is not significant
D. Evaluate x-ray procedures and take steps to reduce unnecessary radiation

180. In normal dental radiographic procedures, the principal hazard to the operator is produced by:

A. Gamma radiation
B. Primary radiation
C. Secondary radiation
D. None of the above

181. Under no circumstances should the operator hold the:

A. Film during exposure
B. BID during exposure
C. Patient during exposure
D. All of the above

182. Traditionally, lead aprons are used _____, though pending Federal guidelines may recommend discontinuance of their use. (This is true.)

A. Only on women of child-bearing age
B. To reassure a pregnant patient
C. To reduce radiation exposure to the operator
D. On all patients

183. In a panoramic radiograph, the right premolars appear widened and are overlapped, whereas the left premolars appear narrowed with the contacts open. This indicates which positioning error?

A. The patient was positioned too far forward.
B. The patient's chin was tipped excessively downward.
C. The patient's chin was tipped excessively upward.
D. The patient's head was twisted or turned.

184. What is the most likely cause of a diffuse vertical radiopacity that obscures the center of the panoramic radiograph and gets progressively wider toward the bottom of the image?

A. The ghost image of the spine that is not erect

B. The ghost image of the hyoid bone

C. The ghost image of the ramus of the mandible

D. Movement of the patient

185. When the patient does not bite in the groove of the bite-block, the most direct result would be that the patient is:

A. Positioned in a rotated or twisted fashion

B. Positioned with the chin too high or too low

C. Positioned too far forward or too far back

D. Slumped, thus producing a ghost image of the spine

186. If you are using a direct digital panoramic machine, which of the following statements is true?

A. You can make all of the same positioning errors.

B. You cannot make darkroom errors.

C. You can immediately view the image on a monitor.

D. All of the above.

E. None of the above.

187. A film-based panoramic machine may be converted to digital by:

A. Installing a CCD sensor adaptor kit

B. Replacing the old screen and film with a panoramic PSP in the cassette and a laser scanner

C. A or B

D. Neither A nor B because panoramic machines cannot be converted

188. Sensors such as the CCD and CMOS types are said to have a narrow degree of latitude with regard to radiation exposure. This means:

A. The image size is narrower than the outside dimension of the sensor

B. Image degradation occurs with very small increments of exposure above or below ideal

C. Background and terrestrial sources of radiation can contaminate the image

D. These sensors are subject to damage with excess exposure to radiation

189. "Blooming" is an undesirable image characteristic seen primarily with CCD and CMOS sensors. It results from:

A. Sensor damage resulting from infection control soaking

B. Sensor protection with latex and polyethylene baggies for infection control

C. Excessive wiping of the active side of the sensor with liquid infection control products

D. All of the above

E. None of the above

190. In digital imaging, "quantum noise" is:

A. An undesirable characteristic produced by too little radiation

B. A series of little black dots much like film fog

C. A more significant feature of the CMOS sensor than the CCD type

D. All of the above

E. None of the above

191. In digital imaging, a laser scanner is needed for:

A. PSP sensors

B. CCD sensors

C. CMOS sensors

D. All of the above

E. None of the above

192. In digital imaging, DICOM is:

A. An abbreviation for bi-functional machines capable of standard and digital imaging

B. A digital imaging system capable of simultaneous communication of the image to two different monitors or computers

C. A contraction of the two Canadian co-discoverers of the CMOS sensor: Disette and Compeau

D. A universal standard for digital imaging software

193. The intraoral digital sensor whose active portion most nearly approximates that of intraoral film is:

A. PSP

B. CMOS

C. CCD

D. None of the above

E. All of the above

194. In a histogram stretch:

A. The contrast histogram is shifted to the darker or lighter side of the scale

B. The density histogram is shifted to the darker or lighter side of the scale

C. The contrast histogram is expanded to include more shades of gray

D. The density histogram is expanded to include more shades of gray

195. In a histogram shift:

A. The contrast histogram is shifted to the darker or lighter side of the scale
B. The density histogram is shifted to the darker or lighter side of the scale
C. The contrast histogram is expanded to include more shades of gray
D. The density histogram is expanded to include more shades of gray

196. The histogram stretch and shift are examples of:

A. Digital image processing
B. Ways of confusing the student
C. Calibration tools needed for digital sensor adjustment
D. A difference between panoramic and intraoral digital imaging

197. Which of the following statements is true?

A. The K orbit is closest to the nucleus, and its binding energy is the lowest.
B. The M orbit is farther away from the nucleus, and its binding energy is greater than the K orbit.
C. The K orbit has the greatest binding energy.
D. The M orbit has the greatest binding energy.

198. X-rays are produced at the:

A. Filter
B. End of the BID
C. Cathode
D. Anode

199. The workload as related to structural shielding design is a measure of the:

A. Time during which a person to be protected is in the vicinity of the radiation source
B. Radiation likely to be produced by an x-ray machine
C. Time during which the radiation is directed at the barriers
D. Parameters of the x-ray tube outside which it will fail

200. Which of the following is not related to heat dissipation in an x-ray tube?

A. Tube rating
B. Duty cycle
C. Copper block
D. Oil around the tube
E. Thermionic emission

201. In an x-ray generating system, turning the mA control adjusts the:

A. Filament temperature
B. Primary-to-secondary ratio of the step-down transformer
C. Primary-to-secondary ratio of the step-up transformer
D. Autotransformer

202. The instruction booklet accompanying an x-ray machine specifies that the unit should not be energized for more than 22 seconds at the maximum kVp and mA. This is referred to as:

A. Tube rating
B. Duty cycle
C. Line focus principle
D. Workload

203. For CMOS and CCD intraoral digital radiography:

A. Timer increments of $\frac{1}{100}$ sec are desirable
B. Constant potential type x-ray machines are preferable
C. Densitometer and sensitometer calibration are needed upon installation of the software
D. A and B
E. A, B, and C

204. Leakage radiation:

A. Originates at the focal spot and leaves the tube head through the shielding
B. Originates at the focal spot and leaves the tube head through the unleaded glass window
C. Is the remaining radiation that passes through the patient
D. Is the remaining radiation that passes through the walls of the x-ray room or operatory

205. In digital imaging, PSP and other sensor holders require infection control procedures because:

A. Digital images do not require chemical processing
B. The image can be immediately viewed on the operatory monitor
C. The image characteristics are similar to those of film
D. They become contaminated as part of the procedure

206. In the exposure phase of intraoral radiography, the following infection control procedures are recommended:

A. Wrap the BID, tube head and yoke, and parts of the chair
B. Wear gloves, and use sterile BID indicators and bite-blocks
C. Isolate contaminated exposed films or PSPs to a defined area
D. Wrap machine adjustment knobs and the exposure switch
E. All of the above

207. In the transportation phase of the film to the darkroom or processor and of the PSP to the laser scanner, the following infection control procedures are recommended:

A. Remove gloves and wash hands, or over-glove
B. Indicate the x-ray room is contaminated
C. Place contaminated films inside daylight loader, or bring them to processing area in the darkroom
D. All of the above

208. In the processing phase, the films are developed or the PSPs are scanned. The following infection control procedures are recommended:

A. Carefully shake out the films or PSPs onto a clean surface
B. Dispose of contaminated wraps
C. Remove contaminated gloves and wash hands
D. Load films or PSPs into the machine
E. All of the above

209. In the clean-up phase, the following procedures are recommended:

A. Don gloves, throw away contaminated paper, and disinfect work area around machine
B. Don over-gloves to open darkroom door or to remove arms from daylight loader
C. Repeat clean-up, and dispose of contaminated wrap in the x-ray room
D. Remove gloves and wash hands
E. All of the above

210. X-rays behave a lot like light. However, they are also different in that they:

A. Are electromagnetic radiation
B. Have more energy
C. Have a greater wavelength
D. Are usually monochromatic

211. The characteristic that makes x-rays most useful in dentistry is that:

A. They are affected by electric and magnetic fields
B. They travel at the speed of light
C. They penetrate opaque objects
D. They are not differentially absorbed by matter
E. They can be focused down to a small area

212. X-rays belong to that large group of radiations known as:

A. Particulate radiations
B. Hygroscopic radiations
C. Alpha radiations
D. Corpuscular radiations
E. Electromagnetic radiations

213. Dense tissues:

A. Permit the passage of x-ray photons and are radiolucent
B. Resist the passage of x-ray photons and are radiolucent
C. Resist the passage of x-ray photons and are radiopaque
D. Permit the passage of x-ray photons and are radiopaque
E. None of the above

214. The unit for measuring x-ray exposure is the:

A. Coulomb per kilogram
B. rad
C. Gray
D. rem
E. None of the above

215. X-radiation is absorbed by different tissues during a diagnostic exposure. The effective dose is expressed in Sv (rems). Sieverts are calculated by using:

A. Roentgens x linear energy transfer (LET)
B. Gy (rads) x radiation weighting factor x tissue weighting factor and summing over the tissues irradiated
C. Gy (rads) x LET
D. R x quality factor (QF)

216. Inside the x-ray tube the anode is inclined at approximately a 17- to 20-degree angle to the vertical plane. This is referred to as the *Benson line focus principle*, which is used to:

A. Increase the efficiency of x-ray production
B. Serve as an x-ray focusing device
C. Produce an effectively smaller focal spot
D. Dissipate heat from energy conversion
E. Immortalize Pete Benson, DDS, MS, OMF radiologist

217. In the processed radiographic image, contrast is defined as the:

A. Differences between black and white areas of the film
B. Overall blackening of the film
C. Degree of overall grayness of the film
D. Capacity to see soft tissues in the image

218. With reference to low kVp versus high kVp, which of the following statements is true?

A. 60 kVp produces short scale high contrast with many shades of gray.
B. 60 kVp produces long scale high contrast with few shades of gray.
C. 90 kVp produces long scale low contrast with many shades of gray.
D. 90 kVp produces long scale high contrast with few shades of gray.

219. "Saturation" is an undesirable characteristic of a digital image and causes image details to "black out." Which of the following can produce "saturation"?

A. Excessive exposure time, kVp, or mA, either singly or together
B. Insufficient radiation exposure
C. Software glitches
D. Sensor exposure to water or saliva

220. In digital imaging, an 8-bit image would have how many shades of gray?

A. 32
B. 64
C. 128
D. 256
E. 512

221. In digital imaging, some manufacturers are developing systems capable of producing 10- or 12-bit images. In normal clinical settings, what is considered the maximum number of shades of gray the eye can discern?

A. 16
B. 25
C. 64
D. 128
E. 256

222. To view a digital image on a monitor, the software programs are designed to reject image bits that can be recognized as noncontributory, such as noise, and will display only the best _____ bits. In addition most high-definition monitors used in dentistry are limited to displaying _____ bits.

A. 6; 6
B. 6; 8
C. 8; 8
D. 8; 6
E. None of the above

223. To satisfy the need for accurate low increments of radiation for wired sensor digital imaging, the x-ray unit should have:

A. Very low exposure times
B. Exposure times in increments of 1/100 seconds
C. Constant potential x-ray generator (constant flow of x-ray photons vs. 60 pulses/sec in traditional machines)
D. B and C
E. All of the above

224. The main reason for using faster films (currently speed F) in the dental office is to:

A. Have exposures lower than digital imaging
B. Improve image quality
C. Decrease radiation dose to the patient
D. Save time taking the radiographs

225. Films used with panoramic and cephalometric cassettes:

A. Are more sensitive to x-rays than to light
B. Are more sensitive to light than to x-rays
C. Fluoresce by means of silver sulfide crystals
D. Are gadolinium oxyphosphate crystals

226. In manual and automatic processing solutions, contrast in the radiographic image is enhanced by:

A. Alum
B. Hydroquinone
C. Sodium acetate
D. Sodium sulfate
E. Sulfuric acid

227. In digital imaging, contrast may be enhanced by an image processing algorithm called:

A. Histogram de-bit
B. Image matrix intensification
C. Histogram shift
D. Histogram stretch

228. The gelatin coating on the film is softened in the developer solution by the addition of:

A. Sodium sulfate
B. Hydroquinone
C. Acetic acid
D. Potassium alum
E. Sodium carbonate

229. When using automatic processors, a softening or swelling of the gelatin coating will cause it to stick to the rollers. Thus _____ is (are) added to the manual developer as (a) hardening agent(s) and to control swelling of the gelatin.

A. Phosphates and sulfates
B. Sodium carbonate and sodium sulfite
C. Glutaraldehyde
D. Glutamic acid and glutaraldehyde

230. In manual and automatic processing solutions, chemical fog is controlled in the developer solution by adding:

A. Elon
B. Acetic acid
C. Sodium carbonate
D. Potassium bromide
E. Sodium sulfite

231. In manual and automatic processing, unexposed silver crystals are dissolved by _____ in the fixer solution.

A. Acetic acid
B. Sodium thiosulfate
C. Sodium sulfate
D. Potassium alum
E. Sodium carbonate

232. In digital imaging, PSPs are manufactured with dark and pale sides. The pale side _____.

A. Must be oriented toward the radiation
B. Must be oriented toward the front of the cassette
C. Must be oriented toward the laser beam in the scanner
D. A and B
E. All of the above

233. In manual and automatic processing, potassium bromide:

A. Is an activator for reducing agents
B. Is an activator for clearing agents
C. Is a component of the developing solution
D. Tends to increase chemical fog

234. In manual and automatic processing solutions, sodium sulfite is a component of the:

A. Developing solution
B. Fixing solution
C. A and B
D. None of the above

235. In manual and automatic processing solutions, which of the following requires an acid pH to function properly?

A. Sodium thiosulfate
B. Potassium alum
C. Potassium bromide
D. Sodium sulfite

236. Which of the following is a function of the rollers in an automatic processor?

A. Transportation of film through the processor
B. Massaging action for uniform distribution of chemicals on the film
C. Squeegee action to remove chemicals from the film when changing baths
D. Stirring action of solutions from roller motion
E. All of the above

237. A panoramic radiograph on which there is an excessive "smile" line of the occlusion and streaking of the hyoid bone across the mandible indicates the:

A. Patient was positioned too far back
B. Patient was positioned too far forward
C. Patient's chin was tipped excessively downward
D. Patient's chin was tipped excessively upward

238. Infection control in panoramic radiology involves:

A. Replace or cover the bite-block with a barrier; patient removes barrier or bite-block after exposure
B. Cover machine parts other than the bite-block, and use of gloves
C. Use of gloves for transporting and processing the radiograph
D. Disinfect contaminated machine parts after each use
E. All of the above

239. Newer standard and digital panoramic machines can:

A. Open the interproximal contacts like bitewings
B. Improve resolution from the traditional 4-6 lp/mm to 9.5 lp/mm (bitewing film about 11-12 lp/mm)
C. Project the panoramic x-ray photons perpendicular to the mandible
D. Autocorrect for some operator errors
E. All of the above

240. The acute radiation syndrome:

A. Invariably results in the death of the exposed person
B. Could be induced in a sensitive individual with a radiation dose of 50 Sv
C. Occurs when the head and neck area is exposed to a radiation dose of 40 to 50 Sv
D. None of the above

241. LD 50 (30d) stands for the:

A. Dose of radiation that kills 30 experimental animals when 50 are irradiated
B. Lethal dose to 25 out of 50 experimental animals within 30 days after an acute exposure
C. Lethal dose to 50% of the experimental animals with the dose fractionated over 30 days
D. Dose of radiation that results in 30 dead animals over a 50-day period

242. A radiation dose of 4 Sv (400 rem) given locally to the arm would most likely cause:

A. Erythema
B. Acute radiation syndrome
C. Carcinoma of the skin
D. Bone marrow death

243. The highest incidence of radiation-induced anomaly production occurs:

A. Immediately after conception
B. During organogenesis
C. In disease-complicated aging
D. When metabolism is reduced

244. When an x-ray photon interacts by the Compton effect, it sets in motion a high-speed electron. This reaction is called the:

A. Target theory
B. Threshold dose
C. Primary interaction
D. Recoil electron

245. In digital imaging, a computer is necessary to _____ the image.

A. View
B. Process
C. Store
D. Transmit
E. All of the above

246. The delta ray is produced by:

A. Interactions along a secondary track
B. A fast-moving secondary electron moving away from the primary electron track
C. The collision of a secondary electron with the primary track
D. The collision of the incident photon with a secondary electron

247. The Bragg peak is an abrupt increase in the LET:

A. Just before the fast-moving electron comes to a stop
B. And involves a decrease in the energy transferred
C. Measured at any point along the primary track
D. And occurs at peak electron velocity

248. RNA differs from DNA in that it consists of a single sugar phosphate chain and that its base uracil replaces:

A. Thymine
B. Guanine
C. Cytosine
D. Adenine

249. The quality assurance procedure that checks for the integrity of the focal spot is the:

A. Spinning top
B. Line pair focal spot device
C. Ionization chamber
D. Sensitometer test
E. Densitometer test

250. The quality assurance procedure that checks the beam to ensure it is collimated to the diameter of the open end of the BID is the _____.

A. Specially designed fluorescent screen
B. Line pair focal spot device
C. Ionization chamber
D. Sensitometer test
E. Densitometer test

251. The quality assurance test that checks for the accuracy of the timer in an x-ray machine is the:

A. Sensitometer test
B. Densitometer test
C. Coin test
D. A and B
E. None of the above

252. The acronym *ALRA* stands for:

A. "**AL**arm: **RA**diation" -type warning device
B. "**A**lpha **L**ong **R**ay **A**cquisition" -type tissue damage
C. "**A**ll **L**ow-let **R**adiologic **A**ctivity" resulting in tissue damage
D. "**A**ctual **L**ow-dose **R**adiation **A**cceptability" for various tissue types
E. None of the above

253. Which of the following statements is true?

A. The spinning top can be used to check the timer accuracy of any intraoral machine.
B. Constant potential machine timers cannot be checked with a spinning top because there are no impulses.
C. Traditional AC x-ray machines can have the timer checked with a pulse oximeter or a spinning top.
D. Constant potential machine timers are capable of small increments of pulsed radiation at intervals of 1/100 of a second.

254. X-rays in the diagnostic range have a wavelength of approximately:

A. 0.01Å
B. 0.10Å
C. 1.00Å
D. 10.00Å

255. One of the easiest ways to check the integrity of the processing solutions either in manual tanks or the automatic processor is:

A. To smell the vinegary odor of depleted solutions
B. A daily check film
C. To observe the accumulation of a surface scum and a soapy feeling
D. To use one of the new electronic probes

256. Which of the following safelight filters is (are) recommended for best results with current intraoral and extraoral films?

A. Kodak Morlite filter
B. Kodak GBX filter
C. Wratten 6B filter
D. Kodak GBX II filter
E. All of the above

257. The kVp can be measured with:

A. An ionization chamber
B. A pocket dosimeter
C. A kVp meter or Wisconsin cassette
D. A kVp meter
E. Fluorescence of thermoluminescent dosimeters (TLDs)

258. A dosimetry badge:

A. Is a plaque on the machine stating radiation dose specs per init time (mR/sec)
B. Is a wall plaque indicating x-ray doses for common examinations
C. Is required on the machine and wall of any room with an x-ray machine
D. Indicates operator exposure to ionizing radiation

259. The processor QA check should be done:

A. Daily
B. Weekly
C. Monthly
D. Yearly

260. Safelight integrity can be checked with:

A. A check film
B. The "coin" test
C. A densitometer
D. A colorimeter

261. The lead foil found in a typical size #2 film packet:

A. Absorbs radiation after film exposure
B. Adds needed weight to the film packet
C. Is used mainly to make the film packet rigid
D. Prevents film packet reversal
E. All of the above

262. The smaller the focal spot or target area, the better is the radiographic:

A. Intensity
B. Density
C. Contrast
D. Detail

263. The waves of x-ray energy that are removed during filtration are characterized as:

A. Short waves
B. Long waves
C. High-frequency waves
D. Bremsstrahlung

264. Adumbration is another term for:

A. Obscured roots
B. The shadow usually referred to as penumbra
C. Compton scatter effects
D. Cervical burnout

265. Primary radiation originates from the:
A. BID
B. Cathode of the tube
C. Autotransformer
D. Anode of the tube

266. Another term for the small spot on the face of the anode where the x-rays originate is the:
A. Focusing cup
B. Filament
C. Benson spot
D. X-ray generator
E. Focal spot

267. Limiting the size of the x-ray beam to that required to expose the film is achieved by:
A. Collimation
B. Filtration
C. Absorption
D. The BID positioning device

268. In digital imaging, a factor referring to image quality is termed *spatial resolution*. This factor is related to _____ and is measured in _____.
A. Constant potential image acquisition; ergs/kg
B. The shades of gray; bits
C. Noise production; grays (Gy)
D. The number of pixels in the image matrix; line pairs per millimeter (lp/mm)

269. In digital radiographic imaging, *JPEG* is a common term. JPEG is classified as a:
A. Lossless compression technique
B. Lossy compression technique
C. Noncompressed image
D. Type of image used in photography only

270. Image compression algorithms are used to:
A. Improve image quality
B. Reduce the size of the digital file
C. Acquire the original image
D. Create special effects like improved caries detection

271. Bridging software is often needed to:
A. Integrate dental imaging into the paperless office
B. Facilitate the recovery of specific image data from multiple sources such as intraoral and panoramic
C. Render imaging sources from different manufacturers easily accessible after storage in the patient's electronic file
D. All of the above
E. None of the above

272. Apart from the master computer and monitors in each operatory, a server may make it possible to:
A. Operate the wireless monitor network
B. Operate the random access memory containing the image data
C. Rapidly sort and recover stored image data
D. Expand the personnel to operate the system

273. One of the differences between the CCD and CMOS sensors is:
A. The low power requirement of the CMOS allows connection to a laptop via BUS
B. The low power requirement of the CCD allows connection to a laptop via BUS
C. The CCD is also known as an active pixel sensor (APS)
D. The significantly lower noise production with the CMOS sensor

274. Digital images can be viewed for diagnostic information on:
A. A high-resolution monitor
B. Ink jet or laser printed photographic quality paper
C. Dye subliminally printed acetate
D. All of the above

275. In dental radiology, the longer the wavelength:
A. The more penetrating are the x-ray photons
B. The less penetrating are the x-ray photons
C. The less absorbed are the x-ray photons
D. The more useful is the x-ray beam

276. One geometric factor that will decrease the penumbra (increase sharpness) of the radiographic image is a:
A. Short source object distance
B. Long object film distance
C. Short object film distance
D. Large focal spot

277. One geometric factor that will increase the penumbra (decrease sharpness) of the radiographic image is a:
A. Short object film distance
B. Short source object distance
C. Long source object distance
D. Large focal spot

278. Using a short BID, the exposure time is 0.2 seconds. If the long BID is used, the exposure time becomes 0.8 seconds if mA and kVp are kept constant. In this scenario the patient will receive:

A. Less radiation dose with the short BID
B. The same radiation dose with either BID
C. More radiation dose with the long BID
D. More radiation dose with the short BID

279. Which of the following demonstrates the indirect effect of x-rays on a biologic system?

A. Chromosomal mutation
B. Chromosomal break
C. Enzyme inactivation
D. Hydrogen peroxide production

280. When an exposed radiograph is placed in the developing solution:

A. Developing time depends on the temperature
B. The unexposed silver bromide is removed
C. Developing time is decreased by cold solutions
D. Developing time depends on the time needed for the image to appear

281. Which of the following film codes would you select for an adult bitewing radiograph?

A. 1.1
B. 1.2
C. 2.0
D. 2.2
E. 3.4

282. In panoramic radiology, the usual adjustment you can make for a small person or child is to reduce the:

A. Exposure time
B. kVp
C. mA
D. All of the above

283. Traditional film-based panoramic radiographic images cannot achieve a resolution (image detail) much above 6 lp/mm. The film-based cassette capable of slightly more detail is:

A. The soft plastic envelope
B. The rigid metal cassette
C. The digital cassette
D. The soft plastic envelope with a fast screen

284. In all panoramic machines:

A. Posterior interproximal contacts cannot be predictably opened
B. The resolution is no better than 6 lp/mm
C. The radiation dose is more than the full mouth survey
D. The exposure switch must be depressed throughout the exposure

285. In current digital panoramic radiology:

A. The dose is about 10 times less than for the full mouth survey
B. Image detail approaches that of intraoral radiography (about 10 lp/mm)
C. Few infection control procedures are needed
D. The interproximal contacts can be opened predictably
E. All of the above

286. In the year 2004, oral and maxillofacial radiology:

A. Has been a recognized specialty for several years
B. Will become a recognized specialty
C. Will not become a recognized specialty in the near or distant future
D. Will be merged with medical radiology by government decree

287. The most effective beam size limiting device(s) is (are):

A. The rectangular collimator
B. A digital sensor
C. A BID alignment ring
D. Aluminum filtration
E. All of the above

288. Proper replenishment of the solutions in the automatic processor can result in diminished patient exposure because it:

A. Prevents overdevelopment of radiographs that are routinely overexposed
B. Ensures a diagnostic image with minimum radiation exposure as weak developer results in light films
C. Routinely develops films to a specific predetermined density regardless of exposure
D. Minimizes film fog from scattered radiation

289. Which of the following factors will reduce the patient's somatic exposure by the greatest amount?

A. Lead apron
B. Short pointed plastic cone
C. Short open-ended BID
D. Long round BID
E. Long rectangular BID

290. The amount of tissue damage after irradiation depends on:

A. The dose rate and intensity
B. The area or volume of tissue irradiated
C. The intensity of the exposure (chronic or acute)
D. The radiosensitivity of the tissue
E. All of the above

291. Which of the following is a major factor in reducing operator exposure?

A. Use high kVp because lower exposures can be used.
B. Use low kVp because these photons are less penetrating.
C. Throw away that old pointed plastic cone (BID).
D. Stand 6 feet away from the tube head and avoid the primary beam.
E. Have the patient wear a lead apron.

292. When x-ray photons are absorbed by silver halide crystals in the emulsion of the film:

A. Nothing happens to the crystal until processing
B. A large grain of metallic silver is formed
C. A minute speck of metallic silver is formed
D. A deposit of solid bromide initiates image formation

293. At the atomic level, x-ray photons from the dental x-ray machine usually lose their energy through:

A. Collisions with the absorbing atom's nucleus
B. Collisions with other photons
C. The Compton effect
D. The photoelectric effect
E. The Bremsstrahlung effect

294. What is the greatest disadvantage of the bisecting-angle technique?

A. Image distortion caused by film bending
B. Lack of definition in the image
C. Superimposition of the zygoma over the apices of the posterior maxillary teeth
D. Shape distortion of anatomic structures
E. Image magnification

295. Most genetic radiation exposure to human beings from human-made sources is the result of:

A. Emissions from nuclear reactors
B. Watching color television
C. Dental radiography
D. Medical radiography
E. Microwave ovens

296. In panoramic radiology, the focal trough is the:

A. Slit where excess radiation is filtered
B. Area where x-rays are generated
C. Zone of sharpest image detail
D. Area that is collimated

297. In digital imaging, the term *electron well* is used in association with:

A. PSP sensors
B. CCD sensors
C. CMOS sensors
D. The computer motherboard

298. The digital image matrix is based on a binary numbering system consisting of:

A. The numbers 0 and 1
B. Numbers to the power of 2
C. Rows and columns alphabetized binomially
D. Numbers divisible by 2

299. What is indirect digital imaging?

A. Image capture from a radiograph on a viewbox with a digital video camera
B. Image capture via scanner with a translucency adapter
C. Image capture from a film using a digital camera
D. None of the above
E. All of the above

300. THE FINAL QUESTION!

What single dental x-ray system delivers the most diagnostic information to the doctor with the least patient dose, the least time and effort, the least infection control procedures, and the most patient comfort and acceptance and is available in a digital imaging format?

A. The constant potential intraoral x-ray unit
B. The constant potential intraoral unit combined with digital intraoral sensors
C. A multifunction, computer-operated panoramic machine
D. The Miles hand-held, digital camera–like intraoral imaging system.
E. You are dreaming; no such system exists!

SECTION 2: RADIOGRAPHIC ASSESSMENT AND INTERPRETATION

Instructions

Look at the illustration and read the questions carefully. The answer being sought may require the selection of the "all of the above" choice or the "none of the above" choice as the correct answer. Also, the reader should be wary of selecting the longest answer or the "C" choice. On the other hand, some of the correct answers are the longest or "C" choice. Also, the correct answer, such as the "B" choice, may occur several or more times in a row.

MULTIPLE CHOICE QUESTIONS WITH A RADIOGRAPHIC IMAGE

301. Select the most appropriate term for the anomaly associated with the 1st (most mesial) molar.

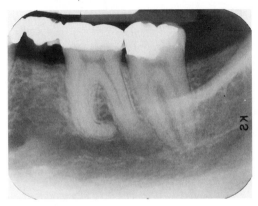

A. Diastema
B. Concrescence
C. Dilaceration
D. Dens invaginatus

302. This patient is a 60-year-old man with markedly shortened crowns. He does not work in an environment where particulate matter or acid-containing fumes can pollute the air. He has no known eating disorders and is healthy systemically. By what process have the crowns acquired this appearance?

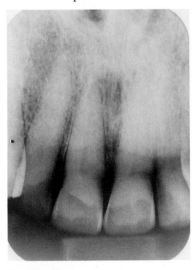

A. Attrition
B. Abrasion
C. Erosion
D. Abfraction

303. Observe the bifurcation area of these three molars. All have the same round, radiopaque, anomalous appearance. Note the overlap of the contacts. What term best describes this?

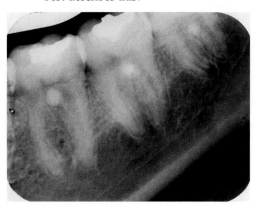

A. Enamel pearl
B. Pulp stone
C. Buccal enamel defect
D. "Faux" enamel pearl

304. We can see at least two errors in this image. Which do you think they are?

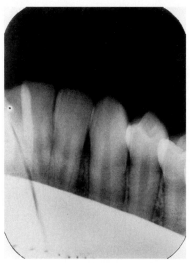

A. Rectangular BID cone cut and film bending
B. Rectangular BID cone cut and static electricity
C. Lead apron and static electricity
D. Lead apron and film bending

305. At least two errors are in this edentulous maxillary posterior periapical view. Select the best choice.

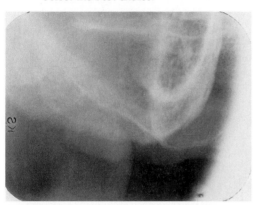

A. Improper horizontal and vertical angulation of the beam
B. Excessive vertical angulation of the BID and round BID cone cut
C. Excessive vertical angulation of the BID and bent film in the processor
D. Round BID cone cut and excessive distal angulation of the BID

306. One major error is in this radiograph. What is the cause?

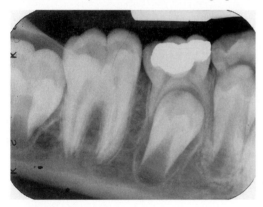

A. Foreshortening
B. Elongation
C. Improper horizontal angulation of the BID
D. Excessive negative vertical angulation of the BID

307. The correct term(s) that best describe the radiopaque objects is:

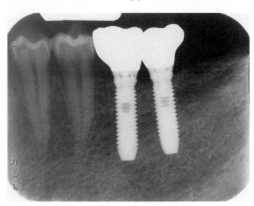

A. Implants
B. Implants and appliances
C. Implants, appliances, and crowns
D. Screw-teeth

308. This patient is a 32-year-old white woman. This was the only lesion she had, and the adjacent teeth were vital. The condition we see here is:

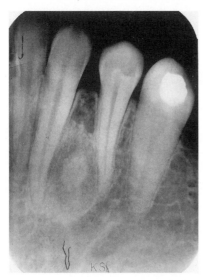

A. Focal cemento-osseous dysplasia
B. Periapical cemento-osseous dysplasia
C. Florid cemento-osseous dysplasia
D. Ossifying fibroma

309. This patient first had the endo done after a long period of abscess and fistula formation. Then the lateral incisor reabscessed and an apicoectomy and curettage were done. Currently the patient is asymptomatic and clinically there is a scar but the area appears well healed. What is your assessment of the periapical radiolucent area at the apex of the lateral incisor?

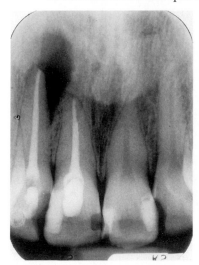

A. Recurrent abscess formation
B. Periapical cemental dysplasia
C. Surgical traumatic cyst
D. Apical scar

310. In this panoramic film, there are at least three positioning errors. They are:

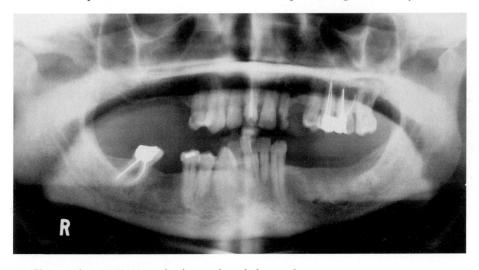

A. Chin too low, patient too far forward, and slumped
B. Chin too high, head twisted, and slumped
C. Chin too high, patient too far back, and tongue not on palate
D. Chin not on chin rest, head twisted, and tongue not on palate

311. In this edentulous patient we can see a number of errors. The most complete and accurate list is:

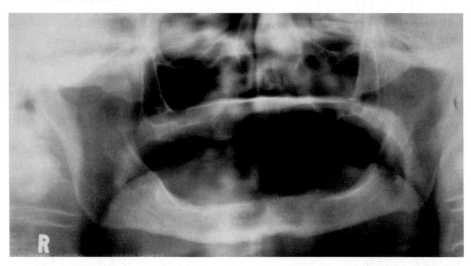

A. Chin too high, head tilted, tongue not on palate, movement, and film crimping
B. Chin too low, head twisted, tongue not on palate, and film crimping
C. Chin too high, head tilted, tongue not on palate, and film crimping
D. Chin too high, head tilted and twisted, tongue not on palate, movement, and film crimping

312. The *arrow* points to a normal anatomic structure. Which one is it?

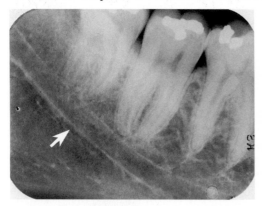

A. Inferior alveolar canal
B. Posterior alveolar canal
C. Lingual canal
D. Mylohyoid line or ridge

313. The 2nd premolar is vital and asymptomatic, and the patient is a black female. Identify the radiolucency to which the *arrow* is pointing.

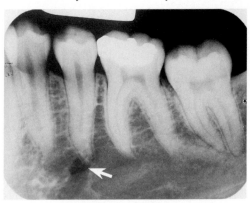

A. Periapical cemental dysplasia
B. Periapical cyst or granuloma
C. Mental foramen
D. Lateral periapical cyst

314. In this edentulous patient we see an oblique shadow to which the *arrow* is pointing. This is:

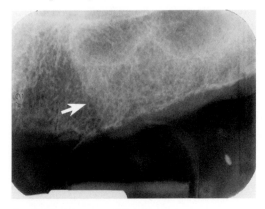

A. A ghost image of the ramus
B. A bend in the film
C. The nasolabial fold
D. Lateral pterygoid muscle, anterior margin

315. We are interested in the central incisors of this 7-year-old boy who has had a lot of fevers during a certain period of his life. What condition affects the central incisors, and when during his life did this occur?

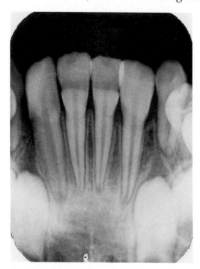

A. Amelogenesis imperfecta; birth
B. Enamel hypoplasia; first 2 years of life
C. Dentinogenesis imperfecta; birth
D. Amelogenesis imperfecta; first 6 months in utero

316. Here we see a very good radiograph of the 3rd molar region. List the anomalies seen in this radiograph.

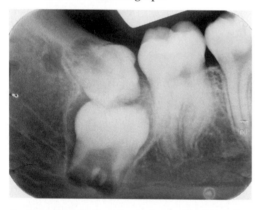

A. Impacted 2nd molar and microdontic 3rd molar
B. Impacted 3rd molar and supernumerary 4th molar
C. Impacted 2nd molar, microdontic impacted 3rd molar, and dilacerated mesial root of the 2nd molar
D. Impacted 3rd molar, impacted supernumerary 4th molar, and dilacerated mesial root of the 2nd molar

317. Notice that there are at least two, possibly three, missing permanent teeth with the retention of at least one or two primary teeth. Among the following list, what is the most likely diagnosis?

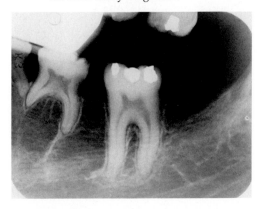

A. Cleidocranial dysplasia
B. Hypohydrotic ectodermal dysplasia
C. Gardner's syndrome
D. Cherubism

318. This patient is a 72-year-old man. Notice that the pulp and root canal spaces are significantly diminished. What is the cause of this?

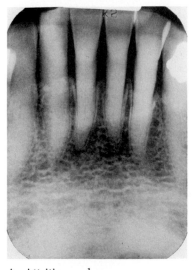

A. Attrition and age
B. Amelogenesis imperfecta
C. Dentinogenesis imperfecta
D. Dentin dysplasia type 1

319. Observe the posterior maxillary tooth. What term(s) best describe(s) this tooth?

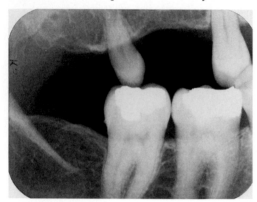

A. Microdont
B. Disto/para molar
C. Macrodont
D. A and B
E. B and C

320. This young adult is missing her 1st premolars; there is also a technique error in this film. Which choice best represents this case?

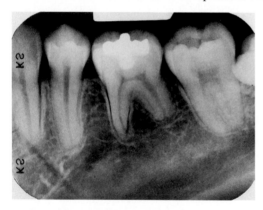

A. Bent film and foreshortening
B. Static electricity and shovel-shaped incisor syndrome
C. Nasolabial fold and taurodontism
D. Bent film and orthodontic root resorption

328. In part *A*, there is a *black arrow* and in part *B* a *white arrow.* Together they depict what anatomic structures?

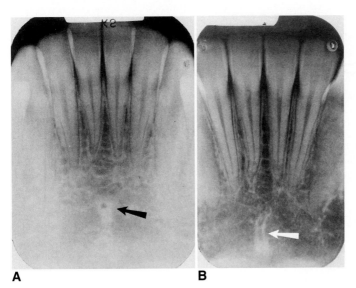

A B

A. Variants of the genial tubercles
B. Variants of the genial tubercles and the lingual foramen
C. Lingual foramen and lingual canal
D. All of the above

329. In this periapical radiograph there are two *white arrowheads.* To what structures do they point?

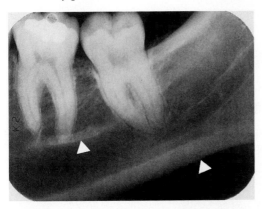

A. Inferior alveolar canal and inferior cortex
B. Submandibular fossa and inferior cortex
C. Inferior cortex and external oblique ridge
D. Mylohyoid ridge and inferior cortex

326. This patient survived a little run-in he had with farmer Brown's shotgun. This is a bit tricky: Identify the metallic objects that have produced (a) ghost image(s).

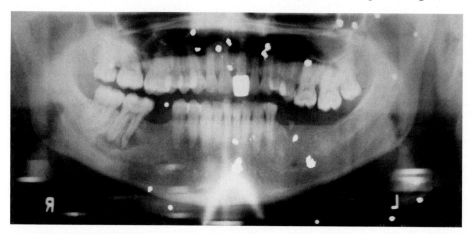

A. Neck chain
B. Left/right markers
C. Shotgun pellets
D. All of the above

327. This radiograph has been cropped. Select the most accurate choice describing what we can see.

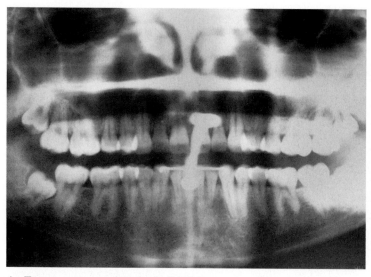

A. Tongue not on palate, barbell left in
B. Tongue not on palate, barbell left in, chin too high
C. Tongue not on palate, barbell left in, chin too high, too far back
D. Tongue not on palate, barbell left in, chin too high, too far back, lingual retainer

324. Note that the lips are slightly open and the tongue is not quite up against the palate; the lead apron may have ridden up very slightly on the shoulder. Several additional errors are in this panoramic radiograph. See if you can find them all.

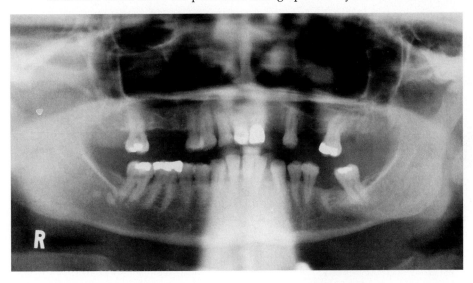

A. Chin too high and slumped
B. Chin not on chin rest and twisted (turned)
C. Too far back, chin too high, and slumped
D. Chin too high, slumped, and twisted (turned)

325. This patient's lips are closed (you can see them), and the tongue is against the palate. There are, however, several errors. What are they?

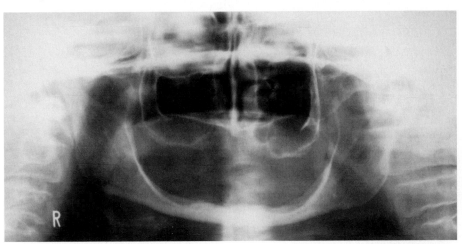

A. Twisted (turned) and tilted
B. Twisted (turned), tilted, and slumped
C. Too far forward, tilted, and slumped
D. Twisted (turned) and too far forward

321. Two technique errors are visible in this image. Identify the cause of the two errors.

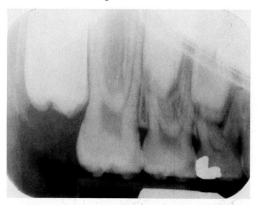

A. Excessive positive vertical angulation and bent film
B. Insufficient vertical film placement and rectangular BID cone cut
C. Insufficient positive vertical angulation and processor damage to bent film
D. Elongation and partial image obscurity

322. Though the contacts are mostly open, what went wrong with this bitewing?

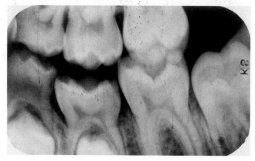

A. Excessive positive vertical angulation
B. Movement
C. Excessive negative vertical angulation
D. Nothing went wrong; it is okay

323. Observe this radiograph. One of the other films in the series was blank. What went wrong here?

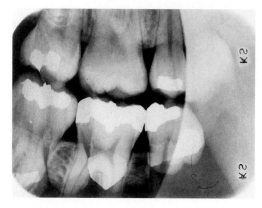

A. Round BID cone cut
B. Fog
C. Double exposure
D. A and B
E. A and C

319. Observe the posterior maxillary tooth. What term(s) best describe(s) this tooth?

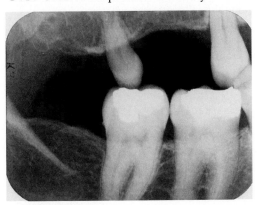

A. Microdont
B. Disto/para molar
C. Macrodont
D. A and B
E. B and C

320. This young adult is missing her 1st premolars; there is also a technique error in this film. Which choice best represents this case?

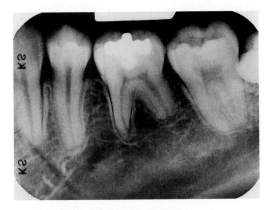

A. Bent film and foreshortening
B. Static electricity and shovel-shaped incisor syndrome
C. Nasolabial fold and taurodontism
D. Bent film and orthodontic root resorption

317. Notice that there are at least two, possibly three, missing permanent teeth with the retention of at least one or two primary teeth. Among the following list, what is the most likely diagnosis?

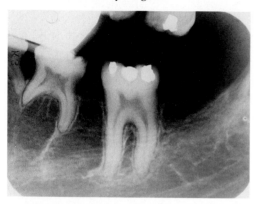

A. Cleidocranial dysplasia
B. Hypohydrotic ectodermal dysplasia
C. Gardner's syndrome
D. Cherubism

318. This patient is a 72-year-old man. Notice that the pulp and root canal spaces are significantly diminished. What is the cause of this?

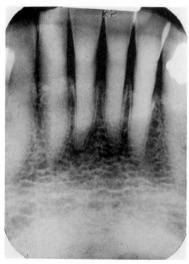

A. Attrition and age
B. Amelogenesis imperfecta
C. Dentinogenesis imperfecta
D. Dentin dysplasia type 1

330. The maxillary lateral incisor (part *A*) and the mandibular central incisor (part *B*) both have periapical radiolucencies in this 59-year-old white man. Read the following question carefully: Select the best choice stating the nature of the periapical lesion and the one tooth with the visible cause identified.

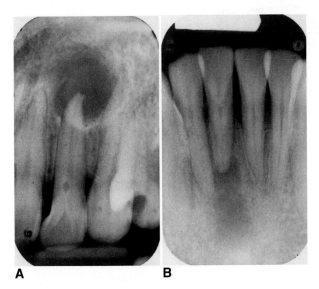

A   **B**

A. Periapical lesion of pulpal origin (abscess, cyst, granuloma) both teeth; trauma to lower central incisor
B. Periapical lesion of pulpal origin (abscess, cyst, granuloma) both teeth; dens in dente maxillary lateral incisor
C. Periapical lesion of pulpal origin (abscess, cyst, granuloma) upper lateral; periapical cemento-osseous dysplasia lower central incisor
D. Periapical radiolucency of pulpal origin (abscess, cyst, granuloma) both teeth; shovel-shaped incisor upper lateral

331. Regarding this image, select the one most accurate choice listing what can be seen in this image.

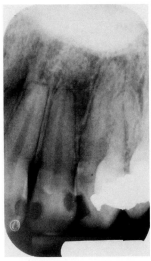

A. Orthodontic root resorption, radiolucent restorations, palatal torus
B. Shovel-shaped incisor syndrome, class 3 caries, film bent and damaged in processor
C. External root resorption, class 3 caries, palatal torus
D. Orthodontic root resorption, radiolucent restorations, film bent and damaged in processor

332. We are considering the radiolucent lesion between the lower premolars. Based on this radiograph, what would be your most likely clinical diagnosis before biopsy?

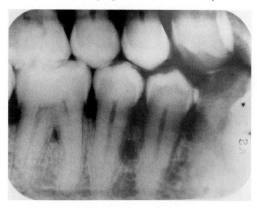

A. Lateral (developmental) periodontal cyst
B. Lateral (inflammatory) periodontal cyst
C. Lateral radicular cyst
D. Odontogenic keratocyst
E. Botryoid odontogenic cyst

333. This patient is a 26-year-old woman with kidney disease. Note the ground-glass pattern of the alveolar bone and loss of the lamina dura. Select the most likely diagnosis.

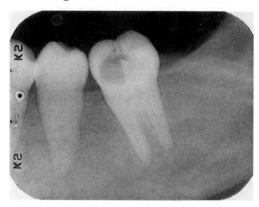

A. Fibrous dysplasia
B. Primary hypoparathyroidism
C. Secondary hyperparathyroidism
D. Paget's disease of bone
E. Nephrotic-induced osteoporosis

334. Okay, forget the bent film and chemical stains. What does the radiopaque lesion represent?

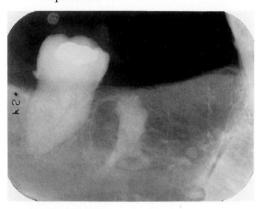

A. Retained root tip
B. Socket sclerosis
C. Postextraction periapical cemento-osseous dysplasia
D. Idiopathic osteosclerosis
E. Parosteal osteoma

335. Observe the radiograph of this fixed 4 unit prosthesis (bridge). What materials is the prosthesis made of?

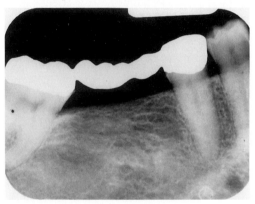

A. All gold
B. Gold with porcelain facings
C. Gold with acrylic facings
D. Acrylic temporary bridge

336. This patient has a history of a fractured mandible. What do you make of what we see at the apex of the 2nd (most posterior) molar?

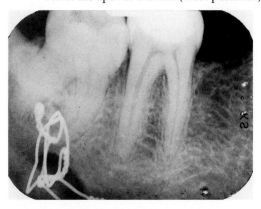

A. Ligature wire
B. Ligature wire and fibrous scar
C. Scratched film and abscessed tooth
D. Some type of double exposure

337. Name two materials associated with taking the radiograph.

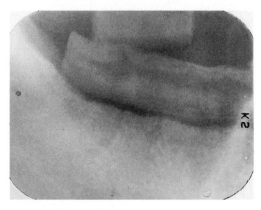

A. Bent film and fog
B. Bite-block and cotton roll
C. Bent film and grainy image caused by depleted developer
D. Bite-block and acrylic stent for implant imaging

338. First let's get oriented. Note the sigmoid notch and coronoid process of the mandible (*black A*) and the maxillary tuberosity (*white B*). Select the correct combination of answers listed from the most posterior (*large arrow*), the middle (*small arrow*), and the most anterior (*arrowhead*).

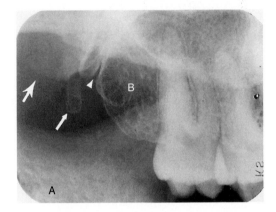

A. Medial pterygoid plate, hamular process of the lateral pterygoid plate, hamular notch
B. Lateral pterygoid plate, hamular process of the medial pterygoid plate, hamular notch
C. Lateral pterygoid plate, hamular process of the medial pterygoid plate, pterygomaxillary fissure
D. Lateral pterygoid plate, hamular process of the lateral pterygoid plate, pterygomaxillary fissure

339. Note the many accessory canals in the lateral walls (anterolateral and posterolateral) of the maxillary sinus and the malar process of the maxilla superimposed on the 2nd molar. This question deals with only the structure indicated by the *arrowheads*. Select the best choice.

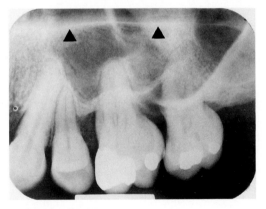

A. Hard palate
B. Floor of the nose
C. Roof of the sinus
D. A and B
E. B and C

340. Look closely at the maxillary sinus. The *arrow* points to a radiolucent line bound by a more radiopaque line on each side that cuts diagonally across the maxillary sinus. This is:

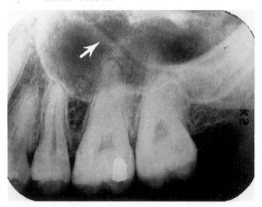

A. The posterior superior alveolar canal
B. The roof of the sinus and floor of the nose
C. A septum of the sinus
D. A fractured sinus wall

341. Because of the blackness of the fingerprints, what chemical do you think contaminated this film?

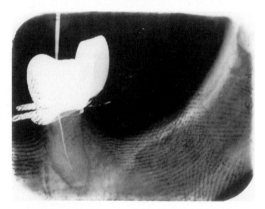

A. Fluoride
B. Developer
C. Fixer
D. Sodium thiosulfate
E. Water contaminated with developer and fixer.

342. For this radiograph, match the descriptive term that indicates the problem; after that, list the cause.

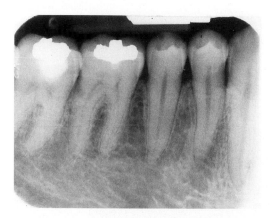

A. Shortened roots; orthodontics
B. Shortened roots; shovel-shaped incisor syndrome
C. Foreshortening of the roots; excessive negative vertical angulation of the BID
D. This is a problem without a cause because there is no problem or error

343. Okay, this is the one you have been waiting for. What happened?

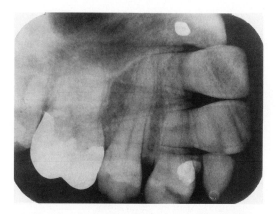

A. Chemical stains
B. Grainy, fogged image
C. Class 4 partial denture with porcelain teeth that have become dislodged
D. Double exposure
E. None of the above

344. Oh yes, you can believe it! Stuff like this happens. Okay, select the most complete list of errors.

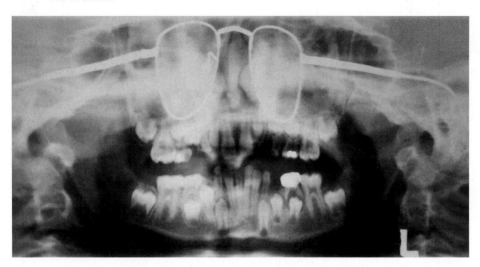

A. Glasses left on
B. Chin too high
C. Tongue not on palate
D. All of the above
E. A and B

345. In spite of the fact that many of the teeth are obscured, three different errors can be noted:

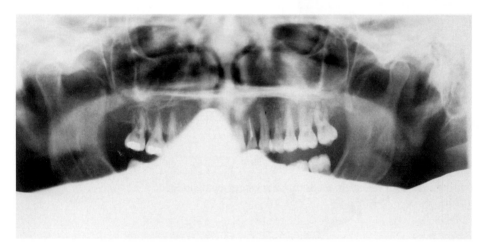

A. Apron shadow, head turned, patient too far back
B. Large fixer stain, head tilted, patient too far back
C. Paper in cassette, head turned, patient too far back
D. Cassette light leak, head tilted, head turned

346. Read this one carefully. The patient is a middle-aged black woman. Match the radiographic findings with the associated disorder.

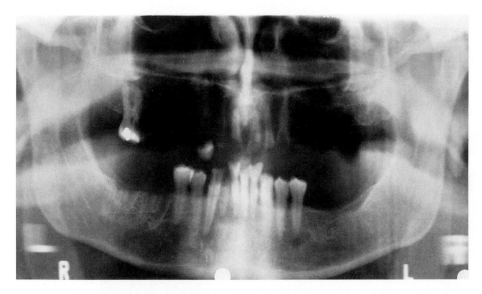

A. Multiple anterior periapical radiolucencies; periapical cemento-osseous dysplasia
B. Multiple anterior periapical radiolucencies and posterior radiopacities; florid cemento-osseous dysplasia
C. Socket sclerosis; gastrointestinal or renal disease
D. Multiple carious teeth; sialorrhea

347. This patient had a tonsillectomy years ago and has the following symptoms: a sensation like a fishbone stuck in the throat on swallowing and occasional lightheadedness when turning the head. The condition depicted here is caused by:

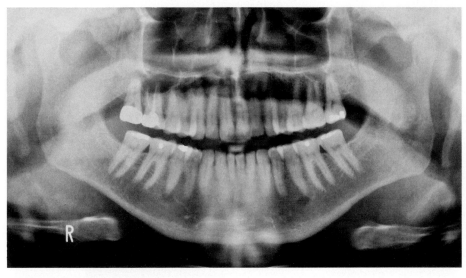

A. Carotid artery calcifications
B. Elongated styloid process and mineralized stylohyoid ligament
C. A large bone stuck in the pharynx
D. Falcon's syndrome
E. Hawk's syndrome

348. This patient is a 47-year-old black woman. There were some periapical radiopacities in the anterior region, which is obscured in this case. The diagnosis is:

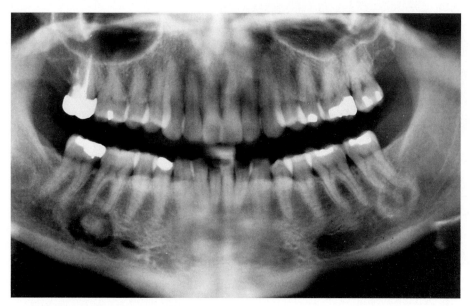

A. Focal cemento-osseous dysplasia
B. Periapical cemento-osseous dysplasia
C. Florid cemento-osseous dysplasia
D. Chronic diffuse sclerosing osteomyelitis

349. Amazingly, three of the four 2nd premolars were non-vital in this 14-year-old Asian teenager. All four 2nd premolars were affected by the same clinical finding. What could this be?

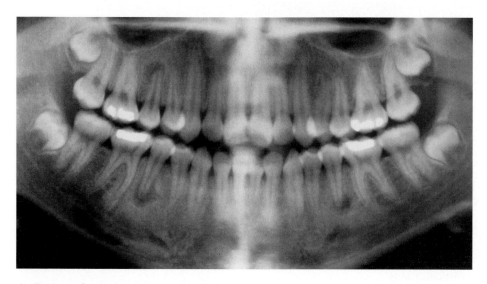

A. Periapical cemento-osseous dysplasia
B. Dentin dysplasia type 1
C. Deep occlusal caries
D. Dens evaginatus

350. Observe these teeth carefully. What condition is present?

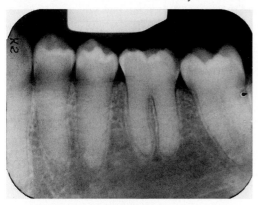

A. Amelogenesis imperfecta
B. Dentinogenesis imperfecta
C. Dentin dysplasia type 2
D. Age-related pulp obliteration

351. An anomaly is present in this patient. It is:

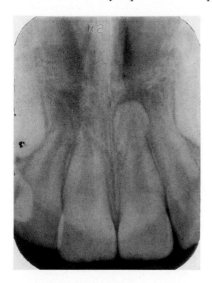

A. Snow-capped tooth
B. Periapical cemental dysplasia
C. Rare double-crowned tooth
D. Mesiodens

352. Note the extruded maxillary 3rd molar. What term(s) best describe(s) the most distal mandibular tooth? Note that the 1st and 2nd molars are present and no teeth have been extracted.

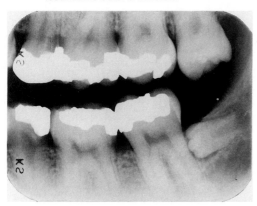

A. Disto molar
B. Microdont
C. Impacted
D. All of the above

353. Note the dilacerated premolar root. The condition that affects this sinus is:

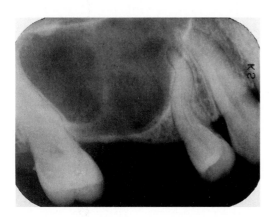

A. Acute sinusitis
B. Chronic sinusitis
C. Sinus elongation
D. Pneumatization

354. In this image you can see the two central incisors and a single lateral incisor. Clinically, there was a notch in the mid-incisal area. The problem here is:

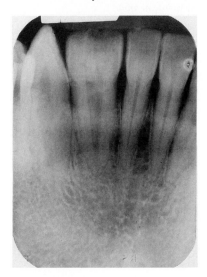

A. Gemination
B. Fusion
C. Dilaceration
D. Twinning
E. Microdontia

355. The maxillary 2nd and 3rd molars have been missing for several years. What has happened to the mandibular 3rd molar?

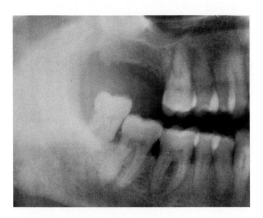

A. Partially extracted tooth
B. Dens evaginatus
C. Supraeruption (extrusion)
D. Eruption sequestrum
E. Floating tooth

356. Notice the soft tissue outline of the nose on roots and lips at incisal edge. We have three structures to identify here. The selections are listed from the left of the photo (*large black arrowhead*), middle (*small black arrowhead*), and right (*white arrow*).

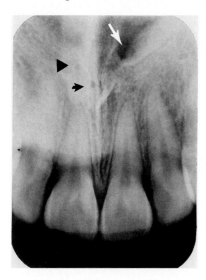

A. Foramen of Scarpa, foramen of Stensen, nasal fossa
B. Foramen of Stensen, foramen of Scarpa, nasal fossa
C. Foramen of Stensen, foramen of Scarpa, superior foramen of incisive canal
D. Foramen of Scarpa, foramen of Stensen, superior foramen of incisive canal

357. Here we are looking at the radiolucent area between the central incisors. This is:

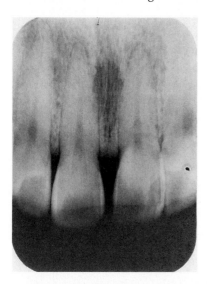

A. Lateral (developmental) periodontal cyst
B. Incisive canal cyst (nasopalatine duct cyst)
C. Nasolabial cyst
D. Incisive foramen

358. Here we want to identify *black letter a* and *white letter b* in that order. Lastly, where are they located?

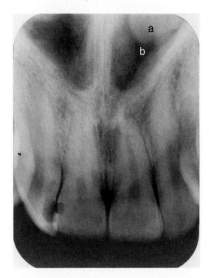

A. Inferior turbinate, inferior meatus, nasal fossa
B. Nasal polyp, air space, nasal fossa
C. Palatal torus, air space, palate and nasal fossa
D. Soft tissue of the nose, air space, nasal fossa

359. The *top arrow* points to a radiopaque structure; the *bottom arrow* points to a radiolucent line. The answer choices are listed from top to bottom.

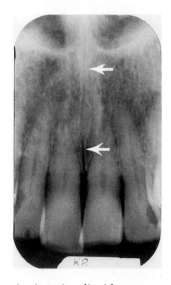

A. Anterior clinoid process; median maxillary cleft
B. Vomer bone; median maxillary fracture
C. Nasal bone; median maxillary cleft
D. Anterior nasal spine; median maxillary suture

360. This #1-size film was pretty well clear. What is (are) the possible cause(s) of this?

A. Unexposed
B. Left in fixer all weekend
C. Fixed before developing
D. All of the above
E. None of the above (it is exposed to light)

361. Here we certainly have a film placement problem, as the bottom of the film is not aligned with the occlusal plane. There is also something else that did not work out too well. What happened?

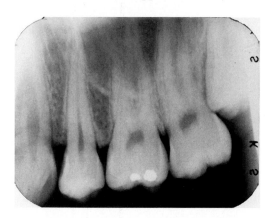

A. Image distortion because of excessive digital pressure
B. Inadequate positive vertical angulation of the beam
C. Patient movement
D. Processor damage to the image

362. It was decided that this film should be retaken. Can you find the reason?

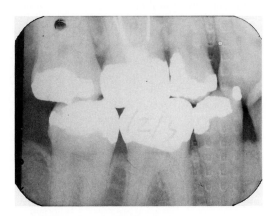

A. Somebody wrote on the film
B. Film packet was reversed
C. Excessive fog
D. Black rectangular BID cone cut

363. A small radiopaque object is in the maxillary sinus. Study the features carefully and see if you can select the correct diagnosis.

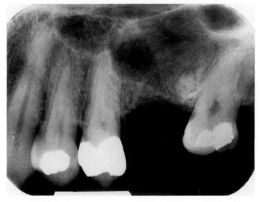

A. Antrolith
B. Antral exostosis
C. Retained root tip
D. Antral osteoma

364. In this image we need to identify four different entities. The choices are listed from top to bottom starting with *(a)*, then *(b)*, then the *white arrow*, and finally *(c)*.

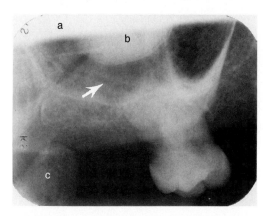

A. Bent film, turbinate, sinus septum, coronoid process
B. Rectangular BID cone cut, sinus osteoma, sinus fracture, soft tissue osteoma
C. Rectangular BID cone cut, palatal torus, posterior superior alveolar canal, coronoid process
D. Streaked fixer artifact, fingerprint with fixer, posterior superior alveolar canal, finger tip (phalangioma)

365. The question was: "How come I have not lost my baby tooth?" Your answer:

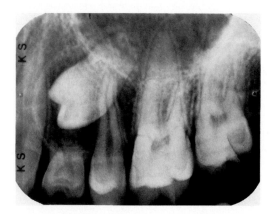

A. Unerupted 1st premolar
B. Possible dentigerous cyst of 1st premolar
C. A and B
D. 1st premolar is erupting; be patient

366. First, this patient's teeth are affected in a generalized way, and second, the *arrows* point to a good-sized radiopacity. Select the best choice.

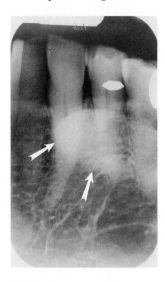

A. Attrition, mandibular torus
B. Erosion, osteoma
C. Abrasion, large exostoses
D. Abfraction, idiopathic osteosclerosis

367. First, a *white arrowhead* is pointing to a radiolucent area in the maxilla; and second, the *number 2* is seen within a radiopaque area bilaterally. Going from inferior to superior, what are the two entities?

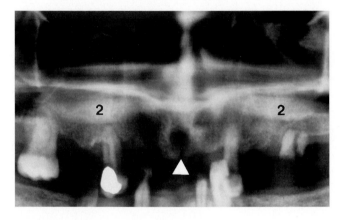

A. Incisive foramen; ghost image of palate
B. Incisive canal cyst; palatal torus
C. Residual lateral periodontal cyst; bilateral buccal exostoses
D. Nasoalveolar cyst; bilateral mucus retention phenomena

368. This patient is an 11-year-old boy; note the premolar is still erupting. What do you think the radiopacity at the apex of the canine represents?

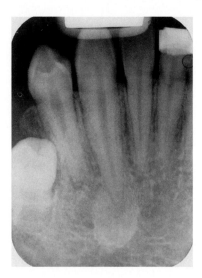

A. Focal cemento-osseous dysplasia
B. Periapical cemento-osseous dysplasia
C. Condensing osteitis
D. Idiopathic osteosclerosis

369. These teeth are restored with temporary acrylic crowns and radiolucent composite. There is a radiolucent area in the root of the lateral incisor. What does this represent?

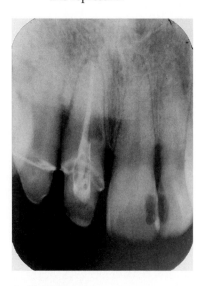

A. Root caries
B. Internal root resorption
C. External root resorption
D. Internal/external root resorption

370. Study the lateral incisor. What features can you note regarding this tooth?

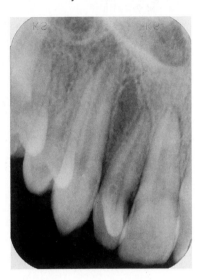

A. Accessory lingual cusp
B. Dens in dente
C. Dilacerated crown
D. Peg lateral
E. All of the above

371. We are interested in the mandibular 3rd molar. Note the lesion at the distal. This is consistent with:

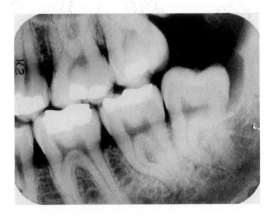

A. Eruption cyst
B. Inflammatory paradental cyst
C. Periodontal pocket/abscess
D. Normal follicular space

372. There's caries in this tooth; it's broken down, and you are contemplating extraction. Which one factor seen here is most likely to complicate the extraction?

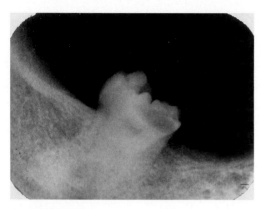

A. Ankylosis
B. Large carious lesion
C. Short crown length
D. Apical osteosclerosis

373. Note the anterior midline diastema. Can you identify a problem sometimes associated with the diastema?

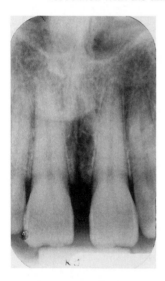

A. Fractured maxilla
B. Anterior median maxillary suture
C. Anterior median maxillary cleft
D. Palatal orthodontic defect

374. You are looking at the posterior mandibular region of a 67-year-old man. He is edentulous, and a full mouth survey was done before making the new denture. He is asymptomatic and has no history of surgery. What is the problem?

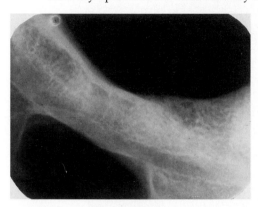

A. Deep submandibular fossa
B. Submandibular salivary gland depression (Stafne defect)
C. Large neuroma or neurilemmoma
D. Large vascular lesion like A-V malformation
E. C and/or D

375. The *black arrow* points to a black, crescent-shaped radiolucent line. This is caused by:

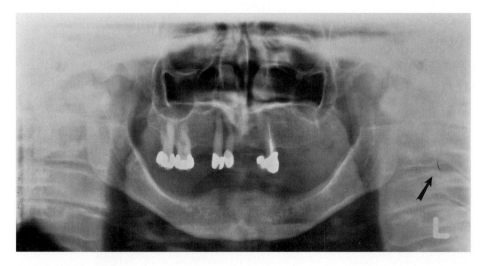

A. Long fingernails
B. Static electricity
C. Developer solution
D. Crimping the film

376. Okay. What was left on before taking the radiograph?

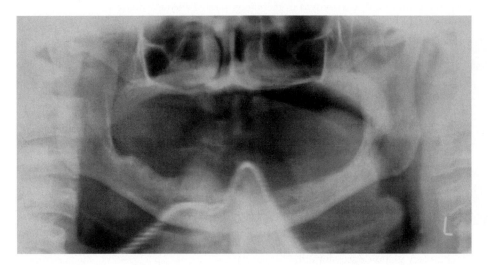

A. Napkin chain
B. Jewelry neck chain
C. A or B
D. None of the above (it was an anti-swallow denture safety chain)

377. This film simply looks too light. The most common cause(s) of this is (are):

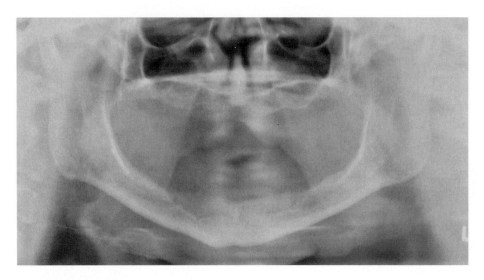

A. Inadequate kVp
B. Depleted developer solution
C. Failure of the autoprocessor heating element
D. All of the above

378. When you can see the turbinates spread bilaterally across the sinus and the shadow of the nose in the maxillary midline as we see here, the positioning error is:

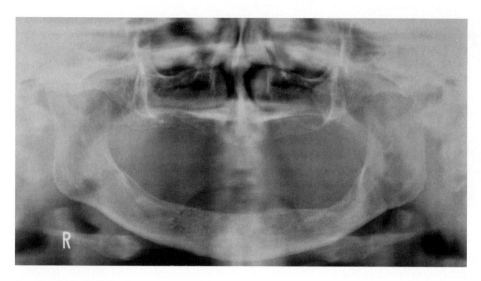

A. Too far forward
B. Too far back
C. Chin too low
D. Slumped

379. There is a dark shadow apical to these three molars. It is not unlike what we saw in Figure 374, yet this one is somehow different. What do you think?

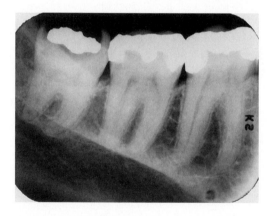

A. Submandibular salivary gland depression (Stafne defect)
B. Submandibular fossa
C. Corner of radiograph partially exposed to light
D. Large periapical cyst as a result of carious 3rd molar

380. Although the stepladder trabecular pattern as seen here was once thought to be a sign of sickle cell anemia, this is no longer believed to be true. The trabecular pattern is, however, interesting. How would you classify this example?

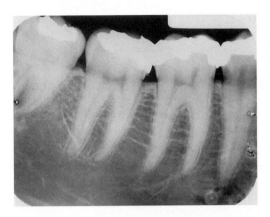

A. Loose
B. Moderate
C. Heavy
D. Trabecular patterns are not classified

381. In this radiograph there is a large triangular radiopaque area labeled *777*. (Why?... There was no "*&*" for the middle "7".) This area represents the radiographic confluence of two structures. Which ones are they?

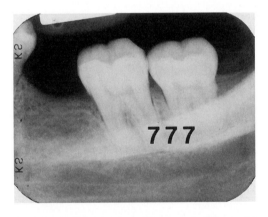

A. Retromolar trigone and external oblique ridge
B. External oblique ridge and internal oblique ridge
C. Internal oblique ridge and the mylohyoid line
D. Internal oblique ridge and a deep submandibular fossa

388. In this radiograph you can see several thin black lines on the maxillary 1st premolar and lower 1st molar. What are these?

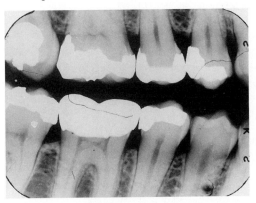

A. Static electricity
B. Scratched film
C. Fracture lines
D. Lint contamination
E. Fibers from the paper wrap

389. If you noticed the water contaminated with developer mark and the bent corner... you are catching on. If you were to look at this area of the patient's mouth clinically, what is the most significant thing you would look for?

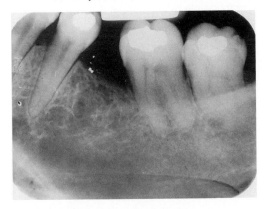

A. Space enough to make a bridge
B. The angulation of the teeth regarding bridge design
C. Whether there is caries on the 3rd molar
D. Correlate pigmented lesion with amalgam fragments for amalgam tattoo

386. Jim has a scar on the right side of his neck. Here is an example of a perfectly acceptable procedure: leave the denture in to assist positioning and to stabilize the patient. However, it looks like something else was left in or on. What is it?

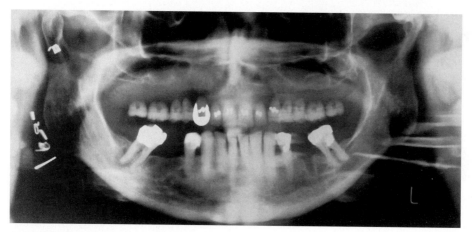

A. Some kind of earring on one ear
B. Scratches on the film
C. Scratched screen
D. Vascular clamps

387. Yep... it's a round BID cone cut! There are heavy radiopaque lines in this radiograph. The one at the cervical area is the external oblique ridge, and the lowest one is the inferior cortex. The opaque line crossing the apices of the molar is:

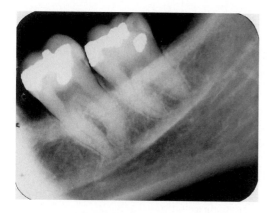

A. Internal oblique ridge
B. Mylohyoid ridge
C. A or B (terms are interchangeable)
D. Submandibular fossa

384. There are several interesting things to see in this radiograph: notice how the root canal of the 1st premolar bifurcates and how bulbous the 1st molar roots are. But what do you see in association with the 2nd premolar?

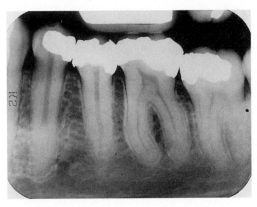

A. Bulbous root
B. External resorption
C. Hypercementosis
D. Idiopathic osteosclerosis

385. This panoramic radiograph is not perfect. Note how the chin is too high and the tongue not against the palate. Now take a look at the large round radiopaque area in the right maxillary sinus. WHOA!!! This is something we readily recognize in dental radiology. Do you know what it is?

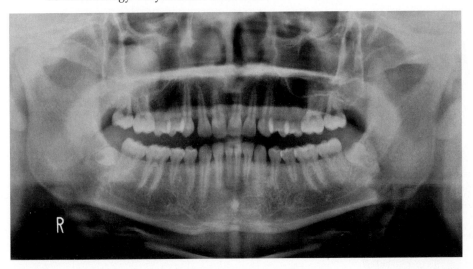

A. Mucous retention cyst (sinus mucocele, sinus pseudocyst)
B. Periapical mucositis (odontogenic mucositis)
C. Palatal torus (unilateral or hemisected)
D. Osteoma (palatal or sinus)

382. Here we see an anatomic landmark at the apex of the canine. It is the:

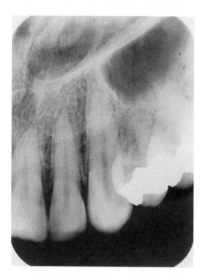

A. Maxillary sinus
B. Nasal fossa
C. Inverted "Y"
D. Ala of the nose

383. There is a prominent radiolucent area at the apex of the central incisor. What do you think this represents?

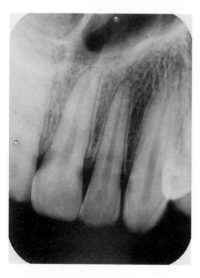

A. Nasal fossa
B. Superior foramen of the incisive canal
C. Periapical cyst
D. Unilateral high incisive canal cyst
E. Inferior meatus

380. Although the stepladder trabecular pattern as seen here was once thought to be a sign of sickle cell anemia, this is no longer believed to be true. The trabecular pattern is, however, interesting. How would you classify this example?

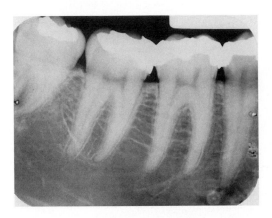

A. Loose
B. Moderate
C. Heavy
D. Trabecular patterns are not classified

381. In this radiograph there is a large triangular radiopaque area labeled *777*. (Why?... There was no "*&*" for the middle "7".) This area represents the radiographic confluence of two structures. Which ones are they?

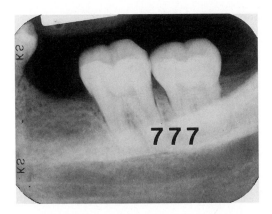

A. Retromolar trigone and external oblique ridge
B. External oblique ridge and internal oblique ridge
C. Internal oblique ridge and the mylohyoid line
D. Internal oblique ridge and a deep submandibular fossa

378. When you can see the turbinates spread bilaterally across the sinus and the shadow of the nose in the maxillary midline as we see here, the positioning error is:

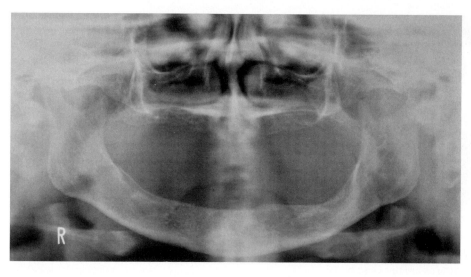

A. Too far forward
B. Too far back
C. Chin too low
D. Slumped

379. There is a dark shadow apical to these three molars. It is not unlike what we saw in Figure 374, yet this one is somehow different. What do you think?

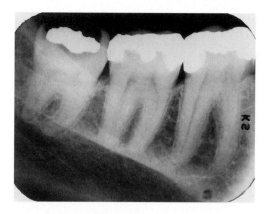

A. Submandibular salivary gland depression (Stafne defect)
B. Submandibular fossa
C. Corner of radiograph partially exposed to light
D. Large periapical cyst as a result of carious 3rd molar

390. This patient has developed discomfort under the bridge. The soft tissues are red and swollen. What problem did you discover?

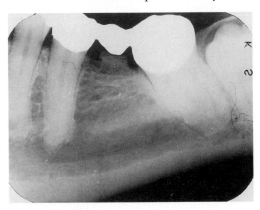

A. Small osteoma
B. Reactive sub pontic exostosis
C. Small wedged chicken bone
D. Osteosarcoma

391. Notice the scratch made on the film by the mosquito forceps used for hand dipping. This 13-year-old female patient is asymptomatic; however, there is a scar in the region. Count the teeth. Now notice the radiolucent area distal to the lateral incisor. What do you think this is?

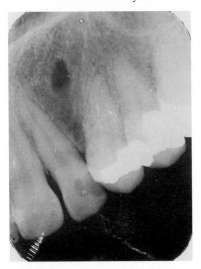

A. Fibrous bone scar
B. Globulomaxillary cyst
C. Adenomatoid odontogenic tumor
D. Residual cyst

392. Here it is, plain and simple: What is the radiopacity between the premolars?

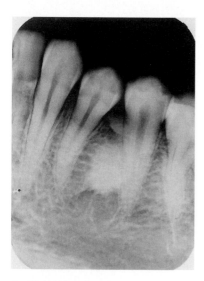

A. Osteoid osteoma
B. Osteoma
C. Mandibular torus
D. Idiopathic osteosclerosis
E. Osteosarcoma

393. A deep periodontal defect was noted distal to the 2nd molar, and the lesion extended around to the buccal. A buccal enamel spur was noted at the bifurcation of the 2nd molar. What condition do you think is present?

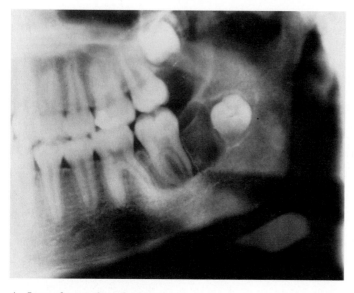

A. Lateral periodontal cyst
B. Botryoid odontogenic cyst
C. Inflammatory buccal cyst (inflammatory paradental cyst)
D. Eruption cyst of 2nd molar
E. Dentigerous cyst of 3rd molar

394. This is an asymptomatic 14-year-old white female. The lesion was noted on a routine radiographic examination. All the teeth were vital. What do you think the lesion is?

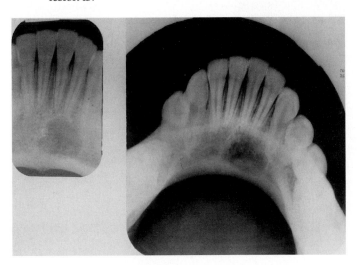

A. Developer solution artifact
B. Focal cemento-osseous dysplasia (radiolucent stage)
C. Simple bone cyst (traumatic cyst)
D. Adenomatoid odontogenic tumor
E. Primordial cyst of a supernumerary tooth

395. Look at the lower 3rd molar. We are interested in the radiolucent space around the crown. What do you think this is?

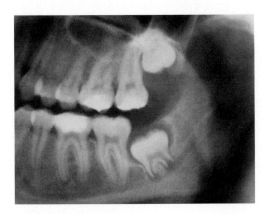

A. Normal follicular space
B. Eruption cyst
C. Dentigerous cyst
D. Inflammatory paradental cyst

396. The *arrow* points to a radiolucency in the sigmoid notch area. This is:

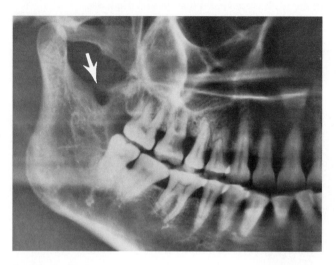

A. Fibrous bone scar
B. Parotid salivary gland depression
C. Foramen of the coronoid process
D. Medial sigmoid depression

397. Yup! You can do vertical posterior periapicals should the need arise. We are interested in the fine, thin, curved, parallel radiopaque structures indicated by the *arrows.* These are:

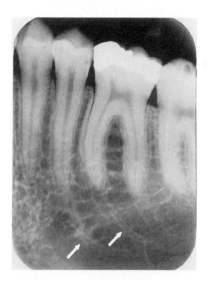

A. A sign of a vascular lesion in the area
B. Normal nutrient or accessory canals
C. Abnormal nutrient or accessory canals
D. The "wormian bone" sign

398. Note the prominent linear radiolucent areas indicated by the *arrowheads.*
These are:

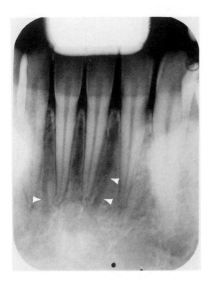

A. Normal nutrient canals
B. Abnormal nutrient canals
C. A sign of susceptibility to destructive periodontal disease
D. B and C
E. Thinned radiolucent interseptal bone

399. Parts *A* and *B* together represent an implant case. Select the most appropriate
answer.

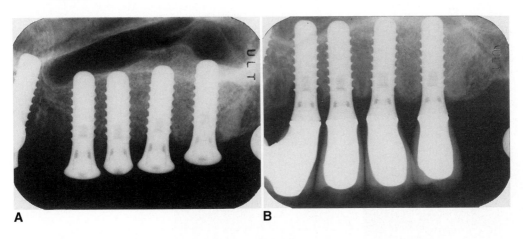

A

B

A. Excellent osseous integration, sulcular bone breakdown
B. Excellent osseous integration, sulcular bone normal for implants, poor crown contours
C. Excellent osseous integration, sulcular bone normal for implants, sinus floor lift being
repneumatized
D. Excellent osseous integration, sulcular bone normal for implants, sinus floor lift being
repneumatized, poor crown contours

400. This is a 14-year-old female who presented with facial swelling on the right side. Select which group of three differential diagnoses would best suit this case.

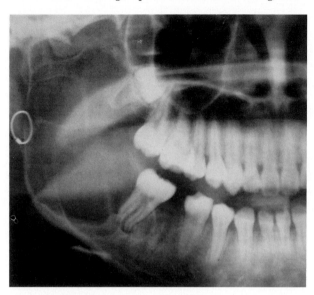

A. Ameloblastoma, mural ameloblastoma, odontogenic fibroma
B. Ameloblastoma, central giant cell granuloma, odontogenic myxoma
C. Mural ameloblastoma, odontogenic myxoma, odontogenic keratocyst
D. Ameloblastoma, mural ameloblastoma, ameloblastic fibroma

401. Parts *A* and *B* are from a 12-year-old female of Greek origin with a bilaterally swollen face. What do you think the problem is?

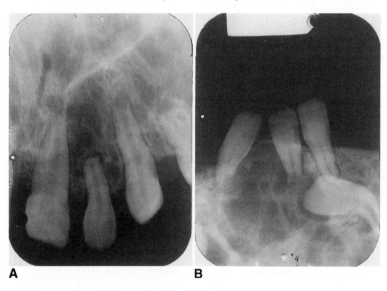

A   B

A. Fibrous dysplasia
B. Mediterranean anemia (thalassemia)
C. Cherubism
D. Greek restaurant syndrome
E. Maffucci's syndrome (multiple hemangiomas)

402. The *arrow* points to a small radiopaque bone fragment. This is:

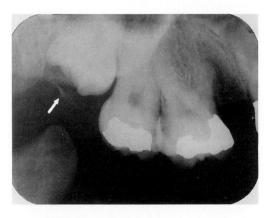

A. A foreign body (chicken bone or similar)
B. An eruption sequestrum
C. An eruption cyst wall
D. Scratched film

403. Assess the anterior region of this child. Select the best choice regarding the findings.

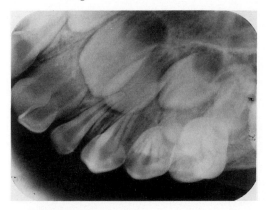

A. Supernumerary incisor
B. Possible fusion between central and supernumerary incisor
C. Lack of resorption of primary lateral apex indicates eruption problems and potential future crowding
D. A and B
E. All of the above

404. Select the most complete answer regarding the lateral incisor.

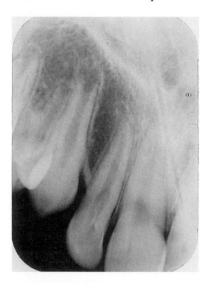

A. Dens in dente
B. Dens in dente with enamel invagination
C. Dens in dente with enamel and dentin invagination
D. Dens in dente with enamel and dentin invagination, lingual pit
E. Dens in dente with enamel and dentin invagination, lingual pit, and possible lingual (palatal) groove

405. We are looking at the molars. Select the most complete description.

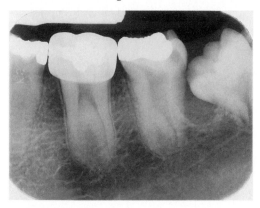

A. Taurodontism
B. Taurodontism, poorly adapted SS crown
C. Taurodontism, poorly adapted SS crown, caries
D. Taurodontism, poorly adapted SS crown, caries, lateral dentigerous cyst 3rd molar
E. Taurodontism, poorly adapted SS crown, caries, lateral dentigerous cyst 3rd molar, rule out genetic abnormality

406. Assess this case regarding the retained primary molar.

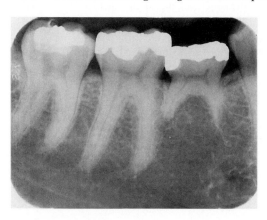

A. Recognize the ankylosis and rebuild the occlusion.
B. Chart the missing tooth.
C. Assess the adjacent teeth for early root caries.
D. All of the above.
E. Leave it alone.

407. Here are two areas from this 47-year-old black woman's mouth. The condition that is present is:

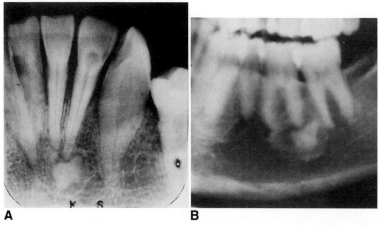

A   B

A. Focal cemento-osseous dysplasia
B. Periapical cemento-osseous dysplasia
C. Florid cemento-osseous dysplasia
D. Idiopathic osteosclerosis

408. This 60-year-old man is a chronic alcoholic and is what you would refer to as a *homeless person*. He has come into the clinic with right facial swelling, pain, and several draining fistulas. The radiographic picture you see here is that of a "moth-eaten" pattern with several small bone sequestrae and possibly a large radiopaque area of infarcted bone anterior to the molar. There is a faint periosteal reaction at the inferior cortex. The most likely diagnosis is:

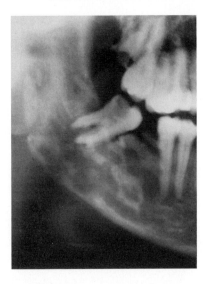

A. Metastatic prostate carcinoma
B. Osteogenic sarcoma (lytic pattern)
C. Acute osteomyelitis
D. Chronic osteomyelitis
E. Garrè's osteomyelitis

409. This patient has a finding at the apical region of the 2nd premolar. What is your assessment?

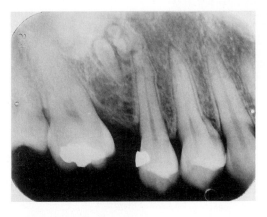

A. Compound odontoma
B. Complex odontoma
C. Idiopathic osteosclerosis
D. Dentinoma

410. This patient came in stating she simply could not tolerate her old denture for another day and wanted to immediately have a new denture made. She never liked doctors or dentists and agreed to have the panoramic radiograph done only because it was "free" with the new denture. What did we discover?

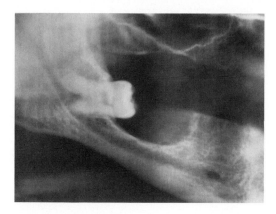

A. Impacted 3rd molar
B. Impacted 3rd molar, dentigerous cyst
C. Impacted 3rd molar, infected dentigerous cyst
D. Impacted and partially ankylosed 3rd molar, infected dentigerous cyst
E. Impacted and partially ankylosed 3rd molar, infected dentigerous cyst, soft tissue swelling at crest of ridge

411. What do we see at the apex of the 2nd premolar?

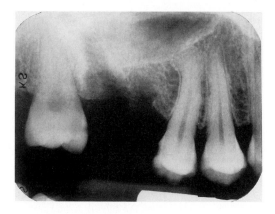

A. Condensing osteitis
B. Idiopathic osteosclerosis
C. Hypercementosis
D. Periapical cemental dysplasia

412. Pick out the one term that best describes the radiopacity between the roots of the maxillary central incisors.

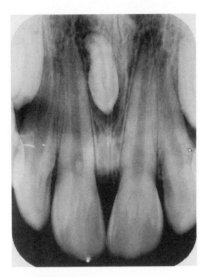

A. Mesiodens
B. Hypodontia
C. Compound odontoma
D. Macrodont

413. Assess this case regarding the retained primary molar.

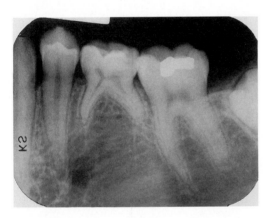

A. Recognize the ankylosis and rebuild the occlusion.
B. Chart the missing tooth.
C. Assess the adjacent teeth for early root caries.
D. All of the above.
E. Leave it alone.

414. Note the linear horizontal radiolucent areas at the cervical of the premolars. Though there is horizontal bone loss, these areas were slightly subgingival. What is your assessment?

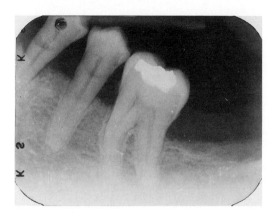

A. Toothbrush abrasion
B. Abfraction
C. Cervical caries
D. Radiolucent cervical restorations

415. Note the occlusal anatomy of the occlusal surface of the mandibular 2nd molar that has just erupted. Now look at the maxillary 2nd premolar and the lower premolars. What is your assessment of these teeth?

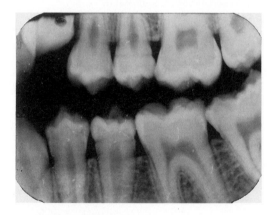

A. Enamel hypoplasia
B. Amelogenesis imperfecta
C. Dentin dysplasia type 1
D. Caries

416. This 14-year-old patient is being worked up for orthodontic treatment. What is your assessment regarding this radiograph?

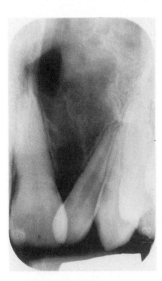

A. Residual abscess or infection
B. Fibrous bone scar
C. Atypical globulomaxillary cyst
D. Cleft palate

417. In your assessment of this case you note that there is resorption of the mesial of the primary canine in association with the eruption of the lateral incisor. This should be considered a sign of:

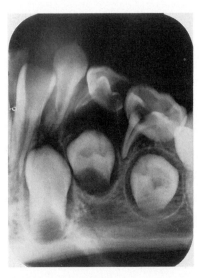

A. Normal eruption
B. Impending crowding of the permanent teeth
C. Macrodontia of the lateral incisor
D. Probable spacing between the permanent mandibular incisors

418. This is the "now you see it and now you don't" question. Notice the small round radiopacity in the furcal area of the molar in the periapical view (*A*). Now look at the bitewing (*B*) taken the same day. What is this?

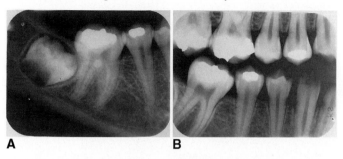

A

B

A. A bitewing from another patient with similar restorations
B. A small drop of fixer in the periapical view (*A*)
C. The "faux enamel pearl" artifact
D. The bitewing (*B*) is the postoperative radiograph

419. Okay, here it is. What is the source of this patient's pain on chewing?

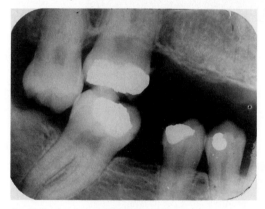

A. Calculus associated periodontitis
B. Caries
C. Extrusion (supraeruption)
D. A problem not visible in this radiograph

420. This 12-year-old boy has very large pulps and a systemic disorder. Select the best choice.

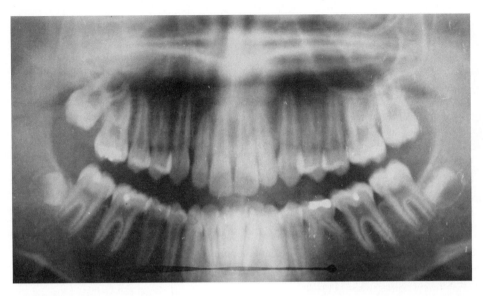

A. Papillon-Lefevre syndrome
B. Renal osteodystrophy
C. Vitamin D–resistant rickets
D. Dentin dysplasia type 2
E. Wilson's disease

421. This is an 8-year-old girl with delayed eruption of the permanent teeth. She has other skeletal defects. What is your assessment of this case?

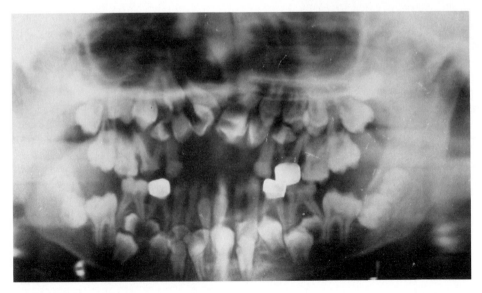

A. Cherubism
B. Cleidocranial dysplasia
C. Gardner's syndrome
D. Hypopituitarism

439. Abfraction is:

A. The loss of tooth structure associated with traumatic occlusion
B. The loss of tooth structure by a traumatic blow
C. Minute craze lines seen in the enamel
D. The root cause of the fractured tooth syndrome
E. Abscess formation after tooth fracture

440. Hutchinson's incisors are associated with:

A. Bertram's molars
B. Congenital syphilis
C. Infantile cortical hyperostosis
D. Pyle's disease
E. All of the above

441. The "phoenix" abscess:

A. Arises from asymptomatic chronic periapical infection like the mythical Egyptian phoenix arising from its own ashes in the desert every 500 years and then consuming itself in fire
B. Was first described by a Dr. Miles Albert Phoenix, later known as a *MAP lesion* and eventually evolved to the term *geographic abscess*
C. Was first seen among desert -dwelling native Americans in Phoenix, Arizona
D. Is a synonym for a Munro abscess
E. Is probably as "mythical" as the above four choices (none of the above)

442. The most significant difference between the ameloblastic fibro-odontoma and the ameloblastic fibroma is that the ameloblastic fibro-odontoma:

A. Occurs in an older age-group
B. Occurs in a younger age-group
C. May demonstrate radiopaque flecks
D. Behaves more aggressively

443. What unusual feature most often characterizes the unerupted or impacted tooth associated with the calcifying epithelial odontogenic tumor?

A. It is a 1st or 2nd permanent molar.
B. It is in an inverted position.
C. It is an anterior tooth associated with "driven snow."
D. The crown of the tooth is partially resorbed.

444. If you see a small cyst-like radiolucency in the mandibular midline region of a panoramic film, what should you do next?

A. Repeat the panoramic radiograph and see if the area can be duplicated.
B. Aspirate the area to check for vascular or cystic lesions.
C. Pulp-test all teeth in the area for vitality.
D. Take a periapical view of the area to see if the area can be duplicated.
E. A, B, and C above.

445. A distinguishing characteristic of the calcification in the early-stage tooth crypt is the appearance of:

A. Flecks, islands, or radiopacities
B. Radiopacities resembling "driven snow"
C. Inverted V-shaped ("circumflex" or ^-shaped) radiopacities
D. Liesegang's rings
E. None of the above

446. How long are postextraction sockets usually apparent on radiographs?

A. 6-8 weeks
B. 2-3 months
C. 6-12 months
D. 1-2 years

447. Focal osteoporotic bone marrow defect of the jaws occurs most often:

A. Below the mandibular canal
B. As an inherited trait in pale-complected females
C. Secondary to hyperparathyroidism
D. After tooth extraction

448. What is the radiographic appearance of the fibrous healing defect?

A. An area of diffuse radiopacity
B. A "punched out" or well-defined "see through" radiolucency
C. A radiolucency at first gradually becoming radiopaque
D. A radiolucency with internal trabeculations

449. A round or ovoid, well-corticated radiolucency located below the mandibular canal in the 2nd-molar ramus area is characteristic of a:

A. Stafne defect (submandibular salivary gland depression)
B. Residual cyst
C. Simple bone cyst (traumatic cyst)
D. Focal osteoporotic bone marrow defect

MULTIPLE CHOICE QUESTIONS WITHOUT A RADIOGRAPHIC IMAGE

426. Which are the most common microdontic teeth?

A. 3rd molars
B. Maxillary permanent lateral incisors
C. Maxillary 1st premolars
D. Primary canines

427. What is gemination?

A. The union between two separate tooth buds usually by dentin and enamel
B. The union of the roots of two teeth by their cementum
C. The aborted attempt of a single tooth bud to divide into two teeth
D. The union of a permanent tooth bud with the roots of a primary tooth

428. What is fusion?

A. The union between two separate tooth buds usually by dentin and enamel
B. The union of the roots of two teeth by their cementum
C. The aborted attempt of a single tooth bud to divide into two teeth
D. The union of a permanent tooth bud with the roots of a primary tooth

429. Dens in dente (dens invaginatus) is most often seen in:

A. Primary maxillary lateral incisors
B. Permanent maxillary lateral incisors
C. Permanent mandibular premolars
D. Primary mandibular molars

430. Dens evaginatus is most often seen in:

A. Primary maxillary lateral incisors
B. Permanent maxillary lateral incisors
C. Permanent mandibular premolars
D. Primary mandibular molars

431. In the hypomineralized type of amelogenesis imperfecta, an unerupted tooth may look radiographically normal. In the hypoplastic type of amelogenesis imperfecta, an unerupted tooth looks radiographically abnormal.

A. The first statement is true, but the second is false.
B. The first statement is false, but the second is true.
C. Both statements are false.
D. Both statements are true.

432. Dentinal dysplasia type 1 has all of the following characteristics except:

A. Normal-size crowns with normal enamel and dentin
B. Very short, blunted molar roots and short, tapered premolar and incisor roots
C. Thistle-tube pulp chambers and root canals
D. Susceptibility to early loosening, exfoliation, and idiopathic periapical radiolucencies

433. What is attrition?

A. The pathologic wearing away of tooth structure by a mechanical process
B. The physiologic wearing away of tooth structure as a result of normal mastication
C. Loss of tooth substance by a chemical process
D. Loss of tooth substance caused by hyperocclusion

434. What is abrasion?

A. The pathologic wearing away of tooth structure by a mechanical process
B. The physiologic wearing away of tooth structure as a result of normal mastication
C. Loss of tooth substance by a chemical process
D. Loss of tooth substance caused by hyperocclusion

435. What is erosion?

A. The pathologic wearing away of tooth structure by a mechanical process
B. The physiologic wearing away of tooth structure as a result of normal mastication
C. Loss of tooth substance by a chemical process
D. Loss of tooth substance caused by hyperocclusion

436. The most common supernumerary tooth is:

A. Mesiodens
B. Mandibular premolars
C. 4th molars
D. Maxillary premolars

437. Which permanent tooth may demonstrate a wider follicular space than other teeth?

A. Maxillary central incisor
B. Maxillary 3rd molar
C. Mandibular 3rd molar
D. Maxillary canine

438. A variant of the dentigerous cyst (follicular cyst) characterized by a bluish, domelike bump on the gingiva over an erupting tooth is properly called a (an):

A. Primordial cyst
B. Traumatic cyst (simple bone cyst)
C. Eruption cyst
D. Mucous retention cyst

424. What error occurred in taking this radiograph?

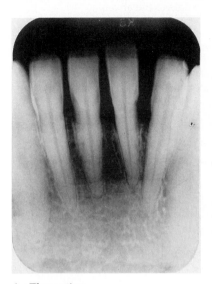

A. Elongation
B. Lips open
C. Film on top of tongue
D. Using a #2 film in this area

425. This 18-year-old has a problem. Can you recognize what it is?

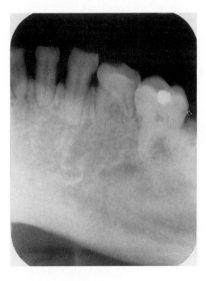

A. Microdontia
B. Hypopituitarism
C. Hypohydrotic ectodermal dysplasia
D. Agenesis of the permanent dentition

422. Note the tongue is not against the palate, the slumped position and the bilateral medial sigmoid depressions in the upper ramus. The *arrow* points to the area of interest. What is this?

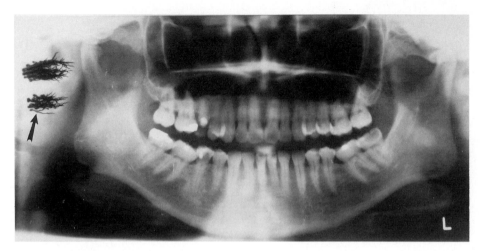

A. Static electricity
B. Developer stain
C. Light leak
D. Scratched emulsion

423. What was left on?

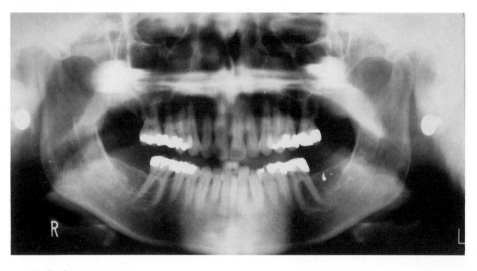

A. Neck chain
B. Bilateral hearing aids
C. Bilateral earrings
D. B and C

420. This 12-year-old boy has very large pulps and a systemic disorder. Select the best choice.

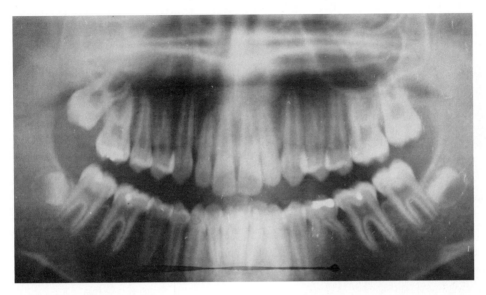

A. Papillon-Lefevre syndrome
B. Renal osteodystrophy
C. Vitamin D–resistant rickets
D. Dentin dysplasia type 2
E. Wilson's disease

421. This is an 8-year-old girl with delayed eruption of the permanent teeth. She has other skeletal defects. What is your assessment of this case?

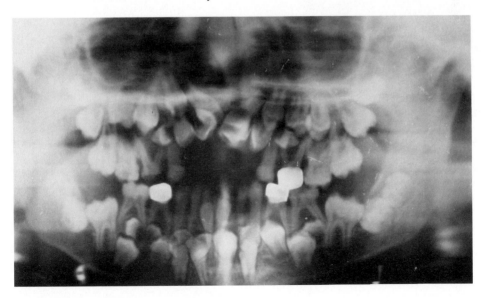

A. Cherubism
B. Cleidocranial dysplasia
C. Gardner's syndrome
D. Hypopituitarism

418. This is the "now you see it and now you don't" question. Notice the small round radiopacity in the furcal area of the molar in the periapical view (A). Now look at the bitewing (B) taken the same day. What is this?

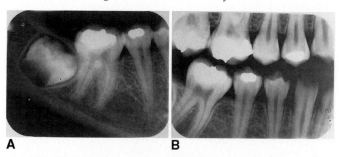

A   **B**

A. A bitewing from another patient with similar restorations
B. A small drop of fixer in the periapical view (A)
C. The "faux enamel pearl" artifact
D. The bitewing (B) is the postoperative radiograph

419. Okay, here it is. What is the source of this patient's pain on chewing?

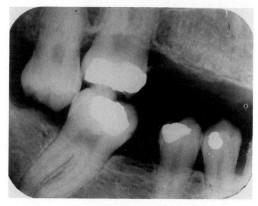

A. Calculus associated periodontitis
B. Caries
C. Extrusion (supraeruption)
D. A problem not visible in this radiograph

450. A developing tooth that undergoes cystic induction before calcification results in a (an):

A. Dentigerous (follicular) cyst
B. Odontogenic keratocyst
C. Residual cyst
D. Primordial cyst
E. B and/or D

451. The lateral periodontal cyst tends to occur in the:

A. Maxillary anterior area
B. Maxillary 3rd molar area
C. Mandibular premolar area
D. Mandibular molar area

452. The most common developmental cyst is the:

A. Incisive canal (nasopalatine duct) cyst
B. Nasolabial cyst
C. Globulomaxillary cyst
D. Median mandibular cyst
E. Primordial cyst

453. The simple bone cyst contains:

A. A low, cuboidal, thin squamous epithelial lining
B. Odontogenic epithelial lining
C. Transitional epithelial lining
D. No epithelial lining
E. None of the above

454. The simple bone cyst usually affects the roots of teeth by:

A. Causing resorption with the apices straddling the lesion
B. Causing resorption with the apices protruding into the lesion
C. Causing root divergence
D. Forming a scalloped margin extending up between the roots

455. The simple bone cyst:

A. May have a "cone" shape at its margin
B. May have a very linear margin
C. Has a wider dimension than the height
D. May be seen with subtle signs of trauma
E. All of the above

456. Which of the following conditions is considered pathognomonic?

A. Ameloblastoma
B. Cherubism
C. Odontogenic keratocyst
D. Dentigerous cyst
E. All of the above

457. Socket sclerosis is a unique form of osteosclerosis:

A. Seen in patients with current or past debilitating intestinal or kidney disease
B. Where there is a lack of resorption of the lamina dura after tooth extraction
C. That occupies only the socket area of a previously extracted tooth
D. That is permanent once it develops
E. All of the above

458. Stones and abdominal groans are associated with:

A. Hypophosphatasia
B. Hypoparathyroidism
C. Hyperparathyroidism
D. Fibrous dysplasia
E. Myotonic dystrophy

459. The cyst that may be associated with a luminal radiopacity is:

A. The residual cyst
B. The calcifying odontogenic cyst (Gorlin cyst)
C. A cystic odontoma
D. B and C only
E. All of the above

460. The radiologically evident "capsular space" is sometimes associated with:

A. The adenomatoid odontogenic tumor
B. Palatal pleomorphic adenoma with calcification
C. Ameloblastoma
D. The wall of the simple bone cyst

461. The lesion said to be attached to the root and obliterates and/or resorbs the root (s) is the:

A. Benign osteoblastoma
B. Benign cementoblastoma
C. Osteoid osteoma
D. Aggressive ossifying fibroma

462. Myospherulosis :

A. Is a developmental anomaly of marrow cells
B. Is associated with the use of petrolatum jelly
C. Associated with the bone marrow effects of sickle cell anemia
D. Is a type of fungal infection of bone most common in South America

463. Neuralgia-inducing cavitational osteopathosis (NICO) is a painful condition that may be associated with:

A. A localized area of osteoporotic bone with vertically oriented lamina dura residues
B. An area demonstrating radiolucent and radiopaque components
C. A "bull's eye" lesion with a radiopaque center surrounded by a radiolucent ring and a radiopaque margin
D. A "hot spot" with a technetium scan
E. All of the above

464. The clinical impression of amalgam tattoo can be confirmed by:

A. A lack of blanching on diascopy
B. Noting a radiopaque metal fragment radiographically
C. Biopsy
D. B and C above
E. All of the above

465. Taurodontism may be associated with:

A. Amelogenesis imperfecta
B. Down's syndrome
C. Klinefelter's syndrome
D. Osteoporosis
E. All of the above

466. In ankylosis there is:

A. A lack of a defined periodontal membrane space
B. No lamina dura
C. Regional sclerotic change resembling osteosclerosis
D. A dull ringing sound in the ears
E. Almost always external resorption

467. The term *antral pseudocyst* has now replaced the former appellation (*mucous retention cyst*) primarily because:

A. Pathologists like to change the names of diseases from time to time
B. The lesion contains a serous, not a mucous, fluid beneath elevated sinus mucosa
C. There is no epithelial lining
D. Most lesions consist of solid soft tissue polyps

468. The lesion that is named after the "blown out" appearance of the bone is:

A. A blow out fracture
B. Reactive proliferative periostitis (Garrè's osteomyelitis)
C. Ameloblastoma
D. Aneurismal bone cyst

469. Which of the following cystic lesions is often multilocular radiologically and also multinodular grossly?

A. Odontogenic keratocyst
B. Botryoid odontogenic cyst
C. Primordial cyst
D. A and C
E. None of the above

470. Cervical enamel extensions are associated with:

A. The buccal bifurcation cyst
B. Mainly primary molars
C. Enamel pearls
D. Amelogenesis imperfecta

471. Radiologically, a tooth in hyperocclusion may demonstrate:

A. Hypercementosis
B. Abfraction
C. Widened periodontal membrane space
D. Widened lamina dura
E. All of the above

472. In Eagle's syndrome, the patient often has had a previous tonsillectomy and current pain on swallowing. Radiographically, we see:

A. Nonspecific calcification in the carotid region
B. Calcification in the tonsillar fossa
C. Elongation of the styloid process
D. Elongation of the styloid process and/or mineralization of the stylohyoid ligament complex
E. All of the above

473. Histologically, which radiologic lesion has tissue very similar to brown tumor:

A. Central giant cell granuloma
B. Periapical granuloma
C. Cherubism
D. Aneurismal bone cyst
E. A and C

474. The lesion characterized as having a "tennis racket" or geometric pattern of bone destruction is:

A. Multiple myeloma
B. Fibrous dysplasia affecting the cranial vault
C. Paget's disease affecting the cranial vault
D. Odontogenic myxoma

475. In the nevoid basal cell carcinoma
syndrome, the odontogenic keratocysts
(OKCs):

A. Recur with greater frequency than other OKCs
B. Are greater in numbers but recur less
frequently than other OKCs
C. Are similar in number and behavior to other
OKCs
D. Are different in that the keratin is
orthokeratinized
E. Are greater in number but similar in behavior
to other OKCs

Answer Key

Chapter **1** Answers

FIGURE 1-1

1. anterior nasal spine
2. interseptal bone
3. crestal alveolar bone
4. inferior turbinate (concha)
5. cartilaginous nasal septum
6. inferior process of ethmoid bone
7. nasal fossa
8. infraorbital foramen
9. zygomatic process of maxilla
10. mental ridge
11. mental foramen
12. external oblique ridge
13. retromolar trigone
14. zygomatico-maxillary suture
15. zygomatic bone
16. zygomatico-temporal suture
17. zygomatic process of temporal bone
18. nasal bone
19. zygomatico-frontal suture

FIGURE 1-2

1. mental ridge
2. mandibular symphysis
3. mental foramen
4. mandibular body
5. external oblique ridge
6. angle of mandible
7. retromolar trigone
8. ramus
9. neck of condyle
10. head of condyle
11. sigmoid notch
12. coronoid process
13. medial sigmoid depression
14. mandibular foramen
15. lingula

FIGURE 1-3

1. coronoid process
2. sigmoid notch
3. head of condyle
4. medial sigmoid depression
5. mandibular foramen
6. angle of mandible
7. inferior cortex of mandible
8. digastric fossa
9. submandibular (salivary gland) fossa
10. mylohyoid (internal oblique) ridge
11. inferior genial tubercle of geniohyoid muscle
12. superior genial tubercle of genioglossus muscle
13. accessory lingual foramen for lingual vessels (lingual foramen)

FIGURE 1-4

1. accessory foramen
2. superior genial tubercle
3. accessory lingual foramen for lingual vessels (lingual foramen)
4. inferior genial tubercle
5. digastric fossa (digastric muscle attachment)

FIGURE 1-5

1. hard palate
2. infundibulum
3. ostium of nasolacrimal canal
4. inferior turbinate
5. middle turbinate
6. nasal bone
7. nasolacrimal canal
8. frontal sinus
9. sphenoid sinus
10. pituitary fossa
11. medial pterygoid plate
12. lateral pterygoid plate
13. hamular process of medial pterygoid plate (hamulus)
14. maxillary tuberosity
15. incisive foramen
16. median maxillary suture
17. palatal process of maxilla
18. palato-maxillary suture
19. shadow of nasolacrimal duct
20. palatine bone
21. greater palatine foramen
22. lesser palatine foramen
23. posterior nares
24. foramen of Stenson
25. incisive canal
26. foramen of Scarpa

FIGURE 1-6

1. interdental groove
2. maxilla
3. vertical process of maxilla
4. floor of nasal fossa
5. vomer bone
6. palato-maxillary suture
7. palatal bone
8. posterior nasal spine
9. sinus recess
10. maxillary sinus (antrum of Highmore)
11. bony septum of maxillary sinus
12. anterior nasal spine

FIGURE 1-7

1. common carotid artery
2. external carotid artery
3. internal carotid artery
4. facial artery

5. inferior alveolar artery
6. internal maxillary artery
7. posterior superior alveolar arteries
8. infraorbital artery
9. labial artery
10. incisive artery

FIGURE 1-8

PART A

1. mylohyoid (internal oblique) ridge
2. submandibular fossa
3. mandibular foramen
4. lingula
5. angle of mandible
6. inferior cortex of mandible

PART B

1. external oblique ridge
2. retromolar trigone
3. mental foramen

FIGURE 1-9

1. accessory foramina
2. genial tubercles (in this example there is only one tubercle on each side)
3. accessory lingual foramen
4. digastric fossa
5. fenestration (loss of bone covering the root without marginal bone involvement)

FIGURE 1-10

1. anterior nasal spine
2. fenestration (with involvement of marginal bone the condition is dehiscence)
3. zygomatico-maxillary suture
4. zygomatic process of temporal bone
5. maxillary tuberosity
6. hamular process of medial pterygoid plate
7. lateral pterygoid plate

FIGURE 1-11

PART A

1. anterior nares (openings) of nasal fossa
2. nasal septum
3. anterior nasal spine

PART B

1. opening to incisive canal
2. incisive foramen
3. median palatal suture
4. accessory foramen (there are many in the area)

FIGURE 1-12

PART A

1. median maxillary suture
2. incisive foramen

PART B

1. median maxillary suture
2. view into the incisive canal
3. foramen of Stenson (usually lateral to foramen of Scarpa)
4. foramen of Scarpa (usually close to the midline)

FIGURE 1-13

1. incisive foramen
2. median maxillary suture
3. palato-maxillary suture
4. greater palatine foramen
5. lesser palatine foramen
6. posterior border of hard palate
7. hamular process
8. zygomatic process of maxilla
9. zygomatic process of temporal bone
10. palatal process of maxilla
11. palatal bone

The following answers for Figures 1-14 through 1-59 are the same for parts *A* and *B*. Note that the diagram in part *A* does uniquely represent the radiograph in part *B*; however, some structural details not pertinent to those being illustrated may have been omitted. Also, some artistic freedom has been used to more clearly illustrate or define the structure to be identified.

FIGURE 1-14

1. accessory canals (from the inferior alveolar canal to the molar root apices containing the artery, vein, and nerve to the pulp)

FIGURE 1-15

1. inferior cortex of mandible
2. inferior alveolar canal
3. lamina dura (radiopaque thin white line)
4. periodontal membrane space (radiolucent thin black line)
5. coronal pulp space (pulp chamber)
6. interproximal contact point
7. dentin
8. enamel
9. interseptal alveolar bone (interradicular alveolar bone)
10. crestal plate (thin white radiopaque line)
11. root canal space (containing the dental pulp)
12. cementum (frequently not distinguishable from the subadjacent dentin unless hypercementosis is present)

FIGURE 1-16

1. soft tissue shadow of upper lip
2. cervical margin (line) of enamel
3. alveolar bone margin (dark band between 2 and 3 is the root)

4. median maxillary suture
5. soft tissue outline of nose
6. incisive foramen

FIGURE 1-17

1. incisive foramen
2. median maxillary suture
3. incisive canal
4. superior foramen of incisive canal (in floor of nose)
5. bony margin of nasal fossa
6. soft tissue of nasal septum
7. nasal septum
8. air space of the common meatus

FIGURE 1-18

1. soft tissue outline of nose
2. median maxillary suture
3. anterior nasal spine
4. bony margin of nasal fossa
5. foramen of Scarpa
6. superior foramen of incisive canal

FIGURE 1-19

1. foramen of Scarpa
2. foramen of Stenson
3. median maxillary suture

FIGURE 1-20

1. median maxillary suture
2. anterior nasal spine
3. bony margin of nasal fossa
4. common meatus (air space in nose) and part of inferior meatus beneath turbinate
5. soft tissue lining of septum
6. soft tissue of inferior turbinate (thin turbinate bones can be seen within)

FIGURE 1-21

1. orifice of nasolacrimal duct (at infundibulum of the inferior turbinate not seen)
2. bony margin of nasal fossa
3. permanent canine
4. permanent 1st premolar
5. permanent 2nd premolar
6. permanent central incisor
7. permanent lateral incisor
8. primary canine
9. primary 1st molar
10. primary 2nd molar

FIGURE 1-22

1. soft tissue outline of nose
2. lateral fossa
3. bony margin of nasal fossa
4. anterior wall of maxillary sinus (3 and 4 comprise the "inverted Y" landmark)

5. air space in maxillary sinus
6. air space (common meatus) in nasal fossa

FIGURE 1-23

1. soft tissue shadow of gingiva
2. crest of alveolar bone (alveolar crest)
3. soft tissue outline of ala of nose
4. "inverted Y"
5. air space in maxillary sinus
6. soft tissue of nasal fossa (darker thin band just above is inferior meatus)

FIGURE 1-24

1. soft tissue outline of nose
2. columella
3. external (soft tissue) naris
4. cartilaginous septum
5. anterior nasal spine
6. nasal air space; superiorly is common meatus (air space) and beneath inferior turbinate is inferior meatus
7. soft tissue of inferior turbinate

FIGURE 1-25

1. embossed dot on all films (should be at occlusal)
2. soft tissue outline of nasolabial fold
3. floor of maxillary sinus
4. bony septum in maxillary sinus
5. air space of maxillary sinus
6. metal part in bite-block

FIGURE 1-26

1. soft tissue shadow of nasolabial fold
2. soft tissue shadow of cheek (buccinator muscle and buccal mucosa)
3. mucosal (gingival) lining of edentulous alveolar ridge
4. bone margin of edentulous maxillary alveolar ridge
5. maxillary sinus

FIGURE 1-27

1. nasolabial fold
2. floor of maxillary sinus
3. posterior superior alveolar canal (in lateral wall of sinus)
4. sinus air space

FIGURE 1-28

1. bony margin of nasal fossa
2. anterior wall of maxillary sinus
3. "inverted Y" landmark
4. embossed dot on all films

FIGURE 1-29

1. metal and plastic parts of bite-block
2. diastema
3. soft tissue outline of nose
4. incisive foramen
5. anterior nasal spine
6. nasal fossa

FIGURE 1-30

1. mamelon
2. lingual pit
3. cervical enamel margin
4. crestal alveolar bone margin
5. anterior nasal spine
6. inferior meatus
7. soft tissue of inferior turbinate
8. soft tissue of bony septum
9. bony septum
10. common meatus

FIGURE 1-31

1. incisive foramen (this area is pear-shaped and darker in the radiograph)
2. soft tissue outline of nose
3. anterior nasal spine
4. soft tissue lining of nose
5. nasal air space (common meatus)
6. bony nasal septum
7. soft tissue (mucosal) lining of septum

FIGURE 1-32

1. mamelon
2. permanent central incisor
3. lingual pit
4. primary canine about to be exfoliated
5. primary 1st molar
6. soft tissue outline of nose
7. permanent lateral incisor
8. developing permanent canine
9. developing permanent 1st premolar
10. developing 2nd permanent premolar
11. anterior wall of maxillary sinus
12. bony wall of nasal fossa

FIGURE 1-33

1. 1st premolar (note the usual buccal and palatal roots)
2. vestigial lingual cusp on canine
3. air space of maxillary sinus
4. bony wall of maxillary sinus

FIGURE 1-34

1. lingual pits in shovel-shaped incisors with heavy marginal ridges
2. lateral fossa
3. nasal fossa
4. maxillary sinus

COMMENT: The bony wall of the nose is generally smoother, straighter, thicker, and slightly more radiopaque than the sinus wall, which is thin and irregular or wavy. The two lines criss-cross to form an "x" (rather than a "Y") in some cases.

FIGURE 1-35

1. zygomatic process of maxilla
2. hard palate/floor of nose
3. nasal mucosa
4. nasal cavity
5. maxillary sinus air space
6. sinus septum
7. floor of maxillary sinus
8. mucosa of alveolar ridge
9. alveolar bone of maxilla

COMMENT: Here we can see how the bony outlines of the nose and sinus criss-cross toward the anterior region. The thin dark lines superimposed on the canine are created by static electricity. There is caries on the distal of the canine and mesial of the premolar, which needs a post and a crown.

FIGURE 1-36

1. inferior meatus (above this line throughout its length is the soft tissue of the inferior turbinate in the nose)
2. posterior superior alveolar canal and branches in lateral wall of sinus (superimposed on the soft tissue of the turbinate)
3. nasal mucosa
4. floor of nose/hard palate
5. floor of maxillary sinus (which is at the alveolar crest because of pneumatization of the sinus whereby the sinus enlarges after adjacent teeth are extracted)
6. sinus air space
7. zygomatic process of maxilla

FIGURE 1-37

1. sinus recess
2. wall of nasal fossa
3. sinus septum
4. floor of maxillary sinus
5. crimp mark and poor image in the area caused by film bending

FIGURE 1-38

(Same patient as in Figure 1-36, B)

1. inferior meatus (above this is the soft tissue shadow of the inferior turbinate)
2. posterior superior alveolar canal and branches (in lateral wall of sinus)
3. nasal mucosa
4. hard palate/floor of nose
5. maxillary sinus air space

6. U-shaped zygomatic process of the maxilla
7. inferior border of zygomatic arch
8. lateral pterygoid plate margin
9. maxillary tuberosity

FIGURE 1-39

1. floor of maxillary sinus
2. sinus air space
3. thickened sinus mucosa (maxillary sinusitis)
4. zygomatic process of maxilla

FIGURE 1-40

1. sinus floor mucosa
2. floor of maxillary sinus
3. zygomatic process of maxilla
4. air space of maxillary sinus
5. bony septum in maxillary sinus
6. sinus mucosa on both sides of septum
7. oral mucosa of hard palate (below hard palate/floor of nose)
8. prominent soft tissue in nasal fossa

FIGURE 1-41

1. upper mandibular ramus
2. margin of maxillary tuberosity
3. enlarged (hyperplastic) coronoid process of mandible (causing notch in zygomatic arch)
4. inferior border of zygomatic arch
5. medial sigmoid depression
6. hamular process of medial pterygoid plate
7. lateral pterygoid plate

FIGURE 1-42

1. maxillary sinus air space
2. zygomatic arch
3. medial pterygoid plate (anterior part of lateral pterygoid plate is also superimposed here)
4. lateral pterygoid plate
5. hamular process of medial pterygoid plate
6. maxillary tuberosity
7. floor of maxillary sinus
8. coronoid process of mandible
9. embossed dot in film
10. *ks* marking indicating "D" speed film
11. bite-block

FIGURE 1-43

1. maxillary tuberosity
2. margin of alveolar bone (buccal and lingual crestal margins superimposed)
3. floor of maxillary sinus
4. interproximal alveolar bone margin (crestal margin)
5. bony septum in sinus
6. margin of zygomatic arch
7. thickened sinus mucosa

8. U-shaped zygomatic process of maxilla
9. zygomatic arch

FIGURE 1-44

1. floor of maxillary sinus
2. hard palate/floor of nose
3. zygomatic process of maxilla
4. follicular space inside bony crypt of developing 3rd molar
5. hamular process of medial pterygoid plate
6. lateral pterygoid plate
7. coronoid process of mandible
8. oral mucosal soft tissue shadow

FIGURE 1-45

1. zygomatic process of maxilla
2. hard palate/floor of nose
3. sinus recess
4. sinus septum and soft tissue mucosa on both sides
5. anterior wall of maxillary sinus (continuous with sinus floor)

FIGURE 1-46

1. lingual foramen
2. genial tubercles (in this view, individual genial tubercles are not usually seen; combined with the lingual foramen, you have the appearance of a donut)
3. unusual accessory foramen with unusual cortication (there appears to be an accessory canal within the bone between this and the lingual foramen)
4. accessory foramens (foramina) of nutrient canals

FIGURE 1-47

1. mental foramen (does not usually have a corticated margin)
2. inferior cortex of mandible

FIGURE 1-48

1. relative radiolucency frequently seen in this area; possibly caused by thin cortical bone and/or large digastric fossa
2. inferior cortex of mandible
3. margin of inferior cortex

FIGURE 1-49

1. mamelons
2. dental papilla of developing teeth
3. genial tubercles
4. lingual foramen (note that there appears to be a corticated accessory foramen below this area)
5. inferior cortex

6. crimp mark caused by # 2 film bending (for this reason # 1 film is often used in this location)

FIGURE 1-50

1. margin of inferior cortex
2. inferior cortex
3. canal space for accessory lingual artery and vein
4. corticated canal wall
5. genial tubercles
6. lingual foramen

FIGURE 1-51

1. inferior cortex
2. margin of inferior cortex
3. genial tubercles
4. lingual foramen
5. canal space for accessory lingual artery and vein with corticated canal walls
6. mental ridge
7. soft tissue shadow of lower lip

FIGURE 1-52

1. soft tissue shadow of lower lip
2. atypical genial tubercles
3. nutrient canals in cross section and/or accessory foramens of nutrient canals

FIGURE 1-53

1. mamelons
2. developing permanent canine

FIGURE 1-54

1. genial tubercles
2. lingual foramen
3. inferior cortex
4. permanent central incisor
5. permanent lateral incisor
6. primary canine
7. primary 1st molar
8. developing permanent canine
9. developing 1st premolar
10. developing 2nd premolar

FIGURE 1-55

1. margin of inferior cortex
2. inferior cortex
3. corticated wall of inferior alveolar canal
4. inferior alveolar canal (mandibular canal)
5. mylohyoid ridge (internal oblique ridge)
6. submandibular fossa

FIGURE 1-56

1. external oblique ridge
2. internal oblique ridge
3. inferior alveolar canal

4. submandibular fossa
5. retromolar trigone

FIGURE 1-57

1. inferior alveolar canal
2. bony crypt wall of a developing tooth
3. follicular space of a developing 3rd molar. This space should not measure more than 2.5 mm on intraoral films or 3 mm on panoramic films. If the size of the follicular space is wider than these measurements, it should be considered as pathologically enlarged—usually caused by cyst formation (follicular or dentigerous cyst) or tumor induction. The maxillary canine follicular space is often larger.
   COMMENT: Notice root formation has barely begun. Much of the root formation occurs after the tooth first erupts into the oral cavity. When root length exceeds crown length and the tooth has not yet begun to erupt into the mouth, eruption is delayed. The usual reasons for delayed eruption are impaction as a result of a lack of space or the presence of a cyst or tumor.
4. developing 3rd molar
5. papilla of developing tooth
6. bulbous root shape (more difficult to extract)
7. tapered root shape (easer to extract)

FIGURE 1-58

1. internal oblique ridge
2. submandibular fossa
3. inferior alveolar canal (mandibular canal)
4. mental foramen
5. anterior branches of inferior alveolar canal (incisive and possibly labial branches)

FIGURE 1-59

1. internal oblique ridge
2. mental foramen
3. submandibular fossa
4. inferior cortex
5. fixer stains (developer stains are radiolucent or dark marks)

FIGURE 1-60

1. Distal mandibular pseudohyperostosis.
2. In situation *A*, a tooth is missing anterior to the tooth in question. The molar has tipped to the mesial and formed a pseudopocket on the mesial pressure side and a pseudohyperostosis on the distal tension side. In situation *B*, a tooth is missing distal to the tooth in question with no missing anterior tooth. Here the original crestal height has been maintained just to the distal of the tooth.

Figure 1-61

1. The radiolucent area is a developing tooth bud with just a hint of the "circumflex" (^) or "accent circonflex en Francais" pattern of calcification of a mesial cusp tip.

Figure 1-62

1. The term is *pneumatization*. ("To pneumatize" means to fill with air... you can coin "pneumohead" if you want... it might just catch on!)

Figure 1-63

1. This is called a "step ladder" trabecular pattern (a variation of normal).
2. It is of no significance though it was once thought to be related to marrow changes associated with sickle cell anemia.

Figure 1-64

1. Part *A*: Loose trabecular pattern.
2. Part *B*: Dense trabecular pattern.
3. The trabecular pattern is a feature of the cortex. You can hollow out all of the spongy bone in the marrow space without seeing any change in the trabecular pattern in a subsequent radiograph.

Figure 1-65

1. Lingual midline: Two enlarged genial tubercles.
2. They are significant in that they may prevent the proper seating of an old (or even new) denture.

   COMMENT: An old denture will impinge on this as the ridge slowly resorbs and the denture becomes more and more hyperextended at the flange or margin.

Figure 1-66

1. *Arrow A*: External oblique ridge.
   Arrow B: Inferior border of cortex.
   Arrow C: Internal oblique ridge.

Figure 1-67

A: inferior meatus
B: common meatus
C: middle meatus
D: soft tissue of inferior turbinate
E: soft tissue of middle turbinate
F: nasal septum
G: floor of maxillary sinus
H: maxillary tuberosity
I: posterior wall of maxillary sinus
J: inferior border of zygomatic arch
K: zygomatic process of maxilla
L: anterior wall of maxillary sinus
M: inferior alveolar canal
N: medial sigmoid depression
O: pterygomaxillary fissure
P: lateral pterygoid plate

Figure 1-68

A: zygomatic process of temporal bone
B: zygomatic process of zygomatic bone
C: inferior orbital rim
D: infraorbital canal
E: real double image of hard palate
F: medial sigmoid depression
G: mandibular foramen
H: real double image of epiglottis (the other side is blurred)
I: right and left mental foramina
J: articular eminence of TMJ
K: glenoid fossa of TMJ (condylar fossa)
L: external auditory meatus
M: zygomatico-temporal suture poorly seen

Figure 1-69

A: common meatus of nose
B: soft tissue of inferior turbinate
C: nasal septum
D: panoramic innominate line; lower half is zygomatic process of maxilla, and upper half is lateral wall of orbit. This line is often mistaken for the posterior wall of the maxillary sinus. The lower portion is destroyed or altered when disease affects the lateral wall of the sinus.
E: anterior nasal spine
F: ghost image of left real image of hard palate (*G*)
G: real double image of hard palate. Note the mirror image can be seen below *F*.
H: diastema
I: body of the hyoid; the two greater horns can also be seen. This is a real double image; *K* is its mirror image.
J: mental foramen
K: body of hyoid. This is the real double image of *I*. One is the mirror image of the other. *K* looks a little different because the patient is twisted in the machine.
L: inferior edge of the ghost image of the contralateral (right) ramus (*G*), which obscures most of the left ramus and makes it markedly more radiopaque above this line; note the same ghost image on the other side. These specific ghosts are the result of placing the patient too far back in the machine.
M: right ramus
N: medial pterygoid plate (somewhat obscure)

FIGURE 1-70

A: coronoid process of mandible
B: sigmoid notch
C: head of condyle
D: posterior border of ramus
E: angle of mandible
F: inferior border of mandible
G: ramus
H: body of mandible (note the shadow of the hyoid superimposed on this area)
I: external oblique ridge
J: floor of maxillary sinus (antrum of Highmore)
K: real double image of left palate
L: ghost image of left palate

FIGURE 1-71

A: outline of base and dorsum of tongue
B: outline of posterosuperior aspect of soft palate; the letter *B* is on the soft palate image. Note the contralateral half-moon shape of the soft palate on the other side.
C: outline of posterior wall of pharynx (throat)
D: air space above tongue (palatoglossus air space) caused by a technique error whereby the patient did not place the tongue against the palate
E: sinus air space; letter indicates upper limit of sinus at the infraorbital margin
F: common meatus. Note the adjacent bony septum and soft tissue lining.
G: nasopharyngeal air space
H: oropharyngeal air space
I: hypopharyngeal air space
J: zygomaticotemporal suture
K: zygomatic process of zygomatic bone
L: zygomatic process of temporal bone

FIGURE 1-72

A: inferior meatus
B: middle meatus. Note the shadow of the double image of the inferior turbinate soft tissue on both sides and obscuring the upper half of the sinus. This is because the patient was positioned too far back in the machine.
C: common meatus
D: nasolabial fold
E: *white* and *black arrowheads*—external oblique ridge
F: *white* and *black arrowheads*—internal oblique ridge
G: air space–like circular radiolucency caused by a cotton roll between the upper lip (*upper arrowhead*) and lower lip (*lower arrowhead*)

H: tip of soft tissue of nose
I: ala of nose (other side can also be seen just above the *D*)
J (black): right and left earlobes because patient positioned too far back
J (white): panoramic innominate line

Chapter 2 Answers

FIGURE 2-1

1. There are several possibilities:
   - Amalgam
   - Gold foil (this was a gold foil)
   - Cast gold inlay
2. Old radiolucent tooth-colored restorative materials:
   - Silicophosphate cement
   - Acrylic
   - Composite resin

   COMMENT: When a tooth has been restored with a radiolucent material, it will have been done before about 1985. The distinguishing feature from caries is the sharp, smooth outline of the cavity preparation. Also, older cavity preparations are much larger than those of current practice.

FIGURE 2-2

1. Possible RPD materials:
   - Chrome cobalt (or other alloy)
   - Gold
2. Radiolucent acrylic
3. Radiopaque cement

FIGURE 2-3

1. Porcelain jacket crown
2. Radiopaque cement outlines the preparation

FIGURE 2-4

1. Lower 1st molar materials:
   - Gutta percha and screw-in post in distal canal
   - Silver points and root canal sealer cement in mesial canals
   - Amalgam in coronal portion

   COMMENT: To complete the restoration of this tooth, a full crown offers the best long-term prognosis.

1. Distal of lower 1st molar: cervical burnout.

   COMMENT: The difference between this and root caries is that cervical burnout disappears when another bitewing is taken at a different horizontal angle. Common locations are the distal of lower canines and the distal of upper molars.

FIGURE 2-5

1. Leaded-glass fragment embedded in the lower lip.
2. Other possibilities:
   - Scratched emulsion
   - Amalgam tattoo
   - Metal fragment such as shrapnel

FIGURE 2-6

1. The two metallic objects are:
   - Ivory #9 rubber dam clamp
   - Root canal file

FIGURE 2-7

1. The x-ray related materials are:
   - Cotton roll
   - Acrylic of bite-block
   - Metal of bite-block

FIGURE 2-8

1. Materials you can see:
   - All porcelain posterior denture teeth
   - Porcelain anterior teeth with metal retention studs
   - Wire mesh to reinforce and strengthen the denture
2. The denture acrylic is radiotransparent; therefore you cannot see it.

   COMMENT: Some prosthodontists hesitate to make a complete upper denture against the natural lower dentition because of the possibility of accelerated resorption of the residual ridge. When they do make one, they often prefer acrylic teeth to prevent wear on the lower teeth by the porcelain and to better absorb the stress from the occlusion. When the acrylic denture base keeps breaking, a thin cast metallic palate usually solves the problem.

FIGURE 2-9

1. The radiopaque object is a wrought wire clasp to retain an acrylic transitional removable partial denture. (In other words, a "flipper.")

FIGURE 2-10

1. The maxillary teeth are the porcelain teeth of a maxillary complete denture.

   COMMENT: It is often desirable to leave in complete and partial dentures with all-acrylic bases because the acrylic is invisible and the prosthesis makes it easier to take the radiographs.

FIGURE 2-11

1. The premolars: Radiopaque composite resin.
2. The molar: Amalgam.

   COMMENT: Note the difference in density between the two materials.

FIGURE 2-12

1. A space maintainer.

FIGURE 2-13

1. Materials you can see:
   - Fresh amalgam restoration on 1st molar
   - Amalgam fragments
   - Rubber dam clamp
2. Items you cannot see:
   - Rubber dam
   - The restoration (if acrylic) in the 2nd premolar
   - The exact nature of the restoration in the 2nd molar

FIGURE 2-14

1. Materials in upper 1st molar:
   - Gutta percha
   - 5 screw-in retentive pins

FIGURE 2-15

1. Lingual pits were routinely filled with amalgam. The radiolucent restorations are most likely on the buccal and consist of the older radiolucent composite material.

   COMMENT: The author has included a number of these older radiolucent restorations because they are still to be found in many patients and nowadays students are prone to interpret these as caries, fractured teeth, and defects like enamel hypoplasia.

FIGURE 2-16

1. Okay, you wanted newer radiopaque anterior composites... you got it!

FIGURE 2-17

1. This is a stainless steel wire habit-breaking appliance for tongue thrusting.

FIGURE 2-18

1. Treatment and materials in primary 2nd molars:
   - Maxillary:
     —Pulpotomy and pulpotomy cement
     —Stainless steel crown
   - Mandibular:
     —Occlusal amalgam

FIGURE 2-19

1. These are implant-related materials:
   - *A:* Implants have been placed within the maxillary alveolar bone such that they are covered by soft tissue. Healing caps are in place at the proximal or "business" end of the implant. Signs of osseous integration include a lack of significant radiolucent

area(s) in the vicinity of the implant and evidence of bone that has grown in between the threads on the implant.
- *B*: Healing caps have been exposed surgically and replaced with the appliance that is screwed into the implant. The appliances have been prepared to receive crowns. Temporary acrylic crowns are in place but cannot be seen; however, the radiopaque cement holding them in place can be seen.
- *C*: Porcelain bonded to gold crowns are in place. These are often screwed into the proximal end of the appliance so that at any time the crown, appliance, and even the implant can be removed by unscrewing the desired part.

COMMENT: Notice the slight V-shaped bony defect in the collar area of the implant at the crest of the ridge. This is normal for implants; however, the depth of the V-shaped notch should not exceed 2-3 mm and the bone in this area should not appear demineralized or more radiolucent than the remaining alveolar bone around the implant.

COMMENT: Smoking compromises the vasculature and oxygen supply to implant-related tissues and almost always results in implant failure.

Figure 2-20

1. Screw-retained stainless steel surgical plates.
2. This patient received trauma. The mandible is fractured in two places. The fracture segments remain slightly displaced on the left side. On the right side, the fracture line can be clearly seen. In the maxilla we see recent extraction sockets as several teeth were avulsed, several others were loose, and the remainder were carious, so all of the remaining maxillary teeth were removed with the patient's consent.

Figure 2-21

1. Comparison of materials:
- *A*: Each of the mandibular canines has a gutta percha endodontic root canal filling plus metallic posts with denture-retaining studs on the proximal ("business") end.
- *B*: Two implants are in place, each with an appliance and a denture-retaining bar.
2. Both patients wear mandibular overdentures against a complete maxillary denture.

Figure 2-22

1. Lower 1st molar restorations:
- *A*: This is a stainless steel crown. Notice that it is somewhat radiotransparent because you can see the outline of the tooth and

possibly a restoration under the crown. Also, note the marginal adaptation is pretty good but not perfect as is seen with stainless steel crowns.

COMMENT: Notice the large pulps, spaces between the premolars and textbook healthy crestal bone. All these indicate a young patient with newly erupted permanent teeth. At this age, stainless steel crowns are commonly used.
- *B*: This is a cast gold inlay. Here the margins are more conservative and there is less tooth coverage than a full gold crown. Here the margins are pretty good but slightly open at the mesial. This area will need to be watched for redecay.

COMMENT: Notice the missing lower 2nd molar and the extruding maxillary 2nd molar. An undesirable collapse of the occlusion has begun. Compare the maxillary premolars with patient *A*. Note the smaller pulp chambers in patient *B*, who is in his early 30s.
2. Patient *B* has the amalgam tattoo. Note the amalgam fragments between the lower premolars. This is how you confirm the pigmented lesion in the mouth is a harmless amalgam tattoo versus a pigmented nevus that should be removed and sent for histopathologic examination.

Figure 2-23

1. Prosthesis comparison:
- *A*: Fixed prosthesis (bridge) with porcelain bonded to metal.
- *B*: Class VI removable partial denture (butterfly) made from cast chrome cobalt or similar material with an invisible acrylic tooth.

COMMENT: In our dental school we will not treatment plan a butterfly partial because patients are known to have aspirated these. This can be life threatening, and, because of the clasps, they can be difficult to dislodge, even with the Heimlich maneuver.

Figure 2-24

1. Left upper central incisor materials:
   A: Gutta percha in the apical ⅓ of the root canal, a puff pf root canal cement beyond the apex, prefabricated screw-in post with cement or remaining gutta percha in the rest of the root canal, porcelain bonded to metal crown.
   B: Gutta percha at the apical end of the root canal, the apex has been sealed via surgical access with amalgam, a cast gold post in the remainder of the root canal, porcelain bonded to metal crown.

FIGURE 2-25

1. Both patients have a bonded lingual wire retainer.
2. Comparison of the two patients:
   - *A*: The composite resin bonding material is an older radiopaque variety; thus it is less well seen; the bonding material cannot be seen on the centrals and is poorly seen on the laterals.
   - *B*: Newer, more radiopaque, bonding material that is well visualized on all of the teeth.

FIGURE 2-26

1. *Restorative materials and restorations:*
   - Anterior composite, radiopaque
   - Anterior composite, radiolucent
   - Amalgam
   Types of restorations:
   - Probably several cast onlays, especially in the right upper 2nd premolar and lower right 2nd premolar and molar
   - Full gold crown upper right molar
   - Lower left posterior full gold crowns retaining a fixed 3-unit bridge
2. We also see ligating wires in three locations. This patient has had bilateral mandibular fractures and a fractured left zygoma that was ligated to the left maxillary tuberosity to prevent medial collapse of the zygoma and interference with the passage of the coronoid process between the zygomatic arch and the skull when the mandible is opened and closed. This type of mandibular fracture is seen with a blow to the chin and possibly a second blow to the left side of the face.

FIGURE 2-27

1. If you said bilateral hearing aids, you are right-on!

FIGURE 2-28

1. Part *D* is a radiograph of the left buccal mucosa. Place the film between the cheek and the teeth and expose with about 65 KV and about 3 or 4 impulses to get the soft tissue and any poorly mineralized bodies in the cheek.
2. Mystery solution: If you said a BB in the cheek, you were right-on once again.

Chapter 3 Answers

FIGURE 3-1

1. thyroid collar
2. lead apron

3. round beam indicating device (BID) or round cone
4. focal spot location indicators
5. tube head
6. yoke
7. articulation of tube head with arm

FIGURE 3-2

1. This instrument is called a *ring alignment device* (also referred to as the *XCP positioning instrument*).
2. Taking bitewings.
3. The film is reversed. The bite-block and ring are correct.

FIGURE 3-3

1. The maxillary central incisors are being radiographed.
2. A rectangular BID or cone.
3. BID not parallel to rod with insufficient vertical angulation.
4. The teeth will be elongated.

FIGURE 3-4

1. *A* is the polysoft packet; *B*, the paper wrapper; *C*, the lead foil; and *D*, the film.
2. The film fits inside the paper wrapper; the lead foil is in back of the paper wrapper; these fit inside the polysoft envelope with the lead foil facing the back side of the packet.

FIGURE 3-5

1. The bite-block is not centered in the ring.

FIGURE 3-6

1. A bitewing is being taken.
2. The BID is not properly centered on the ring.
3. There will be a rectangular cone cut whereby some of the radiograph will not be exposed.

FIGURE 3-7

1. The power-on indicating light.
2. The x-ray light that comes on upon depressing the exposure switch and indicates radiation is being produced. An audible sound is heard when this light is on.
3. The timer shortest setting is $\frac{1}{60}$th of a second. There are 60 impulses in a second with AC-powered machines.

FIGURE 3-8

1. The setup is for the upper right and lower left posterior quadrants.
2. This is #2-size film.
3. The corner of the film is bent.
4. A black line will be seen in this area of the processed image.

5. If the bent edge is fed into the automatic processor first (as the leading edge), there is a possibility the film will be flipped out of the roller assembly into the bottom of the tank and not emerge from the processor upon completion of processing. If films absolutely must be bent, they should be unbent and the bent portion should be the trailing edge in the processor.

Figure 3-9

1. The lower right posterior quadrant.
2. The BID is not parallel to the indicator rod.
3. The lower posterior teeth will be foreshortened, and the inferior border of the mandible (cortex) may appear in the image.
4. This should be avoided when making vertical measurements such as in endodontics.
5. This should be done on purpose if more periapical coverage is desired.

Figure 3-10

1. Paralleling technique.
2. The setup is for the upper right and lower left quadrants.
3. The film is not centered on the bite-block, and someone has written the patient's name on the front of the film packet (with a ball-point pen).
4. The film will be placed more anterior than desired; the patient's name will appear in the image as radiopaque writing.

Figure 3-11

The Off button: This only turns the machine *off*.
The 10-mA button: This turns the machine *on* when depressed and is backlit when the machine is *on*; it sets the mA at 10 milliamperes.
The 15-mA button: This turns the machine *on* when depressed and is backlit when the machine is *on*; it sets the mA at 15 milliamperes. The 15-mA setting allows for shorter exposure times than the 10-mA setting; this is especially useful when using the long BID, which requires 4 times longer exposure times than the short BID if all other factors remain constant.

Figure 3-12

1. The rectangular BID is not parallel to the rod; excessive positive vertical angulation is being used.
2. The maxillary central incisors will be foreshortened.

Figure 3-13

1. *A*: #4; *B*: #2; *C*: #1.
2. #4 is used primarily for occlusal views; #2 is used for bitewings and posterior periapical views as well as anterior periapical views in

some institutions and practices; #1 is used for anterior periapical views.

Figure 3-14

1. The patient's glasses have been left on.
2. There is no protective apron.

Figure 3-15

1. This setup is for imaging the maxillary and mandibular anterior teeth.
2. The film is placed backwards on the bite-block.
3. The image will be pale, and the lead foil pattern will be seen.
4. The film should be discarded because the dot will be reversed. Pathology may be interpreted on the wrong side of the patient. This view should be retaken.

Figure 3-16

1. A cone cut with a long round BID is about to occur.

Figure 3-17

1. The rectangular BID is not parallel to the rod; a mesioangular horizontal angulation is being used.
2. Overlapping of the interproximal areas; possible cone cut at the distal edge of the film; improper projection of the desired teeth on the film.

Figure 3-18

We are looking at the kVp meter, which can be adjusted with the kVp selector knob not seen here. Note, however, that the kVp varies with the two available mA settings. Thus the correct kVp scale must be used when adjusting the kVp according to the previously selected mA. If the wrong scale is used, the processed images will be too light or too dark. For example, if we set the machine at 70 kVp using the top 15-mA scale when the mA has been set on 10 mA, the radiograph will be too dark (on the 10-mA scale the machine is set at 80 kVp). If we set the machine at 80 kVp using the bottom 10-mA scale when the mA has been set to 15 mA, the image will be too light because on the 15-mA scale the machine is really set only on 70 kVp. Remember, too little kVp can produce light images and too much can produce dark images with respect to a given set of mA and exposure time settings.

Figure 3-19

1. The BID is not parallel to the rod; excessive positive vertical angulation is being used.
2. The maxillary premolars and 2nd molars will be foreshortened. The buccal roots of the maxillary 1st molar may be foreshortened and

the palatal root elongated; this is known as *dimensional distortion* and is most prone to occur with the bisecting-angle technique.

FIGURE 3-20

1. The lead foil backing.
2. To absorb remnant radiation after the film has been exposed; to indicate when the film has been placed in the mouth backwards.
3. *A:* fish scale pattern; *B:* tire track pattern; *C:* ping pong ball geometric pattern. The so-called *herringbone pattern* has been retired.

FIGURE 3-21

1. The rectangular BID is not parallel to the rod; excessive distoangular horizontal angulation is being used.
2. The interproximal surfaces will be overlapped; there may be a cone cut at the anterior edge of the film; the desired structures will not be properly projected on the radiograph.

FIGURE 3-22

1. The bite-block is incorrectly placed on the rod; it should be rotated 180 degrees.
2. The profile of the bitewing bite-block when placed correctly on the rod looks like the "tail of a jet plane."

FIGURE 3-23

PART 1

1. A long BID (cone) is specified; this is usually 16 inches unless otherwise specified.
2. The mA setting is 15 mA.
3. Yes, the settings will be okay.
4. The film speed is "F" or Insight film.
5. The kVp is 70.
6. The exposure time for the maxillary anterior periapicals is 18 impulses.

PART 2

1. The exposure time would be 6 impulses. (If you shorten the BID by ½, you can reduce the exposure time to ¼).
2. The molar exposure time would be about 30 impulses. (You can increase the exposure time by one increment for each 20-30 pounds.)
3. For the "D" speed film, the exposure time would be about 30 impulses. ("D" speed film requires about 50%-60% more exposure time than "F" speed film.)
4. For a 10-mA setting, the new exposure time would be 45 impulses. The mAs for the 15-mA setting is 15 mA × 30 impulses = 450 MAI. Therefore if we go to 10 mA, we will

need 45 impulses to equal 450 MAI. Yep! That's how you do it!

5. If you switched to 85 kVp for the molar periapical, you could reduce the timer setting to 15 impulses. The rule of 15 kVp says that if you increase the kVp by 15, you can reduce the exposure time by approximately half; if you decrease the kVp by 15, you must increase the exposure time by about half.
6. No modifications are needed. "F" speed film is the fastest available (2004).
7. The exposure chart specifies the values are the same for the two BID types.
8. The exposure time would be one increment less on the exposure chart; that is to say, 24 impulses.
9. 30 impulses is an exposure time of ½ or 0.5 seconds.
10. Three quarters of a second (¾ sec) is 45 impulses.

FIGURE 3-24

1. The dot is not in the slot at the base of the bite-block.
2. The dot can be superimposed on the apical region of the image and obscure important features.

FIGURE 3-25

1. The region is the maxillary premolar periapical area.
2. The exposure time would be 24 impulses.
3. Part *B* is an error.
4. The error is improper distoangular horizontal positioning of the BID. Note how the interproximals are overlapped and the contact areas are not properly seen in the photograph.

FIGURE 3-26

1. It is a film mount for a full mouth survey.
2. It is a film mount for two #2 films.
3. This full mouth survey includes 4 bitewings using #2 film; 8 posterior periapicals using #2 film; and 8 anterior periapicals using #1 film. The complete survey consists of a 20-film survey. There are many other acceptable full mouth survey configurations using, for example, only #2 film.

Chapter 4 Answers (with Tables 4-1 to 4-3)

FIGURE 4-1

1. Bob's first and last names are written on the front of the plastic film packet before exposure. The ball-point pen ink acted as a radiation barrier to produce the unwanted

TABLE **4-1**   Intraoral Projection or Technique Errors

ERROR	CAUSE	CORRECTION
1. Apices of teeth "cut off"	Film placed too close to teeth in maxillary arch in paralleling technique	Move film away from the teeth
	Too low a vertical angulation, which causes elongation	Increase vertical angulation
2. Overlapping of contact points	Plane of film not parallel to lingual surface of teeth	Place film parallel to lingual of teeth and direct the central ray of the x-ray beam perpendicular to facial surfaces of the teeth and film
	Incorrect horizontal angulation of cone	
3. All of specific region not showing	Faulty film placement	Center the film over teeth to be radiographed
4. Crowns of teeth not showing	Not enough film extending below or above the crowns of the teeth	Increase amount of film extending below and above the crowns of the teeth
5. "Cone cut"	Vertical angulation of cone too high	Decrease vertical angulation
	Beam of radiation not covering area of interest	Make sure cone covers film
6. Shape distortion		
a. Foreshortening	Paralleling technique: Film not parallel with long axes of teeth	Place film parallel to long axes of teeth
	Paralleling technique: Long cone not positioned correctly	Position long cone so central ray strikes film at right angle
b. Elongation	Paralleling technique: Film not positioned parallel to long axes of teeth	Place film parallel to long axes of teeth
	Paralleling technique: Long cone not positioned correctly	Position long cone so central ray strikes film at right angle
c. Dimensional distortion	Inherent error in bisecting-angle technique produces elongation of palatal roots and foreshortening of buccal roots of molars in same view	Use long cone paralleling technique; this method minimizes dimensional distortion
d. Image distortion	Film is bent as patient bites on film holder or bite-block or holds film in mouth	Use more care and less force to retain film; use rigid film backing
e. Fuzzing-out of roots	Seen in maxillary bicuspid region due to improper horizontal angulation of beam	Use correct horizontal angulation
	Film not parallel to teeth in anteroposterior direction	Use proper film placement
7. Magnification	Inadequate control of geometric factors	Use machine with small focal spot
	Usually seen with short cone and excessive object-film distance	Use as long a cone as possible Use as short an object-film distance as possible
8. Herringbone or tire track effect	Back side of film placed toward beam of radiation (film reversed)	Place plain front side of film toward radiation
9. Dark dot in apical region	Right-left identifying depression on film placed toward apical area of teeth	Place dot on film toward the occlusal or incisal surfaces of teeth

TABLE **4-3** Automatic Processor Troubleshooting Guide—cont'd

ERROR	CAUSE	CORRECTION
FILM DENSITY PROBLEMS—cont'd		
	d. Improper safelight	Use 7½ watt frosted bulb in safelight with GBX-2 filter, mounted no closer than 4 feet from working area
	e. Heat fog	Make sure film storage area is not excessively hot
	f. Excessively high developer temperature	Readjust developer thermostat and water to proper temperature
FILM DRYING PROBLEMS		
1. Films are not dry	a. Depleted fixer	Install new fixer solution
	b. Insufficient water flow (film not properly washed)	Check incoming water lines and valves NOTE: The incoming water flow must be a minimum of ½ gallon per minute and a maximum of 1 gallon per minute
	c. Dryer temperature setting too low	Increase dryer temperature
ABNORMAL FILM SURFACE MARKS		
1. Peeling of film emulsion	a. Developer temperature too high	Reduce developer temperature to proper level
	b. Improper fixer strength or depleted fixer solution	Replace fixer solution
	c. Heavy developer deposits on rollers	Be sure to follow recommended cleaning procedures as outlined by manufacturer
2. Pressure marks	a. Foreign material or rough spot on roller	Clean rollers and/or remove rough area on roller
3. Cloudy or smudged appearance of film surface (greenish or yellowish)	a. Depleted fixer	Replace fixer solution
4. White cloudy appearance over film surface	a. No water in wash tank	Check incoming controls and lines. Be sure drain plug in wash tank is inserted in drain outlet
5. Scratches on film surface	a. Foreign material on roller(s)	Clean rollers
	b. Improper handling of film before processing	Proper, gentle handling of film must be practiced
	c. Stalled or sticking roller	Inspect racks, gears, and gear mesh Correct as required
6. Drying pattern on film surface	a. Dryer too hot	Reduce dryer temperature
OTHER PROBLEMS		
1. Lost film in processor	a. Feeding films with bent edges into processor	Unbend films. Bent edge should be trailing edge
	b. Roller assembly defective	Inspect roller assembly
2. Films stuck together	a. Feeding films too rapidly into processor	Feed films more slowly into processor
	b. Failure to separate films in double packets	Identify double films and separate films

Modified from Langland OH, Sippy FH, Langlais RP: *Textbook of dental radiology*, ed 2, pp. 348-351, Springfield, Ill, 1984, Charles C Thomas, Publisher.

TABLE **4-2**   Intraoral Exposure and Manual Processing Errors—cont'd

ERROR	CAUSE	CORRECTION
10. Artifacts from processing		
a. Black crescents	Rough handling of film	Handle film by edges only
b. Fingerprints on film	Fingerprints or finger abrasions	Have fingers dry when handling film (processing and mounting)
Black	Contamination with stannous fluoride compounds	Wash hands before processing
Grey-black	Contamination with developer	Clean area to avoid contamination of hands
White	Contamination with fixer	Handle film by edges
c. Lightning streaks	Static electricity. Too rapid removal of film from packet in air with low humidity	Slow removal of film from packet; humidify darkroom

NOTE: With the infection control procedures in place as recommended by the American Dental Association, some of the above errors will no longer occur.

Modified from Langland OE, Sippy FH, Langlais RP: *Textbook of dental radiology*, ed 2, pp. 331-342, Springfield, Ill, 1984, Charles C Thomas, Publisher.

TABLE **4-3**   Automatic Processor Troubleshooting Guide

ERROR	CAUSE	CORRECTION
FILM DENSITY PROBLEMS		
1. Decrease of film density	a. Developer solution temperature low	Increase heat in the developer NOTE: Check the temperature of the developer solution with a thermometer of known accuracy
	b. Developer solution reaching exhaustion	Drain and thoroughly clean tank; replace developer solution
	c. Developer contamination—the most likely reason for contaminated developer is fixer solution splashed or dripped into the developer	Drain and thoroughly clean tank and rack assembly; replace developer solution
	d. No agitation in developer tank	Be sure the agitator paddle drive belt is in the proper position in the pulleys
2. Increase in film density (overall dark films)	a. Developer solution temperature too high	Water turned off. Check temperature of incoming water supply and adjust to 82°F. Check thermostat control for heating element in developer tank
3. Fogged film	a. Developer solution contaminated with fixer	Drain and thoroughly clean tank and rack: replace developer solution
	b. Processor light leaks	Be sure processor cover is secured firmly in place
	c. Light leaks in darkroom	Check darkroom for light leaks

Continued

TABLE **4-2** Intraoral Exposure and Manual Processing Errors—cont'd

ERROR	CAUSE	CORRECTION
	c. Diluted developer	
	1. Water added to raise level of developer	Add replenisher or replace developer solution
	2. Image too dark	
2. Image too dark	*Overexposure*	
	a. Exposure time too long	Reduce exposure time
	b. kVp too high for exposure time	Reduce kVp
	c. mA too high for exposure time	Reduce mA or exposure time (mAs is one factor)
	Overdevelopment	
	a. Developing time too long	Use time-temperature method with darkroom timer
	b. Developer temperature too high	Lower developer temperature to 70° F
3. High contrast	a. Insufficient penetration of tissues	Increase kilovoltage
4. Low contrast	a. Excessive penetration	Decrease kilovoltage
5. Fog	*Light*	
	a. Light leaks in darkroom	Check doors and walls for leaks
	Improper safelight	Reduce wattage of bulb
	Improper filter in safelight	Check type of filter and examine for cracks in filter. Use GBX2 filters for all films
	b. Prolonged exposure of films to safelight	Reduce exposure time of films to safelight
	Radiation	
	a. Insufficient protection of film from radiation	Store unexposed film in receptacles
	Chemical	
	a. Developer temperatures too high	Reduce temperature of developer to manufacturer's optimal temperature (70° F)
	b. Contaminated developer	Clean developer tank periodically
	Deterioration of film	
	a. Temperature of storage area too high	Store film in a cool place (70° F) or use refrigerator for storage of film
	b. Outdated film	Limit supply and use older films first
6. Streaks on film	a. Failure to agitate film during development	When first immersed in developer, agitate films
	b. Chemical deposits on hanger clips	Keep hanger clips clean
7. Air bubbles	a. Air bubbles trapped on film surfaces, preventing uniform development of emulsion	Agitate racks upon immersion into developer
8. White spots and lines on film	a. Emulsion tears from rough handling of films in processing tank	Do not rub films against sides of tanks or other film hangers
	b. Fixer artifact	Avoid splashing fixer on film before developing
9. Black spots on film	a. Film splashed with developer before being placed in developer tank	Careful handling of solutions and clean work area

TABLE **4-1**   Intraoral Projection or Technique Errors—cont'd

ERROR	CAUSE	CORRECTION
10. Artifacts on radiograph		
a. Writing in image	Writing on film packet with ball-point pen or lead pencil before exposure	Use a crayon-type pencil or plastic marker pen to mark on film packet
b. Dark lines on radiograph	Bending of film to enhance patient comfort	Avoid unnecessary bending of film
c. "Phalangioma" (patient's finger in image)	In holding film, patient's finger placed between film and teeth	Be sure that patient holds film on back side only or use bite-blocks
11. Double exposure	Film exposed twice to radiation	Place exposed film separate from unexposed film
12. Blank image	Failure to fully depress exposure button; failure to turn machine on	Fully depress exposure button, wait for machine to turn on and off before letting go: listen for audible exposure signal
13. Blurred image on radiograph	Movement of film, patient, or tube during exposure	Immobilize patient, film, and radiographic tube
14. Radiopaque objects on radiograph	Leaving prostheses in patient's mouth and/or glasses on patient during exposure	Remove prostheses and glasses from patient before exposure
	Zirconium prophylactic paste in gingival sulcus	Take radiograph before prophylaxis or at another visit: more thorough rinsing of prophylactic paste
15. Tongue image	Placing film on top of tongue	Place film beneath tongue
16. Cervical burnout	Not a true error. Caused by bell-shaped roots, allowing more radiation to penetrate and expose film	Alter horizontal angle; reduce kilovoltage: reduce mAs if possible

Note: The term "Cone" is synonymous with "BID"
Modified from Langland OE, Sippy FH, Langlais RP: *Textbook of dental radiology,* ed 2, pp. 322-330, Springfield, Ill, 1984, Charles C Thomas, Publisher.

TABLE **4-2**   Intraoral Exposure and Manual Processing Errors

ERROR	CAUSE	CORRECTION
1. Image too light	*Underexposure*	
	a. Too short exposure	Hold button for complete exposure. Set exposure time correctly
	b. Too low kVp	Increase kVp by approximately 5 kVp
	c. Too low mA	Increase mA or exposure time (mAs is one factor)
	Underdevelopment	
	a. Improper development	
	1. Time too short	Set darkroom timer correctly (check accuracy)
	2. Low developer temperature	Raise temperature to 70° F
	b. Exhausted and/or contaminated developer	Replace developer

Continued

TABLE **4-1**   Intraoral Projection or Technique Errors

ERROR	CAUSE	CORRECTION
1. Apices of teeth "cut off"	Film placed too close to teeth in maxillary arch in paralleling technique	Move film away from the teeth
	Too low a vertical angulation, which causes elongation	Increase vertical angulation
2. Overlapping of contact points	Plane of film not parallel to lingual surface of teeth	Place film parallel to lingual of teeth and direct the central
	Incorrect horizontal angulation of cone	ray of the x-ray beam perpendicular to facial surfaces of the teeth and film
3. All of specific region not showing	Faulty film placement	Center the film over teeth to be radiographed
4. Crowns of teeth not showing	Not enough film extending below or above the crowns of the teeth	Increase amount of film extending below and above the crowns of the teeth
5. "Cone cut"	Vertical angulation of cone too high	Decrease vertical angulation
	Beam of radiation not covering area of interest	Make sure cone covers film
6. Shape distortion		
a. Foreshortening	Paralleling technique: Film not parallel with long axes of teeth	Place film parallel to long axes of teeth
	Paralleling technique: Long cone not positioned correctly	Position long cone so central ray strikes film at right angle
b. Elongation	Paralleling technique: Film not positioned parallel to long axes of teeth	Place film parallel to long axes of teeth
	Paralleling technique: Long cone not positioned correctly	Position long cone so central ray strikes film at right angle
c. Dimensional distortion	Inherent error in bisecting-angle technique produces elongation of palatal roots and foreshortening of buccal roots of molars in same view	Use long cone paralleling technique; this method minimizes dimensional distortion
d. Image distortion	Film is bent as patient bites on film holder or bite-block or holds film in mouth	Use more care and less force to retain film; use rigid film backing
e. Fuzzing-out of roots	Seen in maxillary bicuspid region due to improper horizontal angulation of beam	Use correct horizontal angulation
	Film not parallel to teeth in anteroposterior direction	Use proper film placement
7. Magnification	Inadequate control of geometric factors	Use machine with small focal spot
	Usually seen with short cone and excessive object-film distance	Use as long a cone as possible Use as short an object-film distance as possible
8. Herringbone or tire track effect	Back side of film placed toward beam of radiation (film reversed)	Place plain front side of film toward radiation
9. Dark dot in apical region	Right-left identifying depression on film placed toward apical area of teeth	Place dot on film toward the occlusal or incisal surfaces of teeth

the palatal root elongated; this is known as *dimensional distortion* and is most prone to occur with the bisecting-angle technique.

FIGURE 3-20

1. The lead foil backing.
2. To absorb remnant radiation after the film has been exposed; to indicate when the film has been placed in the mouth backwards.
3. *A*: fish scale pattern; *B*: tire track pattern; *C*: ping pong ball geometric pattern. The so-called *herringbone pattern* has been retired.

FIGURE 3-21

1. The rectangular BID is not parallel to the rod; excessive distoangular horizontal angulation is being used.
2. The interproximal surfaces will be overlapped; there may be a cone cut at the anterior edge of the film; the desired structures will not be properly projected on the radiograph.

FIGURE 3-22

1. The bite-block is incorrectly placed on the rod; it should be rotated 180 degrees.
2. The profile of the bitewing bite-block when placed correctly on the rod looks like the "tail of a jet plane."

FIGURE 3-23

PART 1

1. A long BID (cone) is specified; this is usually 16 inches unless otherwise specified.
2. The mA setting is 15 mA.
3. Yes, the settings will be okay.
4. The film speed is "F" or Insight film.
5. The kVp is 70.
6. The exposure time for the maxillary anterior periapicals is 18 impulses.

PART 2

1. The exposure time would be 6 impulses. (If you shorten the BID by ½, you can reduce the exposure time to ¼).
2. The molar exposure time would be about 30 impulses. (You can increase the exposure time by one increment for each 20-30 pounds.)
3. For the "D" speed film, the exposure time would be about 30 impulses. ("D" speed film requires about 50%-60% more exposure time than "F" speed film.)
4. For a 10-mA setting, the new exposure time would be 45 impulses. The mAs for the 15-mA setting is 15 mA × 30 impulses = 450 MAI. Therefore if we go to 10 mA, we will

need 45 impulses to equal 450 MAI. Yep! That's how you do it!

5. If you switched to 85 kVp for the molar periapical, you could reduce the timer setting to 15 impulses. The rule of 15 kVp says that if you increase the kVp by 15, you can reduce the exposure time by approximately half; if you decrease the kVp by 15, you must increase the exposure time by about half.
6. No modifications are needed. "F" speed film is the fastest available (2004).
7. The exposure chart specifies the values are the same for the two BID types.
8. The exposure time would be one increment less on the exposure chart; that is to say, 24 impulses.
9. 30 impulses is an exposure time of ½ or 0.5 seconds.
10. Three quarters of a second (¾ sec) is 45 impulses.

FIGURE 3-24

1. The dot is not in the slot at the base of the bite-block.
2. The dot can be superimposed on the apical region of the image and obscure important features.

FIGURE 3-25

1. The region is the maxillary premolar periapical area.
2. The exposure time would be 24 impulses.
3. Part *B* is an error.
4. The error is improper distoangular horizontal positioning of the BID. Note how the interproximals are overlapped and the contact areas are not properly seen in the photograph.

FIGURE 3-26

1. It is a film mount for a full mouth survey.
2. It is a film mount for two #2 films.
3. This full mouth survey includes 4 bitewings using #2 film; 8 posterior periapicals using #2 film; and 8 anterior periapicals using #1 film. The complete survey consists of a 20-film survey. There are many other acceptable full mouth survey configurations using, for example, only #2 film.

Chapter 4 Answers (with Tables 4-1 to 4-3)

FIGURE 4-1

1. Bob's first and last names are written on the front of the plastic film packet before exposure. The ball-point pen ink acted as a radiation barrier to produce the unwanted

label. Students sometimes identify their films so as not to get their patient mixed up with someone else's.

Figure 4-2

1. This is the patient's finger. Some techniques call for using the patient's finger to retain the film.
2. Phalangioma.

Figure 4-3

1. BID (beam indicating device) cut or cone cut.

Figure 4-4

1. The two films were stuck together in the processor.
2. The answer is to not feed the films too quickly one after the other and to use alternating adjacent slots if available.

Figure 4-5

1. This indicates improper horizontal angulation of the beam in relation to these teeth. Note the interproximal overlap.
2. This error may be used to advantage when trying to separate the two roots of this tooth.

Figure 4-6

1. Normally the periapical radiograph should include at least 5 mm to 1 cm of the periapical tissues.
2. To increase the area of apical coverage:
   - Ensure the film is placed as apically as possible.
   - This film seems to be well placed. However, inadequate negative vertical angulation of the beam was used.

Figure 4-7

1. *A*: An unexposed film was processed. Usually this means another film from the same patient will be double-exposed.
2. *B*: An unwrapped, unexposed film was left on the darkroom countertop for 5 minutes and was fogged by an unsafe safelight. A 60-watt bulb was discovered in the safelight instead of the normal 7.5- to 15-watt bulb. If the film is left unprotected in the x-ray area, a similar appearance would be seen.
3. *C*: This film was exposed to light. The same appearance occurs if a film is exposed to a lot of radiation (60 impulses or 1 second).

Figure 4-8

1. The list of possible errors is:
   Patient movement
   Film movement
   X-ray tube-head movement

COMMENT: Here is how you can separate and identify the specific error:
a. Patient movement often results in "double or triple edges" to objects in the image.
b. Film movement because the patient released biting pressure on the bite-block, usually because of discomfort. Thus there would be increased distance between the teeth and the bite-block and the apical coverage would be diminished.
c. Tube-head movement effectively increases the focal spot size. This increases total magnification of the objects in the image with visible penumbra and unsharpness. Note the penumbra (shadow around the shadow or image) around the bottom part of the rubber dam clamp, the magnification, and the unsharpness (fuzziness) of this image. This error mimics the effect of an old, used-up, and pitted focal spot.

FINAL EXPLANATION: Tube-head movement. (This is prone to occur in older, unstable machines and when the student rushes the exposure because of patient discomfort.)

Figure 4-9

1. The appearance is "grainy," and normally this is supposedly caused by "clumping" of grains of silver if the developer is too warm and especially if exhausted.
2. In this case, the film that was found in the bottom of the processor still had the black wrapping paper on it. This caused it to flip out of the developer roller assembly. The recovered film was unwrapped and re-fed into the machine, and this is the result.

   You missed that?.....Anyone would have unless you had seen this before, and even then, would you admit it?

Figure 4-10

1. Radiolucent stain: developer.
2. Radiopaque stain fixer.

   Yes, they were asked in the order used in processing!

   COMMENT: To distinguish chemical stains, use the mnemonic "D-dark-developer." To learn the cause, remember that the fixer removes any unexposed or undeveloped silver grains. So if the film sits in a drop of fixer on the countertop (as happens all the time with "wet reading" manually processed films) before processing, parts of the image can be effaced. The same occurs with a drop of developer on the countertop, especially when the hand processing "quick developer" solutions are used for endodontics. This occurs to varying degrees as water droplets serve to dilute the

droplets of developer and fixer on the countertop. The problems are avoided with neatness and tidiness in the darkroom

FIGURE 4-11

1. Excessive curving of the anterior part of the film. This may be caused by:
   - Excessive finger pressure if the film is being held by the patient's finger
   - Excessive curving back of a bite-block retained film edge because of the curvature of the palate and the patient failing to complain about it (patients want to cooperate and sometimes do not report the discomfort that would signal an error)

FIGURE 4-12

1. The error was caused by excessive vertical angulation of the x-ray beam:
   - *A*: Excessive positive vertical beam angulation
   - *B*: Excessive negative vertical beam angulation
2. The features identifying this error:
   - *A*: Foreshortening of the roots, the molar has foreshortened buccal roots and an elongated palatal root, there is excess separation of the buccal and palatal cusp tips, several cusp tips of lower teeth can be seen
   - *B*: Foreshortening of the roots and excess separation of the buccal and lingual cusp tips
3. The advantage is increased apical coverage.

FIGURE 4-13

1. The chemicals are as follows:
   - *A*: Fixer (notice the developer stain as well)
   - *B*: Developer
   - *C*: Stannous fluoride

COMMENT: The use of stannous fluoride is being rediscovered for patients with severe erosions or demineralized enamel that would be exacerbated by currently popular acidic fluoride solutions. The stannous fluoride does taste awful. The tin in the stannous fluoride causes excessive development of unexposed silver in the emulsion, producing very black marks.

FIGURE 4-14

1. Elongation.
2. With the paralleling technique and the use of a BID positioning device, elongation results from inadequate positive vertical angulation resulting from the BID not being parallel to the positioning rod. In other situations, such as in endodontics, the bisecting-angle technique is

used. Remember that the ala-tragus line or the occlusal plane must be parallel to the floor and then the correct vertical angulation must be selected. Usually this is 45 degrees of positive vertical angulation; less will result in elongation.

FIGURE 4-15

1. Too light:
   - Insufficient exposure time
   - Insufficient milliamperage setting (if adjustable) for selected exposure time (mAs factor)
   - Insufficient kilovoltage (if adjustable)
   - Inadequate development (short time or cold temperature)
   - Weak or depleted developer solution
   - Expired or aged film
2. Too dark:
   - Excessive exposure time
   - High milliamperage setting (if adjustable) for selected exposure time (mAs factor)
   - High kilovoltage relative to selected exposure time
   - Light leak in darkroom

COMMENT: With an increase of 15 kVp, the exposure time can be reduced by 50% to maintain the same density (darkness). With a decrease of 15 kVp, the exposure time will need to be increased by 50% to maintain density. This works best between 60 and 75 kVp but is a good guide for any dental kVp setting.

If you maintain the same exposure time, you will need an increase or decrease of at least 5 kVp to be able to see a visible change in the density.

The most common cause of low-density (light) films is depleted developer solution in the automatic processor.

The most common cause of high-density (dark) films is too high an exposure time. kVp controls contrast, which is the shades of gray in the image: low kVp gives high contrast (few shades of gray); high kVp results in low contrast (many shades of gray).

Fixer solution lasts twice as long as developer solution and thus needs replenishment only every second time. Remember the "6 and 6" rule for developer replenishment: most automatic processors will need 6 oz of fresh developer after processing 6 full mouth surveys (about 120 intraoral films) or 6 panoramic radiographs. Also 6 oz of fixer for every second developer replenishment.

FIGURE 4-16

1. Double exposure.

COMMENT: Remember, it is with this error we usually find one unexposed film in the batch.

FIGURE 4-17

1. Errors:
   - Roller mark (horizontal black line)
   - Static electricity V-shaped black lines on lower molar mesial root
2. Error correction:
   - Roller mark: Clean rollers weekly; pass a blank film through the processor daily first thing after warm-up.
   - Static electricity: Humidify the darkroom with a humidifier or a large open container of water; do not pinch the packet or paper liner when removing the film for processing, and stand on an anti-static pad when processing.

FIGURE 4-18

1. Bitewing *A* was taken with a little too much positive vertical angulation, notice the lower cusp tips are not superimposed; the premolar-canine contacts are overlapped.
2. Bitewing *B* was taken with the incorrect horizontal angulation causing unacceptable overlapping of the interproximal surfaces of the teeth.
3. Both need retaking; in *A* we need to open up the canine-premolar contacts; in *B* we need to open all of the contacts.

FIGURE 4-19

1. Scratched emulsion from rough handling of the film, especially during processing when the emulsion is soft.

FIGURE 4-20

1. The film packet was reversed with the back or printed side of the packet toward the beam of radiation. Thus the embossed lead foil backing filters out some of the radiation and the embossed pattern is recorded on the film. These patterns change from time to time with any film speed.
2. All should be retaken. Remember, the dot will be reversed so this film could be erroneously mounted on the wrong side of the film mount. This can produce a "good news–bad news" situation such as: "we treated the tooth well but we extracted the left molar instead of the right one"!
3. The film speeds are different:
   - *A* is "D" speed or Ultra-speed film (KS embossed marking) about 50% faster than the old "radiatized" or "C" speed film.
   - *B* is "E" speed or Ektaspeed film (EKT embossed marking) about 40% faster than "D" speed film.
   - *C* is "F" speed or INSIGHT film (IN embossed marking) about 20% faster than "E" or "E+" speed film.

   COMMENT: "E" and "E+" films are the same speed. The "E+" uses a flat-shaped silver grain and has PLS embossed on the edge of the film.

FIGURE 4-21

1. The lower edge of the film was not placed parallel to the occlusal surfaces of the teeth. Actually, as often happens, the film was properly placed but was moved by the patient just before exposure.
2. The coronoid process of the mandible. You knew that!

FIGURE 4-22

1. Inadequate fixation. The film was not left in the fixer long enough after development, or the fixer solution needs replenishment.

   COMMENT: The fixer removes all unexposed silver from the image and is said to "clear" the image. Remember: "there's silver in them thar hills"! Only in the dental office it is in the fixer solution. Collection service companies will pay cash for fixer solution or supply a silver recovery unit.

FIGURE 4-23

1. Causes of film fog:
   - Use of outdated film
   - Film storage in a warm place
   - Exposure of film to scatter radiation
   - Light leaks in the darkroom
   - Unsafe safelight:
     —Bulb brighter than 15 watts
     —Distance to countertop less than 4 feet
     —Incorrect safelight filter (Kodak GBX and GBX2 filters are safe for all dental films)
     —Two or more safelights with above specs all okay but too close to each other; the areas of light crossover will be too bright

FIGURE 4-24

1. In example *A* the complete upper denture was left in; in example *B* a cast removable partial denture was not removed.
2. Example *A* is acceptable in some situations because the denture helps to retain and stabilize the bite-block holding the film. Denture acrylic is radiotransparent; that is, it cannot be readily seen in the radiographs; not all plastics are radiotransparent. Example *B* is

usually unacceptable because metallic parts may obscure structures or pathology.

FIGURE 4-25

1. The two errors in both examples *A* and *B*:
   - Foreshortening caused by excessive vertical angulation
   - Overlap of the canine-premolar contact, which should be open to best see the alveolar bone
2. These would not necessarily be retaken, depending on the purpose for which they were taken.

COMMENT: Nowadays, even in training situations, students are not asked to repeat certain imperfect films if the areas of interest can be seen on other films in the series or if the less-than-perfect image suits the purpose. For example, these would not be good to measure root canal length (the crestal alveolar bone and periodontal membrane space are not perfect but perhaps adequate in the absence of disease); the apical regions are well imaged if periapical pathology were being sought.

FIGURE 4-26

1. This is known as consistency. In both instances the film was placed on top of the tongue, wedging it between the film and the mandible.
2. Look at the bottom left corner of the photo. This occurs in automatic processors. Bent film usually produces a radiolucent line. Apparently when a slightly curved film edge is fed into the processor first, the curved edge can somehow become entangled in the roller assembly. The ragged edge is actually torn and has lost emulsion. In this situation the film does not always come out of the processor.

FIGURE 4-27

1. The patient was probably uncomfortable or insufficiently instructed and let go of the bite-block before the exposure was completed.

FIGURE 4-28

1. Two problems:
   - Static electricity and how!
   - "Fingernail" artifact, which is not from anyone's long fingernails but is from bending the film and causing it to crimp

COMMENT: Take a piece of paper. Place it between your thumb on one side and your index and middle fingers on the other side (your index finger is the one you point with and your middle finger is the one... well... you need to properly express yourself in some situations). As you bend

back the piece of paper, watch the crimp mark appear.

FIGURE 4-29

1. The patient's glasses were left on.
2. Glasses material:
   Example *A*: A metal frame and a plastic (radiotransparent) lens
   Example *B*: A metal frame and a glass (porcelain-like density) lens
3. Film sizes:
   Example *A*: Size #1
   Example *B*: Size #2

COMMENT: There are various techniques regarding film size in the full mouth survey. In some cases the anterior teeth are imaged with #1 film and the posteriors and bitewings with #2; others use only #2-size film for the whole survey.

FIGURE 4-30

1. Error: cervical burnout (adumbration).
2. It could be root caries but...note that the horizontal angulation of the beam is incorrect. This is a very common location for cervical burnout.
3. Yes, if the clinical examination cannot confirm the absence of caries or if the interseptal alveolar bone needs to be seen.

FIGURE 4-31

1. Similar film handling errors:
   Example *A*: Film crimping (crescent-shaped radiolucent line)
   Example *B*: Film bending (vertical black line)

FIGURE 4-32

1. Part of the image was exposed to light.

FIGURE 4-33

1. Increased apical coverage:
   - Instruct the patient to keep biting on the bite-block until the beeping sound (signaling x-rays being emitted) stops.
   - Place the film more apically by positioning it more toward the midline of the palate.
   - Increase the vertical angulation of the beam.
2. The dot is at the apex. Remember the "dot in the slot" rule. (The dot is darker than usual because it was inked in so you would not miss it.)

FIGURE 4-34

1. How to get 3rd molar apices:
   - Example *A*: Increase the vertical angulation 10-15 degrees in excess of what the BID positioning device indicates, using the normal technique.

- Example *B*: There are two techniques:
  —*Technique #1*, mesioangular projection: Line the BID up correctly, then turn the cone tip about 10-15 degrees mesially, and then move the tube head and BID distally as one so that you do not cone cut. This will project the coronal portion of the 3rd molar on the 2nd molar but the apical region will be seen.
  —*Technique #2*, distal extension of film: Instead of placing the film centered on the bite-block, move it distally from the centered position by about 1 or 2 cm. Place the film holder and BID indicating rod and ring as per usual. Align the beam as per usual, and then move the tube head and BID distally by the same amount you offset the film on the bite-block.

FIGURE 4-35
1. Cone cut.

FIGURE 4-36
1. Bent film.
2. Film not placed sufficiently apically.

FIGURE 4-37
1. Film too light as a result of factors causing insufficient radiation or depleted developer.

FIGURE 4-38
1. Excess positive vertical angulation. This results in superimposition of the malar process and zygoma on the edentulous alveolar ridge.

FIGURE 4-39
1. Patient movement.

FIGURE 4-40
1. Excess negative vertical angulation of the BID.
2. Notice the shadow of the floor of the mouth crossing the inferior cortex. This is a newly recognized error by Weidman and Warman. The floor of the mouth rises up and gets wedged between the film and the mandible. This is distinguished from the tongue shadow by the straight linear nature of this shadow versus the curved image of the tongue.

FIGURE 4-41
1. Insufficient apical coverage; probably because of pain the child stopped biting on the bite-block.
2. Some film packets are made of paper; these can become soaked through with saliva and

the black paper from the inner wrap sticks to the softened emulsion. With the polysoft film packets this problem does not occur.

FIGURE 4-42
1. Excess biting pressure. Note the black marks at the occlusal of the molar and incisal of the canine. This is a pediatric partial occlusal technique taken with #2 film. This technique offers ease of film retention and comfort for the child.

Chapter 5 Answers

FIGURE 5-1
1. The wired type, which is commonly available in CCD or CMOS subtypes; many brands are available.
2. These are the wireless PSP type; #2 is the Gendex DenOptix; #3, the Sorodex Digora brands.
3. The light side must be positioned to face the radiation.
4. The sensors correspond to film size #2.
5. The PSPs have an image size essentially identical to the film size. The wired type has an active area that is only about 65%-80% as big as the corresponding film size.
6. The wired CCD subtype is the most delicate. Neither the CCD nor the CMOS can be soaked or heated for disinfection.
7. The CCD subtype is the most expensive at about $5000-$7000 each. CMOS sensors are about 20% less. The intraoral PSPs are about $20 each; however, if a 20-image full mouth survey is planned, 20 PSPs will be needed.
8. The image is almost instantaneous with the CCD and CMOS types. PSPs must first be scanned; scanning time is about the same as film processing with the exception of the Air Techniques system, which is significantly faster.
9. Clinically, the PSPs are the most like film to use.
10. The PSPs have the widest latitude regarding exposure time and are thus the most forgiving.
11. The CCD and CMOS sensors have the best resolution over PSPs.
12. PSPs require a laser scanner, currently priced at about $15,000-$18,000.
13. PSPs must be erased before use, and excess exposure to light after exposure but before processing can cause the image to fade.

Figure 5-2

1. There are 8 gray levels in a 3-bit image.
2. A 6-bit image has 64 gray levels.
3. 256 gray levels is an 8-bit image.
4. 13 bits is 8196 shades of gray.
5. The 11-bit image needs the most storage space.
6. The ordinary person is said to be able to separate about 4 bits or 16 shades of gray.
7. Most monitors display 8 bits or 256 shades of gray.
8. The table displays gray scale resolution values in shades of gray and the corresponding bits in the image.

Figure 5-3

1. Image *B* looks best to the author.
2. The maximum lp/mm is 12.
3. Spatial resolution expressed in lp/mm.
4. Image *A* is 6 lp/mm.
5. Image *B* is 10 lp/mm.
6. Image *B* looks best because we see more sharpness and detail, which increases as you go higher on the resolution scale. Therefore image *B* looks better because the resolution is 10 lp/mm, whereas image *A* is only 6 lp/mm.
7. The unaided human eye with 20/20 vision is said to be able to resolve 14 lp/mm.
8. Most high-definition monitors are limited to 8 lp/mm.
9. This device is called a *focal spot checker*. Over time, the focal spot (anode) gets pitted from being constantly bombarded by high-speed electrons from the cathode or filament. The pits increase the surface area of the focal spot, causing it to produce degraded images. Remember, the smaller the focal spot, the better.
10. Machine *A* has a worn-out focal spot. The tube head needs to be rebuilt or the machine replaced. Some clinics place the lowest acceptable lp/mm at a value of 9 or 10 before replacement. In this case, machine *A* has a pitted focal spot, which makes it bigger. The bigger the focal spot, the more is the penumbra, which makes the image look fuzzy. The penumbra (extra shadow outlining the image) increases with focal spot size. The excess penumbra makes the lines run together exactly in proportion to the relative size of the focal spot. Therefore even in digital imaging, the focal spot will need to be checked from time to time.

Figure 5-4

1. In constant potential DC-type machines, the kilovoltage peak (kVp) powers up and stays at the preset kVp for the entire exposure. In ordinary x-ray machines, the AC current is such that x-rays are produced in impulses at the rate of 60 per second in increments of 1/60 second and the time between each impulse when no x-rays are being produced is also 1/60 seconds. In this case, as the kVp powers up to the peak low energy, long wavelength photons as well as longer wavelength photons are all in the beam of radiation, which is referred to as *heterogeneous*. This means some of the longer wavelength, nonpenetrating photons will expose the patient to radiation that is not penetrating enough to contribute to the image. In constant potential machines, the kilovoltage powers up to peak and stays there. The beam here is much more *homogeneous* with regard to the wavelength of the photons. The entire exposure is a single pulse. All other factors like mA, kVp, exposure time, and cone length being equal, the constant potential machine results in exactly the same image with 20% less radiation per exposure.
2. The traditional disadvantage of the DC-type machines was that a kVp more than about 70 would greatly shorten the tube life. With the use of older "D" speed film, many advocated 90 kVp produced the best image contrast for the study of alveolar bone. With the advent of "E," "E+," and "F" speed film, the characteristics of the film are such that 70 kVp produces excellent contrast for bone imaging.
3. Constant potential machines are desirable because the exposure time increments can be set at 1/100ths of a second, a feature desirable with the use of CCD and CMOS sensors. Other advantages are the 20% decrease in radiation dose in addition to the 50% plus dose reduction with digital imaging and 70 kVp produces excellent digital images whose contrast can be further adjusted electronically after image capture.
4. Remember that the tube head is recessed. Thus the full length of the BID is 16 inches with about 8 inches visible outside the tube head and the remainder recessed back into the tube head. The advantage of this is a less awkward tube head for positioning, a shorter support arm connecting the machine to the wall can be used, and therefore less space is needed. It is truly a great design and is highly recommended. Price point is compatible with other standard AC-type machines.
5. Yes, all of these errors will produce identical effects in digital images.

6. These errors for film-based radiography may also produce errors in digital imaging, but the effect can be different:

   - *Overexposure*: Produces "saturation" in which features are lost because of large areas turning irreversibly black. That is to say, it cannot be adequately corrected with image processing. CCD and CMOS sensors are especially prone to this.
   - *Underexposure*: Produces "noise" that cannot be adequately corrected with image processing. CCD and especially CMOS sensors are prone to this.
   - *Leaving film exposed to light*: Wrapped, exposed x-ray film is unaffected by light. PSP sensors are very prone to image degradation when exposed to light after image capture as light erases the image. CCD and CMOS sensors are unaffected by light.
   - *Film bending and crimping*: PSP sensors can be but should not be bent because permanent damage to the PSP plate could, over time, result in clear white non-fluorescing bend and crimp marks in all future images taken with such plates. CCD and CMOS sensors cannot be bent or crimped
   - *Scratched emulsion*: In intraoral films, such marks are a one-time event per film. With PSPs, scratches are permanent and seen in all future images and show up as white areas much like scratches on film. CCD and CMOS sensors cannot be scratched easily.
   - *Film reversed*: This occurs in digital imaging, but the reversed image is not as obvious as on film.
   - *Dot in the slot*: There is no dot on digital sensors; therefore this error cannot occur.

7. No, these are darkroom errors. There is no darkroom or chemical processing of images in digital imaging.

8. Yes, there are some errors unique or more prone to occur in digital imaging. Here is a list, which the author is certain will grow as we work more with digital. This does not imply digital is less desirable than film-based radiography. Digital is simply different and represents the certain future of x-ray imaging in dentistry. Here are a few:

   - *Sensor breakage*: CCD sensors contain very delicate components that can be easily damaged by rough handling, and replacement is expensive. Wired and wireless CMOS sensors are less delicate, and PSPs are most like film. It is virtually impossible to break film by rough handling

though the emulsion can be damaged and the damage is a one-time event for any one film. Sensor damage tends to be permanent, irreparable, and irreversible.

   - *PSP scanning*: Scanning is unique to PSP-type digital sensors. The light side must be placed on the drum or fed into the machine such that it faces the laser beam in the scanner. Otherwise no image or a weak image is the result.
   - *Image orientation in the computer*: Unlike film, digital sensors have no embossed dot to properly orient the film. Some software comes with templates that are like film mounts. If the images are correlated to a location in the template before exposure or if the images are taken in a preset order, the computer will automatically orient the image to the proper arch and side. Sometimes this must be done for each image; that is to say, functions such as rotate left or right 90 degrees or 180 degrees and flip to change over to a right or left side orientation. With the DenOptix drum system, the template is on the drum; however, images will be in the right place only if properly placed on the drum.
   - *Sensor life*: At this time it is believed a sensor of any type will not last forever, though certainly for many thousands of exposures. Thus it is expected a sensor can simply wear out. There is no such possibility with film, though unused film can degrade over time.
   - *Digital image viewing*: Over time, monitors burn out and images become dim and dull. Printers are also subject to wear. Over time, these will need replacement. Film is viewed with a light box. Bulbs and switches may need replacement over time, but the viewbox itself is essentially good for a lifetime.
   - *Digital image loss*: If not properly backed up, digital images can be lost with computer crashes and other catastrophic computer damage. Films can also be lost. Any type of image can be lost as a result of catastrophic events such as flooding or fire.
   - *Viruses*: Digital imaging systems can be attacked by viruses and images rendered inaccessible.
   - *Digital image processing*: Digital images can be altered in innumerable ways after capture. A dark film can be lightened using Farmer's reducer, but that's about it.
   - *Active sensor size*: Because the active part of the wired sensors is smaller than film, it

may in some instances be more difficult to get proper coverage such as getting the apex or 3rd molars in the image.

9. As you know, film processing involves a darkroom with processing tanks or an automatic processor, chemicals, and proper processing conditions such as the safelight or solution temperatures. Digital image processing involves the alteration of the original image, usually to improve the diagnostic features or to highlight in red a feature or structure such as caries for patient education.

10. There are three people in the picture, one of them being the author. The viewbox is not needed.

FIGURE 5-5

1. It is the wired type and is in fact a CCD sensor.
2. Manufacturers like to measure only the thinnest part. In point of practice, it is the thickest part that defines the thickness.

FIGURE 5-6

1. Yes, this is the active side of the sensor.
2. Yes, it is placed behind the teeth and faces the radiation beam just like film.
3. Yes, it can be oriented vertically and horizontally. Perhaps you can now imagine why the computer cannot know in what arch or on what side you placed the sensor in the patient's mouth.
4. The active part of the sensor is about 25% smaller than film.

FIGURE 5-7

1. It is a wireless PSP sensor.
2. The brand is Digora. Note the unique rubberized band around the edges of the PSP. This makes more of the thickness of a film packet for placement into the groove of a standard bite-block and adds to patient comfort at the same time as providing a little needed rigidity.
3. The error is in part B. The light side needs to face the beam of radiation.
   COMMENT: Infection control–wise, neither sensor has been placed in the barrier envelope.

FIGURE 5-8

Part A is incorrect. With this barrier envelope, the tab should be folded back and that side fed into the slot in the bite-block.

Of course gloves need to be worn while capturing digital images.

FIGURE 5-9

Part A: The barrier envelope is on the sensor, but the PSP is not properly centered in the slot.

Part B: Here the barrier envelope can be more readily seen, and the dark side of the sensor can be seen through the clear envelope. However, the dark side of the sensor is the back side; therefore the sensor is back-to-front in the slot.

FIGURE 5-10

The error is in part A; the barrier envelopes are saliva-contaminated and need to be opened with gloves.

FIGURE 5-11

First, note that both pictures indicate the contaminated gloves have been removed and the PSPs are handled with washed bare hands. Remember, hands must always be washed right after glove removal. Part B is incorrect. With PSPs, remember that it is always "face the paleface." Yep, you heard it first right here; who knows where "dot in the slot" originated? So remember, the pale side faces out when loading PSPs into the barrier envelope; it faces out when placing it in the mouth; it faces out when being scanned; and it faces out or the light (light faces the light) when being erased.

So when does the pale side face down? After exposure before scanning, so room lighting cannot begin to erase the image; or place the PSPs in the little box with the top on.

FIGURE 5-12

Items in the DenOptix set up:

1. A panoramic cassette designed to accept a panoramic PSP. That's about all you need to add the film-based panoramic machine to the DenOptix digital intraoral system.
2. Two scanning drums with intraoral film holding template.
3. Behind the drums, the laser scanner commonly referred to as the "bread box."
4. To the right are the computer monitor, keyboard, and mouse; the computer itself is under the table
5. The operator. Did you forget that one? Okay, don't worry.
6. There is a screen open on the monitor that we will look at in more detail.

FIGURE 5-13

By left-clicking the mouse on the top left file icon, the drop box you see here opens. Using the mouse, move the white arrow to the DenOptix scanner line in the drop box. As the arrow touches the line, it turns a darker color. A left click of the mouse on that will open the first scanner screen.

FIGURE 5-14

Upon clicking on the DenOptix scanner field, this is the screen that pops up. Basically, you need to enter the patient's name and other desired data, which is Dr. Diane Flint—one of the contributors to this book. Beneath the patient information field, notice that there are icons for selecting intraoral, panoramic, and cephalometric scans. In this case, the intraoral scan is selected and the default intraoral template can be selected by left-clicking on the icon. Once this is done, scanning can begin and will take several minutes to 5 minutes for a full mouth survey and/or a panoramic image.

FIGURE 5-15

In part A, try to find the little magnifying glass icon just to the left of the lower arrow. In B, you use the mouse and the arrow to click on to a standardized magnification selection, which is 1.5. When you do this, a box appears in the image. With the mouse and the hand icon, which also appears, the box can be moved with the mouse to any desired part of the image. This produces a zoom at the desired area, and now the enlarged region appears on the screen. In part B, the lower arrow points to a sliding scale in which any magnification can be selected. The zoom is, in effect, like looking at an image through a magnifying lens and may make fine details more discernable to the viewer.

If you succeeded, you just processed your first digital image.

FIGURE 5-16

In image B, using the arrow and the mouse, enhancement was selected. The highlighted field in B appears when the arrow contacts the field. If you left-click on that image, C appears and is a mildly enhanced image not very different from the original. This is an important observation since now the operator must decide if further, more specific image enhancements are needed.

FIGURE 5-17

In image A, we can see the highlighted field under the checked enhancement field two lines above it. Now we are going to apply a filter to sharpen the image. Image B is the result in which a significant difference can be seen. Also, filters can be reapplied several times in a row to increase the desired effect in increments. At any stage you can go back a step or two and at any time back to the original image. Processing sometimes messes up the image so much that you simply want to start over with the original image and try something else.

FIGURE 5-18

In image A, the mouse is used to bring the arrow to the negative drop box under enhancement. The histogram to the right shows that the blackest part of the 256 shades of gray are on the left side. Can you see that right beneath the twin peaks? When you left-click on the negative icon, image B appears. Now look at the histogram on the right of the screen. Do you see the blackest part of the image is now toward the right-hand side of the scale representing the 256 shades of gray? In effect, the histogram has been reversed so what was black is now white and what was white is now black. This image looks like an old black-and-white photographic negative. Notice how the radiopaque restorations in A really stand out in B or how the trabeculae of bone stand out in B.

Notice also how the histogram in A (mountain with twin peaks) represents only about one third of the scale. These are the shades of gray in the image. Notice a lone thin peak at the white end of the scale representing the restorations and how in B the thin peak is now at the black end of the scale.

FIGURE 5-19

1. The image is light because it was left out in the open in the room and exposed to the room light after image acquisition.
2. Here is what we see:
   - A: This is the pale original image. Note that it is an image of the maxillary lateral incisor region taken with a #2-size PSP.
   - B: It was decided to see if the image could be brought out with enhancement before going any further. First, enhancement was selected; then a histogram equalization was tried.
   - C: This is the result of the histogram equalization. This brought out the image, but it also enhanced the noise.
   - D: Here the image was darkened but the tools and the histogram on the right side of the screen have been cropped out. Now we need to properly orient the image. So the left 90-degree rotation was selected.
   - E: Now you can see that the image has been rotated to its correct orientation and other parts of the screen can be seen.
   - F: The screen has been cleared of everything except the image.

COMMENT: After all of that and in all probability, this image would be considered non-diagnostic. If, however, the patient was not available, something might be seen that could cause us to contact the patient and schedule another visit. With film in this same situation (equivalent to underexposure) as seen in A, nothing can be done.

FIGURE 5-20

- In *A*, the image is improperly oriented in the computer, thus causing an electronic cone cut.
- In *B*, we see a regular run-of-the-mill cone (BID) cut that occurred at the time of image acquisition.

FIGURE 5-21

- In *A*, we can see the sensor was not well placed, probably because it slipped partially out of the slot. At this time DenOptix sensors fit loosely in film-type bite-blocks because they are thinner than film. Also, excess negative vertical angulation was used, producing foreshortening.
- *B* looks in a way like the same image as *A*, because exactly the same structures are seen. Well, this demonstrates how an image can be altered. The author scanned image *A* into Photoshop Elements and then put it into Power Point and distorted the image to look like elongation.

FIGURE 5-22

The error is in part *B*. Note that the PSP is being removed from the saliva-contaminated barrier envelope with ungloved hands.

FIGURE 5-23

Part *B* is incorrect. Remember the rule: "face the paleface."

FIGURE 5-24

- Part *A, Arrow 1:* The PSP is ready to be scanned, and pressing the touch pad at *A* activated the scan.
- Part *B, Arrow 2:* The scanned PSP falls out of the scanner into the tray below the loading dock. An advantage of this system is the scanned PSP is automatically erased when it comes out of the scanner. In the DenOptix system, the PSPs must be erased by placing the pale side facing a source of bright light for several minutes.

FIGURE 5-25

This is a custom-built PSP image eraser with a bright source of light and an automatic timer.

NOTE TO STUDENTS: Well, now you have done image processing. It is hard to demonstrate photographically and without the computer in front of the author. Perhaps a CD in a future edition will help. That certainly deserves some thought!

Chapter **6** Answers

FIGURE 6-1

1. exit area of the radiation beam
2. CCD digital sensor
3. tube head
4. base for chin rest/bite-block/side guide assembly; also housing for canine positioning light
5. hold-on handles for patient
6. platform for motorized machine adjustment knobs
7. touch screen for machine settings menu
8. primary vertical machine support column
9. support "C" arm for rotating tube head/CCD assembly

FIGURE 6-2

1. chin rest
2. bite-block
3. side guides in closed position
4. base for chin rest/bite-block/side guides
5. support arm
6. support housing for cephalometric assembly
7. center line nasion support/indicator
8. right and left ear rods

FIGURE 6-3

1. left ear rod
2. right ear rod
3. nasion support/indicator
4. CCD sensor
5. soft tissue filter
6. support housing for cephalometric assembly
7. ceph horizontal support arm

FIGURE 6-4

1. open/close side guides control
2. beam alignment controls for tomography
3. beam alignment control for tomography
4. raise and lower machine controls
5. support arm
6. housing for touch screen
7. touch screen machine function/settings menu
8. hold-on handles for patient
9. primary vertical machine support column

FIGURE 6-5

1. base of support arm for special controls and rotating touch menu screen
2. housing for touch screen
3. panoramic program being selected on touch screen
4. touch screen
5. primary vertical machine support column

Figure 6-6

1. There are six (6) program groups.
2. Standard panoramic program (light is on).
3. The exposure time will be 16.1 seconds.
4. The operator is pointing to the auto level adjustment override, which allows the operator to increase or decrease the auto exposure level to darken or lighten the film.
5. This machine has an 8-second exposure time option, which is the fastest on the market and delivers approximately 50% less radiation dose to the patient than most standard 400 speed rare earth film screen combinations.

Figure 6-7

1. The cassette is placed in the machine backwards.
2. The front of the cassette is labeled "tube side" with a drawing of an x-ray tube. Remember, it is the front of the cassette that must face the other side of the machine to properly expose the film.

Figure 6-8

Error: Patient's head is turned or twisted.

Correction: Close the side guides; make sure the vertical midline positioning light is in the patient's midline.

Figure 6-9

Error: Patient is too far forward.

Correction: Use the bite-block or bite stick; make sure the canine light is at the mesial of the maxillary canine for this machine.

Figure 6-10

Error: The chin is positioned too high.

Correction: Tilt the chin down; make sure the positioning light is on the Frankfort plane (orbital rim to tragus of the ear).

COMMENT: Most machines require the chin be tipped a few degrees down from the horizontal plane to compensate for the slightly upward angle of the beam as the beam is projected from under the thick occipital part of the skull toward the film or sensor.

Figure 6-11

Error: Glasses are left on.

Correction: Make certain all extraoral and intra-oral items have been removed.

Figure 6-12

Error: Lips are open, and tongue is not against palate. (Note that side guides are also open and chin is a little high.)

Correction: Instruct patient to swallow or suck on his cheeks or suck on the bite-block. This will usually cause the patient to close the lips and press the tongue against the palate. (Try this by biting on a object about like a pencil eraser.)

Figure 6-13

Error: Patient is slumped. (The neck is not vertical because the patient is not standing up straight.)

Correction: Be sure the patient is standing upright so the neck is vertical with the feet advanced to the point where the patient must hold on to the handles. Some offices place two footprints on the floor for this purpose.

Figure 6-14

Error: Hearing aid is left on.

Correction: Remove the hearing aid. This patient also had a hearing aid in the other ear.

COMMENT: There is no bite-block or bite stick on this Veraviewepocs machine. The patient is simply positioned with the chin on the chin rest with a disposable foam bite-block or cotton roll between the upper and lower teeth. Though the usual positioning lights are available, the auto-focus feature will automatically correct for any malpositioning resulting from the lack of a bite-block. This is an excellent feature because it further simplifies the near-nonexistent infection control requirements for panoramic radiology.

Figure 6-15

Error: Chin is too low.

Correction: Make sure positioning light is on Frankfort plane. (Lower orbital rim to tragus of the ear, which is the little bump in front of the ear opening.)

Figure 6-16

Error: Chin is not on chin rest.

Correction: When you ask the patient to stand up straight, the chin often comes up off the chin rest. Be certain to bring the machine up to meet the chin when this is done.

Figure 6-17

Error: Head is tilted or tipped.

Correction: Close the side guides; ensure the vertical midface positioning light and the patient's midline are aligned.

Figure 6-18

Dad's errors:
1. Glasses are left on.
2. Earrings are left on.
3. Necklace is left on.
4. No protective apron is worn.
5. Positioned too far forward (canine light).
6. Head is turned (midline face light not on midline).

7. Chin is not on the chin rest (special edentulous chin rest has no bite-block because the patient has no teeth).
8. Neck appears slumped.

Figure 6-19

Son's errors:
1. Earrings are left on.
2. Necklace is left on.
3. No protective apron is worn.
4. Positioned a little too far back as teeth do not appear to be in bite groove.
5. Chin is not on chin rest.
6. Neck is slumped.
7. Mouth is open (frequently when the mouth is open, the tongue is not against the palate).

Chapter 7 Answers (with Tables 7-1 and 7-2)

Figure 7-1

1. Error:
   Chin tipped too low.
2. Features:
   Excessively curved "smile line" of the teeth.
   Hyoid bone projected as a horizontal radiopaque band across anterior mandible.
3. Correction:
   Raise chin up a little.
   Check Frankfort plane light parallel to ala-tragus line.

Figure 7-2

1. Error:
   Patient "slumped" or "stooped."
2. Features:
   Lower anterior teeth obscured.
   V-shaped radiopaque ghost image of the spine in midline.
3. Correction:
   Make sure patient is standing upright with back and neck straight.

Figure 7-3

1. *First* error:
   Patient "turned" or "twisted" in the machine.
2. Features:
   Molars wider on right than on left.
   Ramus wider on right than on left.
3. Correction:
   Make sure patient is facing straight forward in the machine.
   Close side guides firmly against patient's head.
   Check anterior vertical midline light; make sure it is aligned with middle of nose and rest of face.

1. *Second* error:
   Patient "slumped" or "stooped."
2. Features:
   Anterior left teeth slightly obscured by radiopaque shadow.
   Ghost image of spine on left midline only as patient is turned in the machine.
3. Correction:
   Make sure patient is standing upright with back and neck straight.

Figure 7-4

1. *First* error:
   Patient positioned too far forward in the machine.
2. Features:
   Excessively narrowed anterior teeth.
   Spine superimposed on ramus on both sides.
3. Correction:
   Make sure patient is biting in groove in bite-block.
   Check that canine light is aligned with middle of lower canine.
1. *Second* error:
   Patient slightly twisted.
2. Features:
   Upper right molar a little wider than upper left molar.
   Right ramus a little wider than left ramus.
   Spine overlaps right ramus more than left ramus.
3. Correction:
   Close side guides firmly against patient's head.
   Check anterior midline light.
   COMMENT: The lower anterior teeth are missing so the patient could not properly bite in the groove in the bite-block, as indicated by the lack of an interocclusal space between the upper and lower teeth. Because the patient was not biting in the groove, he ended up too far forward and possibly contributed to the twisted position as well. A couple of cotton rolls in the edentulous space and careful attention to technique would have taken care of the problem.

Figure 7-5

1. Error:
   Insufficient KVP or depleted developer.
2. Features:
   Image too light.
3. Correction:
   Remember to adjust KVP to patient's size and build.
   Check processor with a pre-exposed radiograph; if it comes out light, replenish the solutions.

TABLE **7-1**   Panoramic Patient Positioning Errors

ERROR AND CAUSE	IDENTIFYING FEATURES	CORRECTION
1. Patient too far forward	Narrow, blurred anterior teeth. Superimposition of spine on ramus	Use bite-block. Line up incisal edge of teeth with notch. Ask edentulous patient to bite about 5 mm behind groove on the block
2. Patient too far back	Wide, blurred anterior teeth	Use bite-block. Line up incisal edge of teeth with groove on the bite-block
3. Chin positioned too low	Excessive curving of occlusal plane; loss of image of roots of lower anterior teeth	Tip chin down, but ala-tragus line should not exceed 5 to 7 degrees downward.
	Narrowing of intercondylar distance and loss of head of condyles at top of film	Use chin rest
4. Chin positioned too high	Flattening or reverse curvature of occlusal plane. Loss of image of roots of upper anterior teeth. Lengthening of intercondylar distance and loss of head of condyles at edges of film. Hard palate shadow superimposed on apices of maxillary teeth	Tip chin down 5 to 7 degrees. Use chin rest
5. Patient twisted	Unequal right-left magnification. Severe overlap of contact points and blurring	Line up patient's midline with middle of incisal bite guide. Close side guides
6. Patient tilted	Mandible appears tilted on film. Unequal distance between mandible and chin rest at a given point on right and left sides	Position chin firmly on both sides of chin rest. Close side guides
7. Slumped position	Ghost image of cervical spine superimposed on midline region of film	Stand-up machine—have patient step forward, or place feet on markers. All machines—be certain patient is sitting or standing erect
8. Chin not on chin rest	Sinus not visible on film; top of condyle cut off; excessive distance between inferior border of mandible and lower edge of film	Position chin on chin rest
9. Tongue not on palate	Relative radiolucency obscuring apices of maxillary teeth (palatoglossal air space)	Ask patient to swallow or suck on tongue and cheeks during exposure
10. Lips open	Relative radiolucency on coronal portion of upper and lower teeth	Ask patient to swallow or suck on tongue and cheeks during exposure
11. Patient movement	Wavy outline of cortex of inferior border of mandible. Blurring of Image above wavy cortical outline	Ask patient to hold still. Explain function of machine to avoid startling patient
12. Prostheses, jewelry	Evidence of prostheses in film. Acrylic denture teeth and bases do not show	Remove all complete and partial dentures, eyeglasses, hearing aids, jewelry, etc.

Modified from Langland OE, Sippy FH, Langlais RP: *Textbook of dental radiology*, ed 2, pp. 342–348, Springfield, Ill, 1984, Charles C. Thomas, Publisher.

TABLE **7-2**   Panoramic Film Handling and Processing Errors

ERROR AND CAUSE	IDENTIFYING FEATURES	CORRECTION
1. Not starting at home base	A portion of film is blank: a portion of anatomy is lost at edge of film	Align machine and/or cassette with starting point
2. Cassette resistance	One or several dark vertical bands on film	Be certain to remove thickly padded items of clothing
3. Paper or lint in cassette	Radiopacity of unusual shape and location	With envelope-type soft cassettes, periodically inspect and clean screens
4. Film crimping	Crescent-shaped radiolucency	Avoid forcefully pushing film into the cassette or bending the leading edge upon removal of film from cassette or box
5. Static electricity	Lightning-like radiolucency; dotlike radiolucencies. Other patterns: tire track, herringbone, starburst, smudge	Dry air in darkroom can be humidified with a humidifier or large bowl of water. Avoid rapid pulling-out of film from envelope-type cassettes. Use antistatic carpet
6. White-light exposure	A portion of the film appears overexposed	Avoid smoking near film. Check other sources of light leaks in darkroom, (i.e., unsafe safelights, etc.); check integrity of cassette, especially plastic ones
7. Double exposure	Two images on same film	Always remove and process films after exposure
8. Underexposed	Film too light	Increase kV and/or mA, depending upon machine. Place film between screens, not to one side of screen
9. Overexposed	Film too dark	Decrease kV and/or mA, depending upon machine
10. No name	Patient's name or identification number not on film	Use film imprinter, special labeling tape, or special pen
11. No right/left marker	No R or L in processed film	Use lead markers on outside

Modified from Langland OE, Sippy FH, Langlais RP: *Textbook of dental radiology*, ed 2, pp. 342-348, Springfield, Ill, 1984, Charles C. Thomas, Publisher.

FIGURE 7-6

1. *First* error:
   Lower partial denture left in.
2. Features:
   Partial denture seen in image.
3. Correction:
   Be sure to ask patient if there is a denture or partial denture, barbell, etc.
1. *Second* error:
   Patient slumped.
2. Features:
   Lower anterior teeth obscured.
   Radiopaque ghost image of spine in lower midline.

3. Correction:
   Make sure patient is standing upright with back and neck straight.

FIGURE 7-7

1. Error:
   Hoop and stud earrings not removed on each side.
2. Features:
   Real and ghost images of earrings.
3. Correction:
   Be sure to check for this in both males and females, especially those with long hair obscuring the ears.

FIGURE 7-8

1. *First* error:
   Tongue not against palate.
2. Features:
   Dark shadow obscuring apices of maxillary teeth.
3. Correction:
   Instruct patient to place tongue on palate; if this fails, ask patient to suck on his or her cheeks while still biting on the bite-block.
1. *Second* error:
   Patient positioned too far back.
2. Features:
   Normally we would expect to see widened teeth, but sometimes this feature is missing, as is the case here.
   Ghost image of the ramus on both sides. This is easy to see because a horizontal line is dividing the ramus from the body; above this line the ramus is excessively radiopaque, and below the line the body is of normal density. The radiopaque shadow is the ghost image of the ramus on the other side and happens only when the patient is too far back.
3. Correction:
   Make sure patient is biting in groove in bite-block.
   Check canine light.

FIGURE 7-9

1. Error:
   Patient positioned too far forward.
2. Features:
   Narrow anterior teeth.
   Spine superimposed on the ramus on both sides.
3. Correction:
   Be sure patient is biting in groove of bite-block.
   Insert upper denture for the exposure if available.
   Check canine light.
   NOTE: The tongue is just slightly off the palate.

FIGURE 7-10

1. Error:
   Tongue not against palate.
2. Features:
   Dark shadow obscuring most of maxilla.
3. Correction:
   Instruct patient to place tongue on palate or suck on cheeks, or suck on bite-block but keep the teeth in the bite-block groove.

FIGURE 7-11

1. *First* error:
   Glasses left on.
2. Features:
   Foreign object seen in image (metal, glass lenses; space between metal and glass lens is a plastic rim).
3. Correction:
   Remove all extraoral objects like glasses, jewelry, etc.
1. *Second* error:
   Patient positioned too far back.
2. Features:
   Teeth not widened again.
   Ghost image of ramus seen on both sides.
3. Correction:
   Instruct patient to bite in groove of bite-block.
   Check cuspid light.
1. *Third* error:
   Patient movement.
2. Features:
   This is usually best noted by a "jiggly" or uneven image of a small portion of the inferior cortex of the mandible. Here we can clearly see this feature starting at the midline all the way to the right 1st premolar area. The movement sometimes causes vertical white streaks, as seen here in the midline.
3. Correction:
   Instruct patient to be still.
   Explain what the machine will do so the patient is not startled.
   Do a practice run if necessary with radiation turned off.

FIGURE 7-12

1. *First* error:
   Chin tilted too far upward.
2. Features:
   "Flat" occlusal plane.
   Heavy radiopaque horizontal line representing the hard palate obscures the apices of all the maxillary teeth. Inferior cortex of mandible gives mandible a "box-like" appearance.
3. Correction:
   Tip chin down 4-7.°
   Align Frankfort plane light (ala-tragus line).
1. *Second* error:
   Patient "tilted" or "tipped" to one side.
2. Features:
   Right condyle above left condyle.
3. Correction:
   Close side guides firmly against patient's head.
   Check midline light.
1. *Third* error:
   Patient positioned too far back.

2. Features:
   Widened anterior teeth not seen (we expect to see widened anterior teeth, but this feature is not reliable).
   Ghost images of the ramus on both sides (this time this feature is not so obvious but is there. The right side radiopaque line is above the one on the left because the patient is tilted.
   The radiopaque inferior turbinates are spread out across the maxillary sinus on both sides immediately above the hard palate. (When present, this is another reliable feature of too-far-back positioning.)
3. Correction:
   Make certain patient is biting in bite-block groove.
   Check canine light.
1. *Fourth* error:
   Patient slumped in the machine.
2. Features:
   Ghost image of spine in anterior area.
   Anterior teeth slightly obscured by ghost image.
3. Correction:
   Make sure patient stands upright with back and neck straight.
   COMMENT: This can be facilitated by asking patients to take baby steps forward once in machine until they must almost have to grasp the handles to avoid falling backwards. You can also paste two footprints on the floor or base of the machine.

FIGURE 7-13

1. Error:
   Double exposure.
2. Features:
   Double set of teeth or too many teeth.
3. Correction:
   Be careful to separate exposed from unexposed cassettes when several patients such as family members are being imaged at once.
   Process the film immediately after the exposure so the cassette is not later mistaken for an unexposed one.

FIGURE 7-14

1. Error:
   Unexposed film.
2. Features:
   Clear, blank image.
3. Correction:
   Separate exposed from unexposed cassettes.
   Be careful when rushed or when multiple family members are being imaged.
   Sometimes this error accompanies the previous double exposure.

FIGURE 7-15

1. *First* error:
   Neck chain left on.
2. Features:
   Ghost image of neck chain in mandibular midline.
   Real image seen on right spine identifies the chain as jewelry versus a napkin chain.
3. Correction:
   Be sure to remove all extraoral items.
1. *Second* error:
   Patient too far forward.
2. Features:
   Narrow anterior teeth.
   Shadow of spine overlaps ramus on both sides.
3. Correction:
   Make sure patient is biting in bite-block groove.
   Check canine light.

FIGURE 7-16

1. *First* error:
   Chin too high.
2. Features:
   The inferior border of the mandible is straight.
   Mandible is box-like.
3. Correction:
   Check ala-tragus light.
1. *Second* error:
   Patient too far back.
2. Features:
   Ghosting of the ramus bilaterally.
   Turbinates spread out across sinus bilaterally.
3. Correction:
   Make sure patient is biting in bite-block groove.
   Check canine light.
   COMMENT: This patient is slightly turned or twisted. See how the ramus is wider on the right and we can only see the epiglottis below the angle of the left mandible.

FIGURE 7-17

1. *First* error:
   Four necklaces left on.
2. Features:
   Note the four curved radiopaque images in the midline: one below the mandible, two superimposed on lower centrals, and one on the maxillary centrals.
3. Correction:
   Remove extraoral items.
1. *Second* error:
   Earrings left on.
2. Features:
   Real and ghost images of earrings.

3. Correction:
   Remove extraoral items.
1. *Third* error:
   Chin too high.
2. Features:
   Flat occlusal plane.
   Mandible box-like.
3. Correction:
   Check ala-tragus light.
1. *Fourth* error:
   Lips open.
2. Features:
   Dark oval shadow partially obscuring the crowns of the upper and lower anterior teeth.
3. Correction:
   Instruct patient to close lips.
1. *Fifth* error:
   Tongue not on palate.
2. Features:
   Dark shadow obscuring apical region of maxillary teeth.
3. Correction:
   Instruct patient to place tongue against palate or suck on cheeks or bite-block.

Figure 7-18

1. *First* error:
   Chin not on chin rest.
2. Features:
   Jaws high up in image.
   Wide space between chin rest just at lower middle edge of image and inferior border of mandible.
3. Correction:
   When adjusting chin, especially in tilting it up, or when asking the patient to stand up straight, the chin will come up off the chin rest. The machine must then be elevated so the patient's chin rests on the chin rest.
1. *Second* error:
   Tongue not on palate.
2. Features:
   Dark shadow above maxillary apices.
3. Correction:
   Instruct patient to place tongue against palate.

Figure 7-19

1. *First* error:
   Leaded apron too high on left shoulder and neck.
2. Features:
   Ghost image of apron below right molar area.
3. Correction:
   Make certain apron does not ride up while positioning.

1. *Second* error:
   Patient positioned too far forward.
2. Features:
   Narrow anterior teeth.
   Anterior tubercle of C-2 superimposed on ramus.
3. Correction:
   Make certain lower teeth are in bite-block groove.
   Check canine light.
   COMMENT: This patient is slightly tilted. Note how one condyle is lower than the other.

Figure 7-20

1. Error:
   Patient movement.
2. Features:
   Wavy outline of inferior cortex of mandible.
3. Correction:
   Instruct patient to hold still.
   Explain function of machine so patient will not be startled.

Figure 7-21

1. *First* error:
   Image too dark (overexposure).
2. Features:
   Image looks dark overall.
3. Correction:
   Reduce KVP.
1. *Second* error:
   Earrings left on.
2. Features:
   You can see only a real image of the right earring. Its ghost image is on the opposite side superimposed on the 3rd molar. We do see a ghost image of the left earring above the right 3rd molar. Therefore we knew there was an earring on each ear.
3. Correction:
   Remove extraoral items.
1. *Third* error:
   Lips open.
2. Features:
   Dark oval shadow obscuring crowns of anterior teeth.
3. Correction:
   Instruct patient to close lips.
1. *Fourth* error:
   Tongue not against palate.
2. Features:
   Dark shadow obscuring apical region of maxillary teeth.
3. Correction:
   Instruct patient to place tongue against palate.

Figure 7-22

1. Error:
   Patient positioned too far back.
2. Features:
   The only sign of this error is that the nasal turbinates are spread across the sinus above hard palate on both sides.
3. Correction:
   Some machines have a special chin rest for edentulous patients. These usually have a bit of a cup and lip configuration so the chin can fit in there snugly.
   Check the canine light; it should be somewhere near the corner of the mouth, depending on the machine.
   COMMENT: In this case we can see the outline of the lips, which are closed around the bite-block.

Figure 7-23

1. Error:
   Patient twisted or turned in machine.
2. Features:
   Right ramus is much wider than left ramus.
3. Correction:
   Close side guides firmly against patient's head.
   Check midface vertical light.

Figure 7-24

1. Error:
   Patient tilted or tipped in machine.
2. Features:
   One condyle is lower than other.
3. Correction:
   Check midface vertical light.

Figure 7-25

1. *First* error:
   Patient movement.
2. Features:
   Note bend, curve, or "chink" in mandibular outline and in turbinate directly above.
3. Correction:
   Instruct patient to hold still.
   Explain machine function and movements.
1. *Second* error:
   Patient positioned too far back.
2. Features:
   Turbinates of nose spread out across sinuses.
3. Correction:
   Place chin properly in special edentulous chin rest.
   Check canine positioning light at or near corner of mouth.
1. *Third* error:
   Patient twisted (turned).
2. Features:
   Left ramus wider than right ramus.

3. Correction:
   Close side guides firmly against patient's head.
   Check midface positioning light.

Figure 7-26

1. *First* error
   Tongue barbell left in.
2. Features:
   Barbell seen.
3. Correction:
   Because these can be superimposed on structures as with this case, these should be removed.
1. *Second* error:
   Film too dark (overexposed).
2. Features:
   Overall image too dark.
3. Correction:
   Reduce KVP.
1. *Third* error:
   Tongue not on palate.
2. Features:
   Dark shadow obscuring apices of maxillary teeth.
3. Correction:
   Instruct patient to place tongue on palate.
   COMMENT: The lips appear to be open as well.
   ABOUT THE BARBELL: The narrowed part is buccal, and the wide part is lingual. This is how you can locate any object. Look for associated fractured and chipped teeth and periodontal defects lingual to the incisors.

Figure 7-27

1. Error:
   Patient positioned very much too far back in the machine.
2. Features:
   Patient so far back or toward the lingual that the whole patient has been widened. As such, anatomy does not fit within boundary of film. Bilateral ghosting of ramus can also be seen. Lower root apices outside the layer and thus not seen in image.
3. Correction:
   Make certain patient bites in bite-block groove.
   Check canine positioning light.
   COMMENT: The bottom of the ghost images of the rami are not symmetrical as to where they cross the mandible; therefore the patient is probably turned as well.

Figure 7-28

1. *First* error:
   Patient's chin tipped too low.

2. Features:
Excessive smile line of occlusal plane.
Apices of lower teeth out of image.
Usually all of hyoid bone is seen as a horizontal radiopaque shadow crossing the mandible; it is not in this case because of the next error.
3. Correction:
Check ala-tragus positioning light.
1. *Second* error:
Patient twisted or turned.
2. Features:
Right ramus narrower than left ramus and toward the buccal or film side of machine.
Hyoid spread out only on left or wide side, which is toward the machine (wide side is lingual; machine or tube head is always lingual).
3. Correction:
Check vertical midline light.

FIGURE 7-29

1. Error:
Cassette resistance probably caused by bulky clothing left on.
2. Features:
Alternating vertical dark lines of overexposure.
Remember, the panoramic beam is collimated to a narrow vertical slit as can be seen here.
3. Correction:
Clothing needs to be removed or adjusted, or bulky apron needs to be properly placed.
Patient and machine should always be viewed through protective leaded-glass window so such exposures can be aborted to avoid injury to patient or damage to machine and to reduce exposure because film will have to be retaken.

FIGURE 7-30

1. *First* error
Nose ring left on.
2. Features:
Observe item.
3. Correction:
Remove extraoral objects.
1. *Second* error:
Some sort of body-piercing object in back of neck or metallic clip on clothing.
2. Features:
Observe item.
3. Correction:
Remove extraoral objects.
1. *Third* error:
Tongue not on palate.
2. Features:
Palatoglossal air space (same dark shadow covering maxillary apices).

3. Correction:
Instruct patient to place tongue against palate.
1. *Fourth* error:
Patient positioned too far back.
2. Features:
Bilateral ghosting of ramus.
3. Correction:
Make certain patient bites in bite-block groove.
Check canine positioning light.
PHEW!!! I guess that was hard work, although the cases were selected to be progressive with lots of repetition of the errors. Hope you are starting to catch on.

FIGURE 7-31

1. Dark stains are developer; whitish stains are fixer.

FIGURE 7-32

1. Fog.

FIGURE 7-33

1. Scratched screen.

FIGURE 7-34

1. Machine not started at home base.
COMMENT: Many of the machines with soft cassettes fitting on a drum can have this error. The drum must be set at a certain starting point before starting the exposure. If this is not done, a sort of panoramic "cone cut" occurs.

FIGURE 7-35

1. Film crimping while removing from box or from cassette.
2. Pits in the screen; each white spot is a small damaged area of the screen.

FIGURE 7-36

1. Static electricity.
2. The problem is from dry air. Humidify the darkroom, especially in winter.

FIGURE 7-37

1. The pattern of the white lines suggests they are physical damage to the emulsion. This can be confirmed when holding the film in your hand. Instead of looking directly at the radiograph, look at the reflected surface of each side of the film. If there are scratches, you will see them this way.
2. In the absence of finding damage to the film emulsion, you then look at the intensifying screen in the cassette. You will see the scratch marks, and every film taken with that cassette will have the same pattern.

FIGURE 7-38

1. Old plastic cassettes tend to split at the seams after a time. This was the case here, with the resulting light leak that produced the black mark.

FIGURE 7-39

1. Cracked screen. The operator would pull the screen and film about one third of the way out of the soft cassette and then flip back the top screen to remove and insert films. Over time, the screen became cracked. In such areas there is no image because it does not fluoresce in these areas.

FIGURE 7-40

1. In some machines (current models also), the cassette can be put into the machine back to front. The result is the same as for intraoral film, only this time things on the back of the cassette are in the image.
2. It is not recommended that it be kept. Having both *L* and *R* markings can lead to "good news–bad news" mistakes. These reversed images should be retaken.

Chapter **8** Answers

FIGURE 8-1

The device is a scanner with a transparency adapter. Note the much-thicker-than-normal top, which is the transparency adapter. You can digitize existing panoramic radiographs by scanning them this way.

FIGURE 8-2

Planmeca is one of the leading manufacturers of factory-installed digital panoramic CCD systems. Others include Morita and Instrumentarium. The DIMAXIS is DICOM-compliant. This machine is also capable of opening the contact points in an interproximal mode with a spatial resolution of about 10 lp/mm and similar to intraoral radiography. There is also a special panoramic projection to better see and study alveolar bone and bone height. With such machines, the need for the traditional full mouth survey (which delivers 10 times more radiation to the patient and involves more operator time, costly infection control supplies, and risk of transmitted infectious diseases such as hepatitis B, hepatitis C, and HIV) needs to be reconsidered. Nevertheless, the intraoral machine still has its place, especially the futuristic hand-held portable machine currently under development by Dr. Dale Miles and colleagues. For the new office, companies such as Planmeca can supply all of the imaging and office software, the imaging hardware, and other items such as chairs and supplies. It is very desirable to have all electronic media capable of intercommunication and be DICOM-compliant. Going the one-manufacturer route helps to achieve this goal in these early days of digital imaging.

COMMENT: The following questions are asked in the order of taking an panoramic radiograph with a film-based machine using the PSP digital system.

FIGURE 8-3

1. These are rigid, flat panoramic cassettes.
2. The DenOptix PSP has a tab on one end for attachment to the scanner drum.
3. Cassette A is for use with film and measures 6 inches × 12 inches. All fluorescent screens are light-colored as can be seen in part *A*. The difference between the two cassettes is as follows: the one in part *A* has rare earth fluorescent screens on the front and back inside surfaces of the cassette and fluoresce a bright-green color when acted upon by radiation; the one in part *B* measures 5 inches × 12 inches and has no screens.
4. The pale side of the PSP must be loaded into the cassette such that it will face the source of radiation ("face the paleface"). Therefore the PSP must be loaded with the pale side facing the front of the cassette. Thus the PSP is being incorrectly loaded in both part *A* and part *B*.
5. If the film cassette is used, the fluorescence would tend to simultaneously erase the PSP as it is being exposed by the radiation. Upon scanning the PSP, the resulting image is lighter than normal and not as sharp.

FIGURE 8-4

1. Yes, there is something odd.
2. In this case we received a 5-inch PSP and a 5-inch PSP cassette for use in a standard film-based panoramic machine. The more usual cassette size is 6 inches × 12 inches. You can see that the cassette does not completely fill the slot. In such cases the cassette should be loaded in the bottom of the slot. Also, if a 5-inch PSP were available only with a 6-inch cassette, the PSP should be loaded in the bottom of the cassette.

FIGURE 8-5

1. The PSP is in the cassette backwards; the image will be light and unsharp if it is scanned instead of being retaken.
2. The scanner drum.
3. The DenOptix scanner, also known as the "bread box."

4. The area need not be darkened. A brief exposure to ambient light will not degrade the latent image. Excessively bright lighting and direct sunlight should be avoided in the scanner area.

FIGURE 8-6

1. The first end of the PSP is being attached to the drum by the tab seen as a light-colored bar on the end of the PSP.
2. Yup! The error is the dark side of the PSP is facing out. Remember, it is the pale side of the PSP that must be exposed to x-rays and be scanned by the laser beam.

FIGURE 8-7

1. The other end of the PSP is being attached to the scanner drum with the use of the tab on the end of the PSP
2. No, there are no errors. The "face the paleface" rule is the clue that all is well.

FIGURE 8-8

1. The drum is being loaded into the scanner.
2. No, there are no mistakes.

FIGURE 8-9

1. The three steps are: enter the patient data in the labeled field provided; select the appropriate template, which in this case was a panoramic image and two bitewings; click on the icon to start the scan.
2. The scanner will not start if you forget to load the drum.

FIGURE 8-10

1. First, note the time remaining is a little over 5 minutes. This timer will count down the time, and as scanning progresses the pale pan and bitewing areas in the template will turn black. This indicated the scan is progressing normally. Notice that there is an abort button just to the right of the time-remaining display. You may have to abort if you hear a funny noise inside the scanner. Sometimes the PSP can come loose or other debris may have fallen into the scanner to disrupt the scan.

FIGURE 8-11

1. The screen indicates 0.01 second is left of the scanning time, and now the scanned PSPs have been fully blacked-in.

FIGURE 8-12

1. No, the upside-down image is not an error. If you are careful in unloading the PSP from the cassette, you can get it onto the drum right-side-up. But just like it's not worth the

effort to keep track of every different intraoral film-type radiograph in the full mouth survey, so too it is not worth the trouble to try to keep track of the orientation of the PSP images before scanning.
2. The operator has selected the "rotate-180-degrees" field by moving the arrow onto the field with the mouse and left-clicking once. This will produce an almost instantaneous result.

FIGURE 8-13

1. If you noticed the image seems pale and unsharp, you are right. Remember how the PSP cassette was being loaded with the PSP back-to-front? Well, the error was not corrected and this is the resultant image.
2. Other errors:
   - The patient's earrings were left on.
   - No bite-block was used.

FIGURE 8-14

We are going to emboss the image.

FIGURE 8-15

This is the embossed image.

FIGURE 8-16

1. This is the histogram for the panoramic image in part *A*.
2. You can make three adjustments: gamma set at 1.00; brightness set at 0; and contrast set at 100. These are the default settings.

FIGURE 8-17

1. The image is brighter, and now you can easily see the ghost image of the ramus on each side.
2. The gamma has not been adjusted. The brightness has been moved from 0 to 11. The contrast has been moved from 100 to 179.
3. The above changes were made by moving the arrow, which is somewhere on the screen, with the mouse to the desired control; left-click on the little button icon, which sort of looks like a car heater control in some cars or the dark/light control on some toasters; hold the left-click down on the mouse, and the control will move to the desired setting. The operator looks at the image while adjusting the control until the image is as good as it is going to get.
4. In Figure 8-17, *B*, you can see the histogram peak is more to the right side of the scale and it has been stretched over more of the gray scale. This is affected by all three controls; the brightness moves the whole histogram

further over to the brighter (right) side of the scale (histogram shift); the contrast adds more shades of gray to the image (histogram stretch). This was responsible for bringing out the ramus ghosts and teeth in Figure 8-17, *A*, which are more apparent as compared with Figure 8-16, *A*.

5. The patient was positioned too far back in the machine. This produces the bilateral ramus ghosts and image of the nose most apparent in Figure 8-17, *A*.

Chapter 9 Answers

FIGURE 9-1

1. The pointed cone is being used. These are now illegal on new equipment; existing equipment should be retrofitted with open-ended BIDs.

COMMENT: The pointed cone causes a wide area of the patient's tissues to be exposed to radiation. This wide area is much more than needed to expose the radiograph. They were nicknamed "scatter guns."

2. Pointed cones were usually 4 inches long.

FIGURE 9-2

1. BID diameter: 2.75 inches.
2. Several of the rules of good technique (accurate image projection) are to have the film (sensor) parallel to the teeth, to have the film (sensor) as close to the teeth as possible to reduce magnification and penumbra, and to have the source (focal spot) as far away from the object and film (sensor) as possible (long BID or cone). For all of the maxilla and to a lesser degree the mandibular anterior region, the film must be placed back away from the teeth to obtain parallelism. The magnification and penumbra are minimized with the long cone. Use of the short cone further contributes to magnification and penumbra and should be avoided in the paralleling technique.

FIGURE 9-3

1. No, the long rectangular BID exposes the patient to the least amount of radiation. Within the next few years it is likely that round cones of any design will not be permitted for intraoral periapical radiography. Rectangular cones will be required. Long round cones will be permitted for taking bitewings.
2. The long round BID provides less exposure than the short BID because the beam is more highly collimated.

FIGURE 9-4

1. The collimator for the long rectangular BID is smaller.
2. No, a cone cut will not occur. There are slots in the round ring for the positioning of the rectangular BID. The ring slots correspond to the correct alignment with the film (sensor) if it is centered on the bite-block.
3. To properly align the end of the rectangular BID with the slots in the ring, the rectangular BID can be rotated. Round BIDs cannot and need not be rotated because they are round.

FIGURE 9-5

1. The collimator is usually at the base of the BID at the point of attachment to the machine.
2. Collimators are made of lead.
3. Refer back to the question. Note that all were said to be current. Therefore all of these collimators are legal.
4. Collimator *D* delivered the least radiation dose to the patient.
5. *A*: 8 inches; *B*: 12 inches; *C*: 16 inches; and *D* is also 16 inches.
6. *D* is the rectangular BID
7. There is no pointed cone because all are current.
8. *C* and *D* are both 16 inches long and have the same exposure times. *D* delivers less radiation to the patient because the collimator is considerably smaller than *C*, the long round cone.

FIGURE 9-6

1. This is used to check the condition of the focal spot (target or anode).
2. Over time, the focal spot gets pitted, effectively making its surface area increase because of the pits. This increases the penumbra. New machines can resolve 11-12 line pairs per millimeter (lp/mm). This old machine is resolving only 6 lp/mm, which is considered unacceptable for an intraoral machine. Such images are said to be less diagnostic because of the blurring of fine details. Non-diagnostic radiographs are a waste of radiation to the patient.

FIGURE 9-7

1. The collimator is being checked to ensure the radiation is limited to the diameter of the BID.
2. As you can see, there is no fluorescence beyond the open-ended BID.

FIGURE 9-8

1. According to current regulations (2003), the protective apron is being put on the patient backwards. Remember, it is the back of the patient that is potentially exposed to radiation in panoramic radiology.
2. By about the year 2004 or 2005, new federal protection guidelines will no longer require protective aprons for patients in dental radiography because of doses delivered with current technology.
3. Wearing gloves is not necessary in panoramic radiology.

FIGURE 9-9

1. The barrier material in the wall is lead. However, two layers of ⅝-inch sheet rock will also absorb any remnant radiation in dental radiographic procedures including intraoral, panoramic, and cephalometric.
2. The glass is leaded, and no radiation passes through.

FIGURE 9-10

1. During exposure, the patient and machine should be observed by the operator. If there is any problem during the procedure, the exposure button can be released to immediately stop the machine. This minimizes unnecessary radiation exposure to the patient, protects the patient from injury by the moving parts of the machine, and can prevent damage to delicate parts of the machine such as the sensor.
2. As with intraoral radiography, the patient must remain under observation through a barrier window during the exposure.

FIGURE 9-11

1. Starting at the top right of the picture we see:
   - Two types of spray surface disinfectant; either one can be used, though the foam type may be preferred on certain machine parts.
   - Barrier wrap for the BID, tube head, and yoke of the machine.
   - A germicidal pre-procedural mouthwash and disposable cup to reduce the number of pathogens in the mouth during the procedure.
   - Two cups for separating contaminated exposed film packets and clean unexposed ones and for transporting the contaminated exposed film packets to the processing area.
   - A sterile ring locator positioning set.
   - One pair of gloves.
   - A patient napkin.
   - Intraoral film.
2. Missing items are as follows:
   - Several more pairs of gloves will be needed: the pair seen in the picture will be used to expose the films; a second pair will be needed in the darkroom or daylight loader because the contaminated gloves cannot be slid through the daylight loader sleeves or to open doors or handle items on the way to or in the darkroom. Alternatively, food handler over-gloves can be used for the transportation of the contaminated film packets. Because the films are removed from the film packets with contaminated gloves, the films must be unwrapped with the gloves on. Then, once all films are unwrapped, the gloves are removed and the films fed into the processing machine or loaded onto the hand processing racks. If retakes are needed, the whole process as just describe must be repeated with either two sets of gloves or one set of gloves and one set of over-gloves. When you are finished, the contaminated wrap on the machine and other contaminated areas must be cleaned with another set of gloves; the items needing sterilization or disinfection also need handling with gloves on.
   - Barrier envelopes for the film packets.
3. A digital panoramic image with a machine programmed to open the interproximal contact points and that has a resolution similar to intraoral radiographs. The dose will be approximately 50% less than the four bitewing radiographs using "F" speed film. Such a machine is the Planmeca ProMax; several other manufacturers will be offering this very desirable feature in the near future.

FIGURE 9-12

Here we see the bite stick of a panoramic machine with a barrier sleeve in place. **This is the only infection control requirement in panoramic radiology.**

A new machine, the Morita Versaview Epocs, does not have a bite stick because it has an auto-focus feature that will automatically adjust the image layer to the final position of the patient; a disposable bite-block or cotton rolls are needed to separate and align the maxillary and mandibular dentition.

FIGURE 9-13

Barrier envelopes have not been widely accepted for use in conjunction with intraoral film. The

thinking is that the film packet is already a barrier and the film packets may be contaminated upon removal from the barrier envelopes. Conversely, barrier envelopes must be used in conjunction with PSP-type digital intraoral sensors.

FIGURE 9-14

1. During the radiographic procedure, the headrest may need adjustment and the chair rotated, depending on the circumstances such as in a small room. In any case, if any part of the chair is to be handled by the operator once the procedure has started, these parts of the chair will need to be covered with food wrap or other barrier material or disinfected before the next patient is seated.
2. No part of the panoramic machine requires wrapping. Some folks like to wrap the side guides and chin rest for sanitary reasons.

FIGURE 9-15

1. Infection control: The operator does not need a mask or gown; the yoke, tube head, and BID have not been wrapped.
2. There are two dose-reduction advantages. First, recessed anode means the effective BID length is 16 inches, which delivers significantly less radiation than the short, 8-inch round cone. Second, the DC constant potential machine delivers 20% less radiation to the patient than does a similar impulse-type AC machine, all other factors being equal.
3. Three people are in the photograph, including photographer extraordinaire Lee Bennack, who seems to have a horrified look on his face!

FIGURE 9-16

1. The cone is being unwrapped after completion of the radiographs. Gloves are not needed for the initial wrap because the machine is not yet considered contaminated. The gloves will be cleaner if they are donned just before beginning to take the radiographs.
2. First, if all other factors are equal, the long rectangular cone requires the same exposure times as the long round cone. However, because the collimator in the rectangular cone is much smaller than the round cone, the dose to the patient is significantly less with the rectangular BID. Data published by the author indicated that on average the rectangular cone delivers 300% or 3 times less patient radiation dose than the long cone with as much as 600% less to the parotid salivary gland, which has been mentioned in the

literature as being susceptible to radiation-induced disease. Collimation represents the single most effective means of reducing patient doses of radiation.
3. New guidelines will in all probability require the use of the rectangular BID for intraoral periapical radiography but not for bitewings.

FIGURE 9-17

1. Infection control measures: operator latex examination gloves; barrier envelope on film; pre-procedural mouthwash; and difficult to see but the headrest is wrapped.
2. The locator ring device is set up for the maxillary posterior left quadrant and the mandibular posterior left quadrant.
3. Federal guidelines will recommend discontinuation of the use of protective aprons.

FIGURE 9-18

1. The spraying of electronic devices such as exposure switches results in damage and the need for repair and/or replacement. At best, they must be covered with barrier material for each examination. Because the floor and shoes are not in the pathway of infection transmission, this switch design is highly recommended. The exception is, of course, those who have the habit of putting their foot in their mouth—the author included!

FIGURE 9-19

1. Infection control problems: the patient cannot wear a mask during the taking of radiographs; the BID is not wrapped, though BID or any x-ray equipment wrapping is not necessary if it is disinfected after every patient.

FIGURE 9-20

1. During transportation, food handler over-gloves can be donned to avoid contamination of clean office areas on the way to the processing area and to negate the need to don a second pair of gloves to unwrap the contaminated film packets.

FIGURE 9-21

1. The sensor is not covered with barrier material.

FIGURE 9-22

1. These are PSP (photostimulable phosphor) plates.
2. *B* is the front side. Remember the rule: "face the paleface."

3. It is a slightly thicker band of soft, rubber-like material for patient comfort, to lend rigidity to the sensor, and for better retention in film-type bite-block slots.
4. These are barrier envelopes.

FIGURE 9-23

1. For wired sensors such as the CCD and CMOS types, a vinyl or plastic sheath (#1) about 12 inches long is used to protect the sensor and the cord. Over this, a latex finger cot (#2) is applied to further protect the sensor. This procedure was reported to result in the least contamination and saliva leakage. Moisture contamination can damage the electronic components of most wired sensors.

FIGURE 9-24

1. Infection control problems: The operator need not wear gloves or a smock; there is, however, nothing wrong with doing this—it is simply wasteful. Difficult to see is the lack of a protective sleeve on the bite stick. If you just checked this but couldn't tell, you would get full credit.
2. Currently in 2004, the protective apron needs to be used and the poncho-type covering the front and back is the best design. New guidelines will, if adopted, drop the protective apron requirement.

FIGURE 9-25

1. The sterilization container is the stainless steel cassette with removable top so it may be used also as an instrument tray.
2. In the background we see the sterilization envelope with a clear plastic, heat-resistant front to be able to see what is in the package, and a paper back to allow penetration by the hot steam or chemical vapors. This package can be heat-sealed.
3. Heat sterilization is recommended for all heat-resistant contaminated items. If, however, this cannot be done, these instruments can be disinfected to high levels with a liquid disinfectant. This is permitted because these instruments are classified as Spaulding *category 2* because they contact only intraoral tissues. *Category 1* instruments penetrate tissues and must be sterilized, and *category 3* contact only contaminated instruments and can be disinfected.

COMMENT: *Sterilization* means the destruction of all microbial contaminants including TB spores, whereas *disinfection* means the destruction of most pathogens but not TB spores. *Sanitization* implies a lower level of decontamination for live human tissues, which can be damaged or poisoned by disinfectants, or for areas such as the floor, which do not require high-level disinfection.

4. All digital sensors are subject to permanent damage or destruction by heat sterilization. In institutions where ethylene oxide gas is available, this may be considered. However, the gas is toxic, special sterilizers with regulated venting are needed, and sterilization takes 8 hours, which is impractical for dental offices and many institutions.

FIGURE 9-26

1. When the symbol changes color, it indicates the packet has reached sterilization-level temperatures in a steam autoclave.
2. Unless otherwise indicated, the packet design and temperature indicators may be used only with the specified sterilizer type as printed on the packet. Similar packets are available for other sterilizer types such as heat and chemiclave.
3. No, the symbol does not indicate sterility of the packet contents. This must be done with a biologic monitor containing bacterial spores specific for the heat-sterilizer type and placed in a similar packet with a full sterilization load. According to the CDC and ADA infection control guidelines, biologic monitoring with the spore test should be done on a weekly basis and the results recorded in a log for each sterilizer.

Chapter 10 Answers

CASE 10-1

1. Excessive orthodontic forces.
2. Iatrogenic root resorption.

CASE 10-2

1. Distal drift; the tooth is also tipped to the mesial.

CASE 10-3

1. Microdont and distomolar. However, it may also be said it is unerupted and impacted.

CASE 10-4

1. Taurodont (bull-like or like the ungulate's dentition; bulls have short legs and big bodies as compared with cows).
2. The pulp chamber is usually elongated with parallel walls; the root canal does not taper from the floor of the pulp chamber. Compare with the adjacent 1st molar.

3. Taurodontism is usually a solitary finding. It may be seen in association with many syndromes and anomalies. Here is a partial list: amelogenesis imperfecta, Down's syndrome, ectodermal disturbances, Mohr syndrome, osteoporosis, tricho-dento-osseous syndrome, and Klinefelter syndrome.
4. Yes, primary teeth can be affected.

CASE 10-5
1. Dentinogenesis imperfecta.
2. *Seen here:* chipped enamel, bulbous crowns, obliteration of the pulp and root canal spaces. *Not seen here:* tapering root form, root fracture.
3. Osteogenesis imperfecta.

CASE 10-6
1. Dilaceration.
2. It got this way because of a tortuous or difficult path of eruption. Remember, the root forms as eruption progresses.

CASE 10-7
1. Image *B*—Billy has the problem.
2. You knew because of Billy's lack of interseptal bone in the anterior region.
3. Do a space analysis and initiate interceptive orthodontic therapy, or refer Billy to the orthodontist.

CASE 10-8
1. Differential diagnosis:
   - Abfraction
   - Toothbrush abrasion
   - Older radiolucent restoration or sealant
   - Cervical caries
   - Erosion
2. This was abfraction.
3. The cause is poorly understood though it is seen in patients with occlusal trauma and bruxism. If occlusal abnormalities exist, they should be eliminated; the defects can be restored with bonded composite tooth-colored material. There is some question that restorations are not well retained in such teeth.

CASE 10-9
1. External root resorption.
2. Prognosis is poor for the ultimate retention of avulsed and re-implanted teeth.
3. Bone quality and quantity allowing and assuming the patient is not a smoker or has any other health impediment, this is an ideal case for an implant.

CASE 10-10
1. Microdont, peg lateral.
2. Place a porcelain veneer. Denyse has one, and it looks great!

CASE 10-11
1. Dentin dysplasia O'Carroll type 1a; subtypes 1b and 1c have varying degrees of increased root formation and the presence of linear horizontal bands of pulpal remnants and periapical radiolucencies. Subtype 1d is different as the teeth are usually fully developed; they also have the horizontal bands of pulpal remnants and huge prominent pulp stones in the root areas.
2. Management involves meticulous home care, occlusal equilibration, and periodontal maintenance at accelerated intervals. In spite of this, type 1a—the most severe form—often leads to premature loss of the teeth.

CASE 10-12
1. Eruption sequestrum.
2. This problem often resolves spontaneously. Sometimes the patient can feel the bone spicule and believes he has an embedded piece of chicken bone or the like. The pain is felt when there is slight infection associated with the sequestration of the spicule. With a little topical anesthetic and sterile cotton pliers, it can be removed.

CASE 10-13
1. Pulp stones; note that they are usually the same density as dentin.
2. The developmental anomaly is dentin dysplasia O'Carroll type 1d.
3. No, it is not present here. You will know it when you see it (I hope).
4. The significance is endodontic therapy. You can imagine that such cases might be best managed by the endodontist.

CASE 10-14
1. To begin, the 1st molar is supraerupted, probably because there is also a missing opposing tooth or teeth. Second, this has altered the contact area, which now favors food impaction. As a result, the patient picked up the habit of using a round toothpick several times a day, thus abrading the 1st molar (toothpick abrasion). The abraded area closely resembles root caries. This case demonstrates the importance of correlating the x-ray findings with a thorough clinical examination and history.
2. *Factitial* is a self-induced injury.

CASE 10-15

1. Transposition is the problem. The 1st premolar and canine have exchanged places.
2. Probably the orthodontist will not be able to help at this point though some realignment may be needed. Esthetically, the two transposed teeth can be made to look like each other with porcelain veneers or full porcelain crowns.

CASE 10-16

1. Note the shovel-shaped incisors. The lingual pit in the central was filled prophylactically, but the lateral was not. The lateral has a dens in dente and invaginated enamel, and dentin can be seen. The prophylactic sealing of a tooth with a dens in dente prevents early carious pulpal involvement. In all probability, this patient did not receive a complete radiographic examination or the dens in dente was not recognized. The patient received a prolonged course of orthodontic therapy, which resulted in iatrogenic resorption of the root apices. *Iatrogenic* means an unintended ill effect as a result of dental treatment.

Did you see all that? If yes . . . you deserve a break.

CASE 10-17

Welcome back.

1. If you noticed there is a tooth there, you are right! If you said this is a migrated tooth, possibly a canine . . . even better. If you also noted the external resorption of the tooth, then you get full points.

CASE 10-18

1. The anomaly is a supernumerary tooth termed a *mesiodens*. It is the most common extra tooth.
2. It should be extracted immediately. Also, Dad should take another radiograph like an occlusal so he can see higher up. The mesiodens is often paired; when only one is seen to be heading south, the other may be heading north and sometimes erupts into the floor of the nose!

CASE 10-19

1. The pulps of the premolars are large, probably at the extreme of normal. There are conditions characterized by large pulps, but this patient is healthy. Should these teeth need restoration, iatrogenic pulp exposure is possible. The mesial pulp horn of the 1st molar

has receded. Note the small radiopaque composite restoration on the mesial surface, which was probably placed as a pit just after the 2nd primary molar exfoliated. Note also the pulp stones in the distal part of the pulp chamber.

CASE 10-20

1. Congenitally missing 2nd premolar.
2. The occlusal plane of the permanent dentition is higher up than that of the primary teeth. Thus when the 1st premolar and 1st molar fully erupt, the retained 2nd primary molar will be below the occlusal plane. This can result in extrusion of the opposing molar. Therefore as soon as the plane of occlusion is established, the retained baby tooth will need a crown to restore the occlusion. In time the deciduous tooth may exfoliate, and then the best prosthesis would be an implant.
3. None. If there were multiple missing teeth affecting other family members, then familial hypodontia may be present. If in addition to multiple missing teeth, the teeth are hypoplastic and misshapen, I would suspect hereditary hypohydrotic ectodermal dysplasia, chondroectodermal dysplasia, or incontinentia pigmenti—all of which may look similar with regard to the dentition.

CASE 10-21

1. Enamel hypoplasia, environmental type.
2. This happened during the first year of life. To figure this out, remember the "1-2-3 rule" for the permanent central incisors and molars: If the defect is on the incisal ⅓ or occlusal of the molar, the problem developed in the 1st year of life; the middle ⅓, the 2nd year of life; and the cervical ⅓, the 3rd year of life. This 1-2-3 rule will serve you well for your entire career.

CASE 10-22

1. Attrition. In such cases, look also for flattening of the interproximal contacts best seen here at the mesial of the 2nd premolar. Here the contact has now been lost and may be the area of food impaction.

CASE 10-23

1. The anomalies are (1) a supernumerary lateral incisor, sometimes referred to as "twinning" in this presentation and (2) microdontia of at least one or both of the laterals, also known as "peg" laterals.

COMMENT: Gemination occurs when one tooth bud attempts to divide; there are no extra

teeth. Fusion is when two tooth buds fuse with an apparent missing tooth. Twinning is seen with an extra tooth, as this case illustrates.

CASE 10-24

1. The non-vital tooth is the canine.
2. Features: obliterated pulp space (pulp chamber and root canal) without any apparent cause. Most likely this tooth was traumatized at one time.
3. No treatment. Nature has done the job of filling the canal; the periapical area looks acceptable. Note that the apical lamina dura is absent, but this alone is not a reason to initiate a "mission impossible" in trying to do endo on this tooth.

CASE 10-25

1. Ectopic eruption.
2. Probably prophylactically seal the lingual pits of all the maxillary incisors because they are shovel-shaped. However, the lateral definitely needs sealing because of the dens in dente there. Did you see that?

CASE 10-26

1. Anomaly: Dentin dysplasia Shields type 2.
   COMMENT: Shields was the one who first recognized that there are types 1 and 2 dentin dysplasia. O'Carroll classified the radiographic appearance as previously discussed.
2. Restorative material: amalgam. UGH!

CASE 10-27

1. Treatment: Endodontics and a stainless steel crown.
2. Enamel hypoplasia, Turner environmental type.
3. The connection: Turner type enamel hypoplasia occurs in the developing enamel of the permanent tooth replacing a primary tooth that has abscessed or has been intruded or devitalized as a result of trauma. In this case, the primary molar was abscessed but the damage occurred before treatment could be initiated. This underlines the need for frequent dental checkups in children and the need for radiographs when indicated.

CASE 10-28

1. The anomaly is fusion between the developing left incisors; the clue is that no teeth have been extracted.
2. Clinically, you would call this an example of macrodontia, which means "a big tooth" but does not specify the exact cause.

3. Fusion is a single enlarged, joined, or double-appearing tooth, and when this tooth is counted as one, there is a missing tooth.
   COMMENT: If an incisor had been extracted, then gemination would be the answer; that is to say, it could have been gemination of the central and extraction of the lateral. Thus it is history and tooth number rather than appearance that distinguish fusion and gemination. Even then, it is hard to identify fusion between a tooth of the normal complement and a supernumerary tooth from gemination of a tooth of the normal complement in the presence of a supernumerary tooth.

CASE 10-29

1. The clinical appearance suggests lateral incisor is non-vital though this should be confirmed with pulp tests. If it is non-vital, the periapical lesion can be referred to radiologically as a periapical radiolucency of pulpal origin associated with external resorption of the root apex.
   COMMENT: This lesion consists of one of the following: periapical abscess, periapical cyst, or periapical granuloma; and all are periapical responses to pulpal inflammation or infection. Radiologically, this looks like a periapical granuloma because the apex is resorbed and the lesion does not exceed 1 cm in diameter. But the lesion is not densely radiolucent as it would be for a granuloma, and there is a hint of a thin sclerotic margin as would be seen in a radicular cyst. Periapical lesions of pulpal origin may abscess, then granulate in, and finally become cystic, thus alternating histologically over time. It is for this reason it is imprudent to be too assertive clinically about the specific pathologic process and why features of transition between one reaction and another can sometimes be seen, as in this case. Radiologically, it would be accurate to say the lesion appears to be a periapical radiolucency of pulpal origin.
2. Treatment would be to get the periodontal disease under control the crown-root ratio of this tooth is diminished. An occlusal analysis should be initiated to rule out occlusal trauma. Then the tooth is treated endodontically, followed by internal bleaching, and ultimately with one or more porcelain veneers, depending on if the patient wants to eliminate the diastemas.

CASE 10-30

1. The tooth is ankylosed as evidenced by the lack of any visible periodontal membrane space. Ankylosis involves fusion of the

cementum of the root with alveolar bone. Extraction will be difficult.

2. On percussion, such teeth are said to make a different kind of a sound, such as a hollow or "thunking" sound. In any case, it is different from adjacent non-ankylosed teeth.

Case 10-31

1. The problem is a supernumerary incisor or mesiodens impeding the eruption of the central incisor.
2. Treatment involves removal of the primary central and probably the lateral and the supernumerary tooth.
3. The eruptive potential of the central incisor is excellent because the apex is wide open and root formation is less than the length of the crown. With about 3 or so weeks to go before Christmas, I wouldn't make any promises but I would assure mom the tooth should be well on its way and certainly visibly catching up to its mate by Christmas.

Case 10-32

1. There is a supernumerary cusp or tubercle on the occlusal of the 2nd premolar. This is called *dens evaginatus* or *Leong's premolar.*
2. These tubercles can result in a pulp exposure as there may be a pulp horn within the tubercle. Pulp exposures may occur from wear or iatrogenically when preparing the tooth for a restoration.

Case 10-33

1. The best terms are *supraeruption* or *extrusion*.
2. The generalized condition is attrition, easily seen on the occlusal surfaces caused by physiologic wear.

Case 10-34

1. This is dentin dysplasia type 1d. That is to say, Shields type 1 and O'Carroll subtype 1d with the prominent pulp stones and signs of pulp obliteration in several teeth.

Case 10-35

1. So-called *internal resorption.* The problem is that there is no way to determine that the resorption is not external without physically examining the tooth.
2. This must be managed by endodontic therapy even if the tooth tests vital. Once the canal has been prepared thoroughly, the dentist can look for a perforation in which an area on the canal wall bleeds. If there is no perforation, the prognosis is relatively good. If there is

perforation, the tooth must be exposed surgically and the perforation sealed with amalgam while still maintaining the root canal space, which must be filled. The prognosis here is guarded but worth a try.

Case 10-36

1. These teeth are microdonts and appear somewhat hypoplastic because of radiation stunting.
2. Teeth in a field of radiation treatment have been known to erupt though it is often delayed. In this case, root formation appears complete; thus eruption is not expected.
3. The maxillary irradiated bone is subject to complications of osteoradionecrosis. When oral micro flora are allowed to enter into the bone, unmanageable infection can result. Thus orthodontic traction and oral surgery should be avoided.

Case 10-37

1. There is a supernumerary tooth called a *paramolar* either buccal or lingual to the 2nd molar. Note the dark lines representing the follicular sac and root canal spaces outlining the little microdont.

Case 10-38

1. It looks like an enamel pearl, not a pulp stone, because it is both in and out of the pulp cavity and pulp stones tend to remain within the confines of the radiographic pulp space.
2. We can call this a "faux pearl" like real-life faux pearls and furs. *Faux* simply means "false" in French. So what happened? The angulation of the x-ray beam causes overlapping of portions of the mesial and distal roots above the furca, creating the illusion of a faux pearl. Look closely and you will also note the interradicular bone and furcal area of the tooth are somewhat obscured by the improper horizontal angulation of the beam.
3. The significance is that this is important to anyone responsible for management of a furcal problem and thinking it might be associated with an enamel pearl. Imagine initiating a surgical or curettement procedure and finding nothing!

Case 10-39

1. The generalized pulp obliteration in an older individual with otherwise unremarkable teeth is a normal part of the aging process.

CASE 10-40

1. The problem is called *ectopic root resorption*. The distal root of the maxillary 2nd primary molar should not be resorbed in association with the eruption of the permanent 1st molar. Compare with the lower molar, which is okay.
2. The significance is that this person is probably going to have crowding of his permanent teeth and should be followed closely to confirm this.

CASE 10-41

1. The problem is *erosion,* which is a loss of tooth structure caused by chemicals.
2. This patient was actually *bulimic*. Her behavior was characterized by periodic bouts of binge feeding followed by vomiting. Erosion caused by exposure of the teeth to the gastric acids is called *perimolysis*. Common causes of perimolysis are anorexia nervosa, vomiting associated with chronic alcohol abuse, hiatal hernia, or gastrointestinal reflux.
3. Aside from the medical and psychologic help available, the dental hygienist can suggest to bulimics and anorexics that they rinse thoroughly with antacids or bicarbonate of soda as a mouth rinse after vomiting; and make them aware of the damage the habit is causing.

CASE 10-42

1. The anomaly is a *supernumerary 4th molar* that has erupted. Don't tell me you missed that!
   Okay, time for a break. When fatigue sets in, you start missing the easy things!

CASE 10-43

1. The lateral incisor, canine, and 1st premolar all have at least a bifurcated root canal space. The main sign of this is a sudden narrowing of the root canal space. This is seen in all three teeth. Second, the root canal can be seen to bifurcate or branch right where the narrow part starts, as can be seen in the canine. Third, you can sometimes see a double periodontal membrane space down one or both sides of the root, indicating a bell-shaped root that is seen on the distal of the lateral. Last, you can actually see a second root as is seen in the canine.

CASE 10-44

1. Macrodontia.
2. Gemination.

3. Gemination is a single, large, joined or double tooth in which the tooth count is normal when the large tooth is counted as one.

CASE 10-45

1. The primary 2nd molar is submerged and ankylosed.
2. There appears to be a periodontal defect developing distal to the primary tooth and possible root caries on the mesial of the 1st permanent molar. Rule out cervical burnout with a bitewing or physical probing of the area if accessible.
3. The treatment is to crown the primary molar to reestablish the plane of occlusion and to restore proper interproximal contact. The 2nd premolar will probably need orthodontic uprighting. The 2nd molar may also need ortho.

CASE 10-46

1. This is the typical collapse of the occlusion caused by not replacing the missing 1st molar. The maxillary 1st molar has supraerupted; sometimes there is associated root caries and a periodontal defect. The lower 2nd and 3rd molars are tipped mesially.
2. Treatment involves extraction of the lower 3rd molar if it is not needed; uprighting the 2nd molar; root canal therapy on the upper 1st molar followed by a reestablishment of the maxillary plane of occlusion with a crown and then a bridge or implant to replace the original missing molar.

CASE 10-47

1. This patient is about 16 to 18 years old.
2. There is diffuse calcification of the pulp.
3. There is no significance except when endodontic therapy is needed. Notice that this finding does not appear to be age-related or to represent any type of reactive response of the pulp.

CASE 10-48

1. The sign of future crowding is a lack of resorption of the primary incisor root in association with the eruption of the lateral incisor.

CASE 10-49

1. The anomaly looks like fusion of two supernumerary teeth, mostly because it almost looks like there are two roots and separate pulp and root canal chambers.

CASE 10-50

1. The condition is cleidocranial dysplasia.
2. The clavicle or collar bone; this allows the shoulders to be brought together in front of the patient.
3. Hypertelorism is when the eyes are far apart. Specific measurements are when: the distance between the inner canthi exceeds 45 mm; the interpupillary distance exceeds 75 mm; and the distance between the outer canthi exceeds 95 mm.

CASE 10-51

1. There are abnormally large pulps for his age. Note the more densely radiopaque band of dentin surrounding the pulps, giving a "tooth within a tooth" appearance. This is a very rare example of this latter finding. Note also the osteoporotic and even "burnt out" appearance of the alveolar bone characterized by enlarged marrow spaces and thickened, poorly mineralized trabeculae.
2. The patient has vitamin D–resistant rickets (hereditary hypophosphatemia).

CASE 10-52

1. The entity is an impacted, ankylosed mandibular molar, probably a 3rd molar, with no evidence of associated inflammation or connection to the oral environment.
2. This is a "leave me alone" situation. Embedded teeth under dentures may be left in if there is no associated pathology. In this case the ankylosis may require a lot of bone removal to get the tooth out, which can only diminish the support for the denture. All edentulous patients should be examined periodically and receive a panoramic radiograph if indicated by the dentist.

CASE 10-53

1. Dentinogenesis imperfecta (*A*).
2. Osteogenesis imperfecta (*B*). Note the current fracture of the tibia and the deformity at the distal end of this bone from previous fractures.
3. Blue sclera of the eyes. The sclera of the eyes is the part we know as the white part. Remember the expression from the civil war: "Don't shoot till you see the whites of their eyes!" The white, or sclera, of the eyes surrounds the colored iris. The sclera sometimes appears blue because it is thinned by a disease process.

CASE 10-54

1. A single unerupted supernumerary premolar in each quadrant.
2. Because these teeth will most likely attempt to erupt, the erupted teeth may become displaced. At this stage of development they often shell out easily, and their removal is recommended.
3. The most common supernumerary tooth is the maxillary mesiodens, followed by the upper 4th molars, mandibular 4th molars, premolars, canines, and lateral incisors, in descending order of prevalence.

CASE 10-55

1. Ghost teeth.
2. Focal dermal hypoplasia syndrome (Goltz-Gorlin syndrome). The jaw cyst basal cell nevus syndrome is also known as the Gorlin-Goltz syndrome.

CASE 10-56

1. If you said concrescence... right on!
2. The joining of two teeth by cementum; thus they are united to each other by their roots.

CASE 10-57

1. Two microdontic supernumerary teeth in the maxillary left anterior area.
2. Multiple endosteal and parosteal osteomas.
3. Gardner's syndrome.
4. Malignant polyposis mainly affecting the large bowel and rectum. I would strongly recommend prophylactic removal of these structures as the polyposis begins at about age 30 and virtually affects all patients by age 50.

CASE 10-58

1. Technically you could call this hereditary (vs. environmental) enamel hypoplasia and, specifically, amelogenesis imperfecta hypoplastic subtype.
   COMMENT: There are four basic types of amelogenesis imperfecta: type I hypoplastic, type II hypomature, type III hypocalcified, and type IV combined variants of hypoplastic and hypomature with taurodontism. To date there are some 15 variants among the 4 subtypes with clinically smooth, pitted, rough, stained or discolored, and snow-capped presentation. The patterns of inheritance include autosomal dominant, some of which are X-linked; and autosomal recessive, some of which are X-linked. The least severe cases tend to be the dominant ones, and the most severe are the recessives.

Case 10-59

1. Microdontia of the incisors, canines, and premolars characterized mainly by shortened roots and shovel-shaped incisors, which are susceptible to lingual pit and interproximal caries.
2. This is known as the "shovel-shaped incisor syndrome."
3. Pits at the cusp tips, which tend to develop class VI caries.

COMMENT: This syndrome is not yet well recognized but is seen very frequently in regions where the Hispanic population is high. Recognition is important because these patients are more susceptible to certain types of caries and early tooth loss should periodontal disease develop. When tooth loss occurs for any reason, the remaining affected teeth are poor abutments for prosthetic appliances because of the poor crown-root ratio. For these reasons and perhaps others as yet unknown, this syndrome needs to be recognized by dentists and learned by students so patients like Henry and his parents can have important counseling from the hygienist so that his teeth can be retained for a lifetime.

Case 10-60

1. This patient has numerous enamel pearls.

COMMENT: These are known more broadly as ectopic enamel and subdivided into enamel pearls and cervical enamel extensions, which are sometimes associated with the buccal bifurcation cyst. Enamel pearls are sometimes removed because they may become associated with furcal periodontitis when located here. Enamel pearls may consist entirely of enamel; however, they may also include dentin and a pulpal extension. The latter possibility should be evaluated and endodontic treatment considered and presented to the patient if the pearl is to be removed. Ultimately, pearlectomy may be needed for the best periodontal prognosis of affected teeth. Each case must be considered individually, and the role of the hygienist and patient compliance must be part of the consideration.

2. The author has never seen so many enamel pearls in one patient. The author has counted 10 pearls and possibly as many as 16 or more though several may not show up in the printed version. This case may represent a record for the most enamel pearls in a single patient. Here's the author's score sheet:
   - Maxillary left 3rd molar: maybe at mesial developing apex.
   - Maxillary left 2nd molar: 1 distal.
   - Maxillary left 1st molar: 1 furcal.
   - Maxillary right 1st molar: maybe 1 mesial and 1 furcal.
   - Maxillary right 2nd molar: 1 mesial and 1 distal.
   - Maxillary right 3rd molar: maybe at distal developing apex.
   - Mandibular right 3rd molar: 1 or 2 at developing apex.
   - Mandibular right 1st molar: 1 or 2 furcal.
   - Mandibular left 1st molar: 1, 2, or 3 furcal.
   - Mandibular left 2nd molar: 2 furcal.
   - Mandibular left 3rd molar: 1 or 2 at developing apex.
3. Other anomalies include: malformed maxillary incisors; apparently maxillary 3 erupted premolars bilaterally or the canines have supernumerary lingual cusps; bulbous crowns with shortened roots; some dilacerated roots and pulp calcifications.

Case 10-61

1. Ectodermal dysplasia. There are a number of variants; this one probably represents hereditary hypohydrotic ectodermal dysplasia.

Case 10-62

1. Amelogenesis imperfecta type III hypocalcified and is probably a recessive subtype based on the expression, though this cannot be known without a genetic work-up.

COMMENT: Note that the developing 3rd molars appear normal; however, the enamel chips off the teeth soon after eruption.

Case 10-63

1. This question involves an assessment of eruptive potential. When the wide-open "blunderbuss" apex is seen, the root is still developing; thus there is some eruptive potential. However, if the crown length exceeds root length, eruption can be considered delayed and in this case the delay is because lower 3rd molars appear impacted. The uppers look like they will erupt. If a tooth has not erupted and root formation is complete, further eruption is unlikely. The lower and upper 3rd molars should be extracted. The uppers should be extracted also because they can extrude, resulting in a periodontal defect distal to the 2nd molar and distal root caries on the 2nd molar may develop.
2. The extraction of 3rd molars to avoid orthodontic regression is controversial. In theory (growth and development of the

mandible) and in the orthodontic literature, this should not be expected.

CASE 10-63.1

Class 1, position C, vertical.

CASE 10-63.2

Class 1, position C, horizontal.

CASE 10-63.3

Class 2, position B, mesioangular.

CASE 10-63.4

Class 2, position B, horizontal.

CASE 10-63.5

Mandibular: Class 1, position B, mesioangular.
Maxillary: Class C, mesioangular, NSA.

CASE 10-63.6

Mandibular: Class 2, position B, mesioangular.
Maxillary: Class C, mesioangular, SA.

CASE 10-64

1. Figure 10-64, *A* and *B*—the impacted 3rd molar is toward the buccal.

COMMENT: Remember, the lingual object including the lingual cusp is usually a little more radiopaque than the buccal cusp because it is closest to the film. The lingual cusp is also usually a little more inferior and a little flatter. Now in part *A*, look at the mesio buccal cusp of the 2nd molar. It is less radiopaque and a little higher than the mesio lingual cusp. So now you have the known object, the mesio buccal cusp of the 2nd molar (is on the buccal right?). Okay, now look at this same cusp in part *B*. Which way did it move? It moved toward the mesial with respect to the lingual cusp, right? Now look at the unknown object, the 3rd molar. It moved toward the mesial as it is now superimposed on the distal of the 2nd molar, right? So the 3rd molar moved in the same direction as the known object (the buccal cusp of the 2nd molar); therefore the impacted 3rd molar is also toward the buccal. You can reverse *A* and *B* and the rule still works.

CASE 10-65

1. Figure 10-65, *A* and *B*—the enamel pearl is toward the lingual.

COMMENT: In this case we have two known object locations: the malar process of the maxilla and coronoid process of the mandible are both buccal to the 2nd molar. In part *A*, note the position of the enamel pearl superimposed on the mesial root of the 2nd molar and the positions of

the known buccal objects. In part *B*, the known buccal objects have both moved toward the distal with the coronoid process moving right out of the image. However, the enamel pearl moved toward the mesial—the opposite direction as the two known objects. Therefore the enamel pearl is toward the lingual. You can reverse *A* and *B* and the rule still works.

CASE 10-66

1. Canine: Horizontal bone loss; moat periodontal defect (3-walled infrabony pocket); prominent periodontal membrane space, loss of lamina dura, and adjacent reactive sclerotic bone consistent with periodontitis and unrelated pulp calcification.
2. 1st premolar: Horizontal bone loss; moat periodontal defect; prominent periodontal membrane space and a zone of adjacent reactive sclerotic bone consistent with periodontitis; a horizontal radiolucent line indicating toothbrush abrasion or abfraction; class VI cusp tip enamel caries; distal drift and unrelated pulp calcification.

CASE 10-67

1. Supragingival calculus.
2. Calculus bridge or calculus splint.
3. Individual tooth mobility.
4. Vertical and horizontal bone loss.
5. Periodontitis; note prominent periodontal membrane space, loss of lamina dura, and the more radiopaque reactive bone in the area.
6. The soft tissue outline of the floor of the mouth as the film has been superimposed over this area. If it was the tongue, the shadow would be convex.

CASE 10-68

1. "Floating tooth."
2. Malignant disease can cause a floating tooth appearance; this possibility must be ruled out as part of clinical assessment of patient.
3. The defect completely surrounds the tooth. There is a thin remaining wall of bone either on the buccal or lingual side of the apical ⅓ of the root. The slight jog in the distal root contour may be a root fracture, which may be the cause of the problem. A wide zone of sclerotic reactive alveolar bone surrounds the defect, strongly suggesting an inflammatory process rather than a malignant one.

4. Long-term mobility is indicated by the flattened contact point between the two molars; this is a form of attrition.
5. The cause of the mobility may be associated with the flattened mesial cusp tips of the 2nd molar caused by hyperocclusion and which may have been the earliest finding in the chain of events leading to the present condition.
6. Note the thickened periodontal membrane space; this may represent the early signs of a class 1 furcal involvement, which must be localized and confirmed by the clinical examination with a periodontal probe.

CASE 10-69

1. 1st molar:
   - Leaky restoration margin at the distal, indicated by a step defect and the softened dentin made radiopaque by the leaching of tin (Sn) from the amalgam into the dentinal tubules. This more radiopaque dentin is usually flame-shaped, with the tip of the flame pointing to the pulp.
   - Vertical and horizontal bone loss with a lack of trabecular pattern at the cervical third of the root, indicating a loss of alveolar bone in this area.
   - Periodontitis as suggested by the loss of the lamina dura.
   - Focally thickened periodontal membrane space at the mesial furcal area and centered on an unusually high lateral root canal and may represent the beginning of a periodontal abscess of pulpal origin.
   - Pulp calcifications that may affect access to the root canal space needed for endodontic treatment.
   - 1-cm diffuse radiolucent area at the mesial apex, indicating a non-vital pulp representing a periapical abscess, cyst, or granuloma; however, tooth vitality must be confirmed by clinical pulp tests such as electrical, hot, cold, and percussion.
2. 2nd molar:
   - Redecay at the mesial and distal margins of the restoration.
   - Vertical and horizontal bone loss with a lack of trabecular pattern at the cervical third of the root, indicating a loss of alveolar bone in this area.
   - Periodontitis as suggested by the loss of the lamina dura.
   - The tooth appears to be vital radiographically.

CASE 10-70

1. Three posterior teeth findings:
   - *2nd premolar:* Rough contour and overhang, both of which can discourage flossing. Probe the area beneath the restoration for soft redecay, which is most likely present, and compare with the bitewing findings; in this situation the best treatment is to redo the restoration.
   - *1st molar:* Between the 1st and 2nd molar there is evidence of ramping at the crestal bone; this is a type of vertical defect and is often a single-walled infrabony defect.
   - *2nd molar:* Look at the dome-shaped radiopaque band of soft tissue within the sinus at the apex. This is known as *periapical mucositis.* It is often caused by either pulp infection or periodontal disease. In this case I would suspect a deep bony defect along the buccal of this tooth secondary to calculus formation adjacent to the opening of Stenson's duct of the parotid gland. This impression must be confirmed with a clinical examination. In the absence of an odontogenic origin, the soft tissue in the sinus may represent polyp formation secondary to especially allergies and sometimes chronic sinus infection.

CASE 10-71

Take a look at these two molars:
   - In the 1st molar there is a poor distal contour to the restoration and a poorly adapted distal margin of the restoration; mild to moderate horizontal bone loss; a suggestion of a class 1 furcal involvement; and possible ankylosis as a result of the missing periodontal membrane space around most of the root.
   - For the 2nd molar there is moderate horizontal bone loss with an apparent class 3 (through and through) furcal defect, which must be confirmed clinically; there is a suggestion of partial ankylosis.

COMMENT: Ankylosis can be further assessed by the dull wooden sound of such teeth on percussion as compared with other teeth. With auscultation (listening with the blood pressure diaphragm) of the jaw during percussion, a louder sound can be heard when ankylosed teeth are percussed and compared with normal adjacent teeth.

CASE 10-72

1. A vertical lingual groove is often found here and results in an associated infrabony defect. Sometimes the groove can be seen on the lingual enamel running from the central pit

area vertically onto the root. Radiographically, this is suggested by the prominent lingual groove in the lateral and the vertical faint hairline radiolucency in the same area of the central incisor. A developing palatal (lingual) periodontal defect may be indicated by the focal loss of the lamina dura around this tooth.

CASE 10-73

1. Defective restorations; description; management:
   - *Maxillary 1st molar:* Very tiny amalgam fragment on distal and two more almost invisible fragments on mesial; correlate with clinical finding of amalgam tattoo.
   - *Maxillary 2nd premolar:* Overhang on distal; remove with hand instruments or redo restoration.
   - *Mandibular 2nd molar*: Overhang and redecay on distal and poorly contoured mesial; redo restoration.
   - *Mandibular 1st molar:* Rough contour and overhang on distal; poor contour, inadequate contact, and overhang on mesial; correct with hand instruments and abrasive strips or redo restoration.
   - *1st premolar:* Poor contour, poor contact on distal; poor marginal fill on mesial; redo restoration.

CASE 10-74

1. Periodontally significant findings:
   - Calculus, especially in association with molars.
   - Molar hyperocclusion, as indicated by the grossly widened periodontal membrane space and widened lamina dura around both molars; needs to be confirmed clinically.
   - 2nd premolar extrusion; note the altered and deficient contact points, which often encourage food impaction.
   - 2nd premolar ankylosis; note the almost absent periodontal membrane space and lamina dura.
   - Horizontal bone loss associated with all three teeth, especially the molars; the calculus and hyperocclusion may be etiologic factors.
   - The external resorption at the distal apices of the 1st and 2nd molar roots may represent iatrogenic effects of previous orthodontic treatment and which may be the root cause of the ongoing hyperocclusion.

CASE 10-75

1. Caries classification:
   - 1st primary molar: Distal class II deep dentinal caries with pulpal recession; possible pulp exposure
   - 2nd primary molar: Mesial class II deep dentinal caries with probable pulpal involvement

   COMMENT: Actual caries progression is usually more advanced clinically than what is seen on radiographs.
2. Turner's enamel hypoplasia should one or both of these teeth become abscessed. Primary teeth often abscess at the furcation area, causing a "gum boil" (parulis) clinically and damage to the enamel of the subadjacent developing premolar.
3. These teeth will exfoliate between the ages of 10 and 12 years.
4. The 1st molar may not have a pulp exposure and if so may be restored with an amalgam restoration; the 2nd molar probably has a pulp exposure and will need a pulpotomy and a stainless steel crown. There are many other approaches to the restoration of primary teeth; however, their preservation is important especially to the proper maintenance of space for the permanent dentition.

CASE 10-76

1. The 3rd molar is partially erupted with a mesial pseudopocket and significant calculus formation; a moat defect appears to surround the tooth.
2. Root caries distal of 2nd molar with probable pulpal involvement. This is based on the symptoms associated with irreversible pulpitis and the widened periodontal membrane space at the apex of both roots—a sign of early abscess formation.

CASE 10-77

1. The one surface not to be sealed would be the lower 1st molar because there is occlusal caries into dentin. In such cases, combinations of sealant, fissureotomy, and caries removal and restoration can be used.
2. Cervical burnout can be seen on the mesial and distal of the mandibular 2nd premolar.

CASE 10-78

1. Arrested caries.
2. Cervical burnout.
3. There is occlusal caries on the lower 1st premolar.
4. Class II more than halfway through the enamel; for some clinicians this indicates the

surface should be restored rather than be remineralized. However, diligent probing could prove this to be arrested caries as with the molars. Arrested caries may need restoration for esthetics or function.

CASE 10-79

1. Class III dentinal caries.
2. Radiolucent tooth-colored filling material.
3. Amalgam.

CASE 10-80

1. Classification of caries:
   - *Maxilla:*
     —1st premolar: Distal class II full-thickness enamel caries; note typical V shape.
     —2nd premolar: Mesial superficial class II enamel caries; distal class II full-thickness enamel caries.
     —2nd molar: This was a large buccal caries involving the buccal cusp and wrapping around to the distal surface.
   - *Mandible:*
     —1st molar: Mesial class II full-thickness enamel caries; occlusal class I pit.
     —2nd molar: Early occlusal caries spreading horizontally at the DEJ just beneath the occlusal enamel. Look for the horizontal radiolucent band at the cervical of the lower 2nd molar; this was arrested buccal subgingival caries that was not seen in the clinical examination of this patient until the radiograph was studied.
     —3rd molar: Occlusal redecay or recurrent caries.
2. Cervical burnout can be seen on the distal of the lower 1st molar.

CASE 10-81

1. These are both relatively deep root caries, especially the molar.
2. The etiology for the lower molar is extrusion with the altered contact, probable food impaction, and development of the distal root caries. The etiology for the lesion on the distal of the maxillary 1st premolar is not obvious but may be associated with a clasp of a maxillary removable partial denture though the patient was obviously edentulous in the area for a long time for the extrusion of the lower molar to have occurred.

CASE 10-82

1. Recurrent caries: distal maxillary canine; distal mandibular 1st molar; mesial mandibular 2nd molar.

CASE 10-83

1. The patient has a fractured mesio lingual cusp.
2. Restore with an amalgam or composite buildup and a crown.
   COMMENT: Note the poor margins and contour on the adjacent crown, which should be replaced.

CASE 10-84

1. Take a look at the mesial of the maxillary 2nd premolar. Can you see it now? Note the flame-shaped radiopaque area beneath the restoration, with the tip of the flame pointing toward the pulp. Note also the very slight radiolucent shadow at the gingival margin of the restoration. Note also the open contact. Thus the cause is a leaky margin and redecay associated with demineralized dentin with radiopaque tin ions leached into the dentinal tubules from the amalgam in association with the leaky margin. This finding has been confirmed in the literature with the use of spectroscopic analysis of the affected dentin.
   COMMENT: A very slight similar finding appears to be present beneath the restoration on the distal of the maxillary 1st premolar. It is probably not yet symptomatic though both restorations need replacement and the caries removed.

CASE 10-85

1. We wish to prevent the development of Turner's enamel hypoplasia in the developing 2nd premolar.
2. Because the infection is persistent, the 2nd primary molar should be extracted and a space maintainer placed. The 1st primary molar should normally be restored now with a permanent material to help support the space maintainer. However, there is deep root caries on the mesial and deep caries on the distal with a caries control temporary restoration. If this tooth is non-restorable, it also should be extracted and the additional space incorporated into the space maintainer design.

CASE 10-86

1. The 2nd molar shows deep caries that may be arrested. However, there is evidence of early abscess formation at the apices of both roots. Note the widened periodontal membrane space and loss of the lamina dura in the apical areas. There is also a suggestion of pulp calcification.
2. The 2nd molar needs endodontic treatment, a buildup, and a crown. If an implant or implants cannot be used to fill the space, the

molar may serve as a distal abutment for a fixed bridge as is or the 3rd molar may be extracted and the 2nd molar uprighted before making the bridge.

CASE 10-87

1. There is no problem. Though traumatized teeth can become non-vital and abscess, in this case we are looking at the air space within the nares of the nose at the apices of the central incisors. Also, it is the soft tissue outline of the nose crossing the roots of the central incisors—not a fracture line.

CASE 10-88

1. This tooth appears to be non-vital.
2. Because of its location to the side of the apex of the tooth, it is referred to as a lateral apical periodontal cyst, abscess, or granuloma (you cannot with certainty distinguish these radiographically). The granuloma is usually densely radiolucent with a punched-out look, less that 1 cm in diameter, and may have resorbed the apex. The cyst usually is delineated by a thin radiopaque line and may be small or fill an entire jaw. The abscess has diffuse margins with evidence of reactive bone at the periphery. All will resolve with successful endodontic treatment.
3. Stainless steel crown.
4. Taurodontism.

CASE 10-89

1. Caries: Mesial class II involving the pulp.
2. Root shape: Bulbous caused by the presence of hypercementosis at the apical ⅓. Note the dentinal outline within the cementum.
3. Periapical reaction: Periapical mucositis secondary to pulpal infection.
4. Management: Check occlusion because hypercementosis sometimes develops in association with tooth mobility. Caries removal, endodontics, a cast or manufactured post, buildup, and an esthetic crown. Extraction: The now bulbous root shape makes extraction more difficult than normal.

CASE 10-90

1. Close relationship suspected: yes.

CASE 10-91

1. The superior wall of the inferior alveolar canal cannot be seen as it crosses the 3rd molar.

CASE 10-92

1. Radiolucent band on mesial and distal roots where the canal crosses the roots; slight interruption of the superior canal wall where the canal crosses the dilacerated mesial root; possible slight narrowing of the canal just anterior to the mesial root.

CASE 10-93

1. Pneumatization seen on radiograph: yes.

CASE 10-94

1. As is, things look bad for implants.
2. There is a retained root tip; notice the root canal and periodontal membrane space. Other possibilities for similar radiopacities include antrolith, antral exostosis, small antral osteoma, and foreign body or object.
3. Pneumatization.
4. A sinus floor lift can be done by transplanting autogenous bone from a donor site such as the iliac crest (hip). Some patients undergo re-pneumatization failure of the implants. A fixed bridge would be an alternate choice.

Chapter **11** Answers

CASE 11-1

1. **Left** side.
2. **Stafne defect** (sublingual salivary gland depression).
3. **No treatment** is necessary; biopsy or an oral and maxillofacial radiologist's report may be needed to rule out other conditions if the radiologic diagnosis is uncertain.

Case 11-2

1. Differential diagnosis:
   - **Lateral periodontal cyst** (developmental)
   - **Lateral radicular cyst** (inflammatory, in this case from periodontal disease)
   - **Odontogenic keratocyst**
2. **Lateral periodontal cyst.**
3. **Surgical removal and biopsy**. Because the patient has obvious periodontal disease, the lateral radicular cyst resembling a lateral periodontal cyst and occasional odontogenic keratocyst cannot be ruled out. All three conditions are histologically distinct.
   COMMENT: This was a lateral periodontal cyst.

CASE 11-3

1. **Ground-glass** alveolar bone pattern; **loss of lamina dura**; probable extension into the maxillary sinus.
2. **Fibrous dysplasia** (craniofacial type based on involvement of zygoma).
   Paget's disease (alkaline phosphatase is very elevated, especially before treatment).
   Hyperparathyroidism (serum calcium is elevated in the primary type; urinary calcium is elevated in the secondary type).
3. **Fibrous dysplasia (craniofacial type).**
4. Some patients receive **surgical reduction** of the fibro-osseous mass for esthetic reasons.

CASE 11-4

1. The radiolucent lesion is about 2 cm in diameter and is surrounded by a thin, well-corticated, radiopaque margin. The inferior margin is interrupted with a somewhat more diffuse radiopaque margin, indicating inflammation in this area. The mylohyoid ridge is superimposed on the lesion horizontally, and there is a 3-mm roundish radiopacity in the center of the lesion.
2. Because of the history and ascribing to the adage that "common things occur commonly," **residual periapical cyst (residual cyst)** with slight infection is the diagnosis; the central radiopacity is seen with some frequency with this cyst.
3. Other possibilities in this age-group include **calcified odontogenic cyst** (Gorlin cyst) and **calcifying epithelial odontogenic tumor** (Pindborg tumor).
4. **Biopsy and follow-up.**

CASE 11-5

1. There is a **torus palatinus**, which will probably need to be removed before denture construction.

CASE 11-6

1. The pain is probably caused by **trauma** of the soft tissue of the lower ridge from the cusp of the upper 1st molar.
2. A **radiopaque pericoronal mass** about 2 cm in diameter surrounded by a thin radiolucent band that is delineated by a diffusely thickened radiopaque zone of reactive bone. The mass consists of areas of varying density radiopaque and radiolucent zones. The soft tissue overlying the lesion appears thickened and in contact with a cusp of the maxillary molar. The reactive bone surrounding the lesion is an indication of infection within the lesion.
3. Differential diagnosis:
   - **Complex odontoma**
   - **Dentinoma**
   - **Ameloblastic fibro-odontoma**
   - **Odontoameloblastoma**
4. **Complex odontoma with secondary infection** was the diagnosis.
5. **Yes**, assuming treatment is not delayed, the eruptive potential of the 1st molar is excellent since root formation does not exceed crown length.

CASE 11-7

1. **African-American.**
2. **Periapical cemento-osseous dysplasia.** (One of several cemento-osseous dysplasias; the other two are focal and florid.)
3. The teeth are **vital.**
4. The stages consist of: early **osteoporotic stage,** wherein the area becomes slightly more radiolucent with diminished and sometimes prominent trabeculae; the second **osteolytic stage,** with little evidence of the formation of a cemental mass.
   COMMENT: These two radiologically distinct stages are often combined into a single osteolytic stage. In this case, a slight rim of sclerotic bone is associated with the right canine, indicating the lesion is active in this area, and absence of the sclerotic rim indicates dormancy in the other areas.
5. **No treatment** is needed although periodic observation is recommended.
   COMMENT: There are now three recognized subtypes of cemento-osseous dysplasias: *focal,* seen mostly in whites; *periapical,* seen mostly in blacks; and *florid* (multiple quadrants of involvement), seen mostly in blacks.

CASE 11-8

1. Well... if you said **bilateral mandibular torus removal**, you would be right-on! Note the several round radiopaque lobes on this left side and, yes, the condition is almost always bilateral. Regarding prognosis, they **may occasionally recur,** especially if teeth are still present in the area.

CASE 11-9

1. A large **multilocular radiolucency** extending from the left 1st molar crossing the midline to the right canine area; there is one large crenation at the inferior margin and several wispy trabeculae within the lesion. There is multiplanar root resorption of many of the adjacent teeth, and the thin radiopaque line superimposed on several teeth indicates

expansion to the lingual on a panoramic radiograph.
2. Differential diagnosis:
   - **Central giant cell granuloma**
   - **Central odontogenic fibroma**
   - **Ameloblastoma**
   - **Odontogenic myxoma**
   - **Odontogenic keratocyst**
3. Diagnostic impression: This was a **central giant cell granuloma.**
4. Prognosis:
   - **Central giant cell granuloma**: Probability of this diagnosis is high because of age, sex, location, and radiographic appearance. Probability for recurrence is highest when the age is younger than 17 years and when there is pain, rapid growth, evidence of perforation, and size over 2 cm.
   - **Odontogenic fibroma**: Has a predilection for females; may occur in young persons but mean age is in 40s; is multilocular when large; and may resorb and displace teeth. Recurrence is rare.
   - **Ameloblastoma**: More common in males; may occur in young persons but mean age is in late 30s; many in mandible with sparing of the posterior angle area; larger lesions are multilocular with well-defined, rounded loculi; knife-edge pattern of root resorption; may displace teeth. Recurrence of multilocular lesions is high. Multiple retreatment may rarely result in metastasis of histologically benign tumors.
   - **Odontogenic myxoma**: Equal sex predilection; average age is 20s and 30s; septa forming the loculi; loculi are straight and often at right angles to each other and form geometric shapes like squares, rectangles, diamonds, and triangles; may displace teeth. Recurs most frequently in larger multilocular lesions breaking out into the soft tissues (fish skeleton pattern).
   - **Odontogenic keratocyst**: May be seen in younger persons; slightly favors males; more scalloped at the margins rather than multilocular; rarely expands bone or resorbs teeth; mostly in the posterior mandible and ramus. About one-third will recur, and higher if associated with the basal cell nevus syndrome.

COMMENT: Any radiologically multilocular lesion must be considered benign but locally aggressive with a marked tendency to recur.

CASE 11-10

1. This lesion is classified as a **pericoronal radiolucency with radiopaque flecks.** The

lesion is large, extending from the mandibular right 1st molar up into the ramus almost to the level of the coronoid process. There is buccal expansion as indicated by the downward projection of the inferior margin and lingual expansion with trauma from the maxillary 2nd molar. The lesion contains dense, rounded radiopaque flecks with a radiolucent component, resorption of the distal root of the 1st molar, and downward displacement of the inferior alveolar canal, indicating the lesion may be odontogenic.
2. Differential diagnosis:
   - **Ameloblastic fibro-odontoma**
   - **Developing odontoma**
   - **Cystic odontoma**
   - **Odontoameloblastoma**
   - **Calcifying odontogenic cyst**
   - **Calcifying epithelial odontogenic tumor**
   - **Ameloblastic fibrodentinoma**
3. The diagnosis was **ameloblastic fibro-odontoma.**
4. Treatment is **surgical removal; recurrence is rare.**

CASE 11-11

1. **Surgical ciliated cyst of the maxilla** (postoperative maxillary cyst).
2. Variations in presentation:
   - **Entirely within the maxillary sinus**
   - **Entirely within the maxilla just beneath the sinus**
   - **Partly in the sinus and in the maxilla**
   COMMENT: Lesions may be less than 1 cm in size or so large as to fill the entire sinus.

CASE 11-12

1. **Reactive subpontine exostosis** (subpontic hyperostosis).
2. **Surgical removal** but may recur after a time. Removal of the bridge may result in spontaneous regression.

CASE 11-13

1. **Hypercementosis.**
2. The radiology consists of a **dense material that partially or completely surrounds the root(s) of a tooth through which the dentinal outline can be seen.** The periodontal membrane space and lamina dura are usually seen, and either or both may be slightly thickened on one side of the tooth. The cementum may display denser cemental spikes, especially at the apex. Overall, the appearance is that of an enlarged bulbous root. Rarely it appears as a localized ball-like density at the apex of the root.

3. **Paget's disease of bone** (specify "of bone" because there is also Paget's disease of the breast). This case is unlikely to be associated with the disease because Paget's is most frequently seen with generalized hypercementosis.
4. One etiologic factor in hypercementosis is reported to be **traumatic occlusion**. In this case we see two possibilities. First, the 1st premolar is splinted to the canine, probably because the root is short and would make a poor distal abutment. Second, the splinted tooth probably serves for the clasp that helps retain and stabilize the partial denture, which is old and may be unstable. Thickening of the periodontal membrane space and/or lamina dura are further evidence of traumatic occlusion; the lamina dura appears thickened on the distal side of the root.
5. **No**, the dilacerated root is developmental and is an indication of an obstructed or altered path of eruption.

CASE 11-14

1. The right mandibular body appears somewhat **rarefied** with several crisscrossing **radiolucent tracts,** two of which terminate at the inferior cortex. There is a small **bony sequestrum** at the 3rd molar alveolar crest. A small, densely radiopaque area in the 2nd molar area may also be a sequestrum. There is a V-shaped notch in the inferior cortex, and the diffusely denser bone above this may represent a **partially healed fracture** site or **infarcted non-viable bone**. Recent **extraction sockets** are in evidence throughout.
2. The diagnosis was **chronic rarefying osteomyelitis.**
3. The lamina dura is resorbed in **4 to 6 weeks**.
4. Prescribe **clindamycin stat,** and obtain **aerobic and anaerobic culture and sensitivity tests,** including clindamycin, from the pus or exudate or from curetted material from within the bone such as a fistulous tract. Upon receipt of the test results, modify the antibiotic Rx if necessary.

CASE 11-15

1. The mandibular right 1st molar has a **deep occlusal caries** with evidence of **abscess and reactive bone formation at both root apices**. An apparent through-and-through **class 3 furcal defect** indicates a probable **coronal fracture** line (which may be visible in this case) terminating in the floor of the pulp chamber above the furca. Apical to the 1st molar, the cortex is thinned but

somewhat more opaque with a radiolucent line within which an "onion skin"–pattern **periosteal reaction** occurs. This consists of several alternating radiolucent and radiopaque bands of reactive new bone formation beneath and probably buccal (remember the bony hard clinical swelling) to the cortex.
2. **Osteomyelitis with proliferative periostitis** (periostitis ossificans; Garrè's osteomyelitis).
3. In this case, **extract the tooth** because of the fracture. In a sound tooth, endodontic therapy will bring about resolution.
4. Resolution of the swelling takes **2 to 6 months and up to 1 year**. Thus patience, parental reassurance, and radiographic evidence of resolution are key to the follow-up plan.
5. In resolution, the **laminations first become indistinct**; the subperiosteal new bone blends with the inferior border of the mandible. This is followed by remodeling, which produces **regression of the bony enlargement** and a **return of the normal appearance** of the cortex and bone in the region.

CASE 11-16

1. **Pulp test** both teeth adjacent to the radiolucency. The **lateral incisor was non-vital.**
2. The so-called **"globulomaxillary cyst"** is not a diagnosis but is a clinical term for this often pear-shaped lesion causing divergence of the adjacent roots and occurring in this location only. Most cases are a radicular cyst of an adjacent non-vital tooth, followed in frequency by lateral periodontal cyst, odontogenic keratocyst, or a number of other rarer cysts or solid lesions like calcifying odontogenic cyst, adenomatoid odontogenic tumor, and giant cell granuloma.
3. **Good question!** The lateral will receive endodontic treatment. The tooth may return to its normal position without orthodontic treatment. However, orthodontic treatment may be needed.

CASE 11-17

1. **Stafne defect** (submandibular salivary gland depression) is the diagnosis.
2. **No treatment** is necessary.
3. Tooth parallelism assessments are **relatively accurate** with panoramic radiographs. This is a basic physical principle of the geometry of panoramic imaging.
COMMENT: Salivary gland depressions are now reported in association with all three major

salivary glands, and all are on the lingual or medial side of the mandible. Thus the associated gland should be specified as part of an accurate radiologic diagnosis.

CASE 11-18

1. There is a **multilocular radiolucent lesion** in the mandibular right posterior quadrant at the crest of the edentulous ridge. The **inferior margin blends** with the adjacent host bone with a broad but distinct 1-cm **transitional zone**; the superior margin appears to be perforated with a **peripheral cuff of bone** at the mesial margin. Within the lesion there are **wispy trabeculae** of bone.
2. This was a **peripheral giant cell granuloma.**
3. **Surgical removal**; radiographic **follow-up** because about 1 in 10 recur; obtain serum calcium tests to **rule out the brown tumor** of hyperparathyroidism, which is histologically identical and which can on rare occasions present as a peripheral lesion; **reline, rebase, or fabricate a new denture** once healing is complete.

CASE 11-19

1. This lesion is a **pericoronal radiolucency**. It is large, extending from the left 1st molar area to the upper ramus. The fully developed 2nd molar is displaced mesially and inferiorly to an area apical to the 1st molar, and the developing 3rd molar is displaced posteriorly and superiorly to the upper posterior ramus. The 1st molar displays a pattern of knife-edge root resorption. The inferior margin consists of a thickened, sclerotic, smoothly curved line; the remaining margins are corticated but less distinct. The extended superior margin represents lingual expansion on a panoramic radiograph; a buccal component of expansion cannot be discerned here. Within the lesion there are several faint trabeculae; the inferior alveolar canal appears to be displaced inferiorly, indicating a possible odontogenic origin. There is soft tissue swelling at the superior margin, which appears to contact the maxillary 2nd molar.
2. Differential diagnosis:
   - **Unicystic ameloblastoma**
   - **Ameloblastic fibroma**
   - **Calcifying epithelial odontogenic tumor**
   - **Odontogenic keratocyst**
   - **Atypical dentigerous cyst**
3. Diagnosis: This was a **unicystic or mural ameloblastoma.**
4. **Surgical excision and follow-up.**

COMMENT: Here the surgical and pathology findings are important as well as the preoperative radiologist's report. If the lesion separates easily at surgery and if histopathologically the mural nodule does not extend much into the connective tissue wall of the original dentigerous cyst, probability of recurrence is very low. If, however, the lesion separates with difficulty from the adjacent bone and if the ameloblastomatous proliferation extends into the adjacent bone histologically, higher recurrence rates, up to 25%, have been reported. Suspecting the nature of the lesion presurgically with the aid of an oral and maxillofacial radiologist's report can lead to more aggressive surgery in areas of bony adherence and ultimately improve the prognosis. Radiologic signs of transcapsular penetration might include knife-edge root resorption, both buccal and lingual expansion, perforation of a thinned expanded margin, and the appearance of trabeculae within the lesion and/or scalloping at the margin.

CASE 11-20

1. The lesion is a **large radiolucency with radiopaque foci in the right posterior mandible**. It extends from the 2nd premolar to the angle area with posterior displacement of the developing 2nd and 3rd molars. On this panoramic radiograph there is a characteristic downward bowing of the inferior cortex, indicating inferior and buccal components of expansion, and an upward projection of the crest of the ridge, indicating both lingual and superior expansion; thus the three-dimensional shape of the lesion would be **"ball-like."** At the crest of the ridge there is soft tissue swelling that appears to contact the erupting maxillary 2nd molar. Within the lesion the mineralized component appears to consist of an admixture of both a spicular osseous component and smooth, rounded, calcific spherules of cementoid-like material, the latter tending to clump toward the center of the lesion. There is a downward bowing of the inferior alveolar canal, and the distal root of the 1st molar appears to project into the lesion. Interestingly, there is a single, thin, radiopaque margin of condensed bone bisecting the lesion at the distal 3rd forming a second lacuna beyond which there is little indication of a distal margin; the remaining margin appears thinly radiopaque.
2. Differential diagnosis:
   - **Ossifying fibroma (cemento-ossifying fibroma)**
   - **Juvenile ossifying fibroma (aggressive ossifying fibroma)**

- Ameloblastic fibro-odontoma
- Ameloblastic odontoma
- Cystic odontoma
- Calcifying odontogenic cyst
- Calcifying epithelial odontogenic tumor

3. The diagnosis was **ossifying fibroma.**
4. Management consists of **surgical removal with radiographic follow-up**. Recurrence is not anticipated; however, if the lesion is aggressive, rapid regrowth would be observed.

COMMENT: This lesion is radiographically characteristic of ossifying fibroma with the exception of the distal indistinct margin. Loculation has been seen in several large lesions. The concern is the possibility that this could be a juvenile ossifying fibroma with both trabecular and psammomatoid patterns radiographically. The most typical juvenile ossifying fibroma would be seen in the first or second decade, be fast growing, be painful, be located in the maxilla, and have histologic signs including lack of a significant capsule and specific cellular components. This case did not, to our knowledge, recur; however, one of our most aggressive juvenile cases was in this location in the mandible of a boy the same age.

CASE 11-21

1. The pathognomonic radiographic sign that strongly suggests the diagnosis is the **"fingerprint pattern"** observed within an area of ground-glass bone replacement and enlargement. If you spotted this . . . bravo!
2. The diagnosis is **fibrous dysplasia**. If you knew this too, you have serious potential!

COMMENT: There are three types of fibrous dysplasia: monostotic occurring in one bone only; craniofacial affecting the maxilla and one or more facial bones; and polyostotic affecting two or more bones. There are two subtypes of polyostotic fibrous dysplasia: the Jaffe-Lichtenstein syndrome, having irregularly outlined "coast of Maine" café au lait skin pigmentations; and the McCune-Albright syndrome with the skin pigmentations and endocrinopathies.

CASE 11-22

1. Diagnoses:
   - **Socket sclerosis.**
   - **Stafne defect** (parotid salivary gland depression; round radiolucency in upper ramus).
2. Significance:
   - **Socket sclerosis** indicates continuing or past systemic disease at the time of the tooth extraction, especially **gastrointestinal or renal disease**; we have frequently

observed this finding in **diabetes**. Significantly, it is important to find out if these systemic problems are of a continuing nature because they may have an impact on patient management.
   - **Parotid Stafne defect** is recognized for what it is; there is **no other significance.**
3. **Male.**

COMMENT: Both of these findings can be helpful in forensic cases seeking to identify an unknown victim, because they suggest systemic disease and gender (most salivary gland depressions are in males and increase in size with age).

COMMENT: There are three types of Stafne defect. These are depressions on the lingual side of the mandible made by each of the major salivary glands: submandibular, sublingual, and parotid. These depressions are associated with resorption of the lingual cortex adjacent to a lobe of the associated salivary gland.

CASE 11-23

1. Radiologic pattern: **Multilocular.**
2. Most significantly, the small, well-defined, very-round radiolucent areas, some of which are outlined by a thin, distinct, radiopaque margin in the area of the 1st molar. These represent **corticated vascular canals** seen in cross section and suggest some type of vascular lesion. In addition, the lesion is multilocular and almost displays the typical "ballooned-out" appearance. The history of age 20, rapid growth, pain, and a "welling up" of blood at surgery are typical. Finally, the patient's name "Sang" is the simple common French word for "blood"! The English word *sanguinous* means "blood-associated."
3. Diagnostic impression: **Aneurysmal bone cyst.**

COMMENT: Vascular lesions are perhaps the most important category of jaw pathology to clinically suspect radiographically because perioperative bleeding can lead to exsanguination and death. This is not a common sequel of aneurismal bone cyst; however, the risk increases with some hemangiomas and especially arterio-venous malformations. Preoperative recognition of vascular lesions leads to a thorough workup and preparedness for all possible eventualities, thus greatly improving the prognosis.

CASE 11-24

1. Overall pattern: **Multilocular.**
2. Clinically, this pattern suggests a **locally aggressive benign lesion** having a significant propensity to **recur.**

3. The multilocular radiolucent lesion is large, extending from the mandibular left 2nd premolar region into the upper ramus. The superior margin is expanded, indicating superior and lingual expansion of the lesion, and this margin also appears perforated. Internally, two patterns are seen: first, the **loculi form angular or geometric shapes such as rectangles, triangles, squares, and diamonds**; second, in the more mesial, less-loculated part of the lesion, faint thin bony septa can be seen at right angles to a more prominent septum (**fish skeleton appearance**), indicating the lesion is breaking out of the bone and extending into the soft tissue. The angle area is involved.

4. Differential diagnosis:
   - **Odontogenic myxoma**
   - **Ameloblastoma**
   - **Central odontogenic fibroma**
   - **Desmoplastic fibroma**
   - **Hemangioma**
   - **Arterio-venous malformation**
   - **Aneurismal bone cyst**

5. Diagnosis: **Odontogenic myxoma.**

6. The 2nd premolar is **extruded** and appears to have **eroded the opposing maxillary ridge**.
   COMMENT: Odontogenic myxomas have linear trabeculae that meet at right or sharp angles, unlike any other lesion. Second, if the "fish skeleton" pattern can be seen, it can help. Finally, when treated the lesion consists of a pale brownish "gelatinous mass," which further helps suggest the specific diagnosis at surgery. These are characteristic clues.

CASE 11-25

1. Radiographic pattern: **Interradicular radiolucency.**

2. The lesion is large, extending from the canine to the 3rd molar area in the left body of the mandible. Superiorly, the lesion **scallops up in between the roots** of the posterior teeth with resorption of the lamina dura and possibly slight root resorption of the mesial root of the 1st molar; inferiorly, there is resorption of the endosteal surface of the mandibular cortex. The margin appears well defined in most areas but is less well defined mesially and is non-corticated in most areas. The lesion is wider mesio-distally than it is superior-inferiorly. The teeth appear vital.

3. Diagnosis: This was a **simple bone cyst** (traumatic cyst, solitary bone cyst).
   COMMENT: This is a typical example. However, the recently reported cone shape, whereby one or more margins are very straight and linear sometimes forming a cone shape, is absent in this case. The greater width mesio-distally is also a new finding for jaw lesions. The history of trauma, although helpful, is frequently impossible to confirm because of the active lifestyle of most kids and is not necessary for this diagnosis.

CASE 11-26

1. Same condition? **No.**

2. If you said **yes,** you probably thought this is a case of periapical cemento-osseous dysplasia—one area being in the lytic stage and the other in the mature phase.

3. If you said **no,** you probably said the 2nd premolar radiolucency represents the **mental foramen**. The lesion apical to the 1st premolar is a case of **focal cemento-osseous dysplasia**.
   COMMENT: In the cemento-osseous dysplasias, any single individual lesion resembles the others; the specific diagnosis is a radiographic one but must also be correlated with location, sex, and race. The focal variant may be solitary, and the vast majority are in white women in their 30s and 40s. This case demonstrates the mature stage characterized by a crescent-shaped radiopaque mass at the root apex; surrounding this is a mixed radiolucent area within which are characteristic tiny, rounded, calcific spherules and at the periphery there is an irregular band of reactive sclerotic bone, indicating the lesion is active. No treatment is normally recommended.

CASE 11-27

1. Differential diagnosis:
   - **Cystic odontoma**
   - **Calcifying epithelial odontogenic tumor (Pindborg tumor)**
   - **Calcifying odontogenic cyst (Gorlin cyst)**
   - **Odontoameloblastoma**
   - **Adenomatoid odontogenic tumor**

2. Root resorption: There are two things about root resorption: first, it is usually associated with a **slow-growing benign lesion** such as a tumor, cyst, or reactive lesion. Root resorption is rare in malignant lesions though it can be seen especially in chondrosarcoma and osteosarcoma. Second, roots resorbed or not tend to **straddle cysts** and **penetrate into tumors** though this is not a hard and fast rule.

3. The diagnosis was **calcifying odontogenic cyst**. Note the resorbed root of the central incisor straddles the lesion. The only other cystic lesion on our list, the cystic odontoma, is seen in much younger persons. Odontoma can also be associated with the calcifying odontogenic cyst. Confused? In the calcifying

odontogenic cyst the mineralized material can be clumps of dentinoid or an odontoma.

COMMENT: There was a big hint once again in the name of the patient! *M. Phantome* in French means "Mr. Ghost"... and in English a phantom is an illusive apparition like a ghost ...still mystified? The Gorlin cyst is also referred to as the *odontogenic ghost cell tumor,* and the characteristic cells in all Gorlin cysts are called *ghost cells.*

CASE 11-28

1. The lesion is a **periapical radiopacity**. It is approximately 2 cm in diameter and is round in shape. The lesion is **intimately associated with the apices of the 1st molar** with about one half of the root length obscured by the lesion. The lesion is mainly radiopaque with small radiolucent foci throughout. Surrounding the lesion is a **thick radiolucent band**. The roots of the adjacent teeth appear to be displaced by the lesion.
2. Diagnosis: **Cementoblastoma.**
3. Mandibular left 2nd molar: **Reactive periapical radiolucent lesion** with **resorption of both root apices**; class 3 **furcal involvement** associated with probable tooth fracture and secondary carious destruction. The periapical lesion is a radicular cyst, granuloma, or abscess. The infection appears to have caused **rarefaction of the bone** between the cementoblastoma and the reactive periapical lesion; the infection may be associated with an unusually wide radiolucent zone circumscribing the cementoblastoma.
4. Maxillary teeth are obscured because the **tongue was not against the palate** when the radiograph was taken.

CASE 11-29

1. Diagnosis: **Cherubism.**
2. Note the involvement of the sinus and the apparent extension beyond the infraorbital rim. The roof of the sinus is the orbital floor; **pressure and upward expansion of the orbital floor** cause the eyes to appear to look upward in some cases. The normal position of the lower eyelid is that it should be just touching the limbus, which is the margin of the colored iris (covered by the transparent cornea) and the white sclera.
3. **Simple observation**. The swollen cherubic appearance and radiographic changes usually regress spontaneously around age 20 to 30 years.

CASE 11-30

1. Diagnosis: **Adenomatoid odontogenic tumor**.
   COMMENT: In this age, sex, and location, especially with the radiopaque flecks looking like figures such as snowflakes, paw prints, or donuts and the thick radiolucent rim representing the thick capsule found with this lesion, this diagnosis is strongly suggested. Also, in this location the lesion tends to grow inward and occupy the sinus rather than cause significant facial swelling. In other locations the lesion may resemble a number of conditions and the radiologic diagnosis is much less certain.
2. Management is by **surgical removal**; the lesion shells out easily and **does not tend to recur**.

CASE 11-31

1. **Primordial cyst**. It would be hard to miss this diagnosis once you discover one of the 3rd molars is missing. Remember, a primordial cyst develops instead of a tooth.
2. **Odontogenic keratocyst (OKC).** Just about all primordial cysts are OKCs.
3. Case management. Remember that these cysts recur in about 10% to 50%, usually within 2 to 5 years after treatment. However, some have suggested **radiographic follow-up** should be for at least 10 years.
   COMMENT: The following features may be helpful in predicting OKC recurrence:
   - **Clinical findings:**
     —Cysts are a component of the jaw cyst basal cell nevus syndrome.
   - **Radiographic findings:**
     —Radiologically, if the cyst is large and multilocular with internal spiculation.
     —Radiologically, if there is evidence of perforation.
   - **Surgical findings:**
     —Surgically, when separation from the bony wall is difficult.
   - **Pathologic findings:**
     —Histologically, if "abtropfung" or a "dropping down" of epithelial cells in the connective tissue capsule is present.
     —Histologically, if "daughter cysts" are seen in the connective tissue capsule.
     —Histologically, if the epithelium is separated from the connective tissue cyst wall.

CASE 11-32

1. Diagnosis: **Osteoporosis.**
2. Radiologic features:
   - **Thinning of the inferior cortex** and adjacent **lamellations with endosteal detachment** in the premolar region.

- Markedly **thinned cortex at the angles** of the mandible.
- The **alveolar bone is more radiolucent** than normal.
- The **trabeculae** are coarser, less numerous, and not as radiopaque as normal.

COMMENT: The observation of osteoporotic change in the mandible is not seen in the early stages and is more suggestive of well-established disease.

CASE 11-33

1. The diagnosis is **florid cemento-osseous dysplasia.**
2. There are two complications of this condition. One is **secondary infection and sequestration of a cemento-osseous mass,** as can be seen here in the mandibular left premolar area. The second complication is the development of associated **simple (traumatic) bone cysts,** which may be multiple and tend to recur after surgical curettage (not present here).

CASE 11-34

1. *Café au lait* is a French expression for **"coffee with milk."**
2. **Polyostotic fibrous dysplasia, Jaffe-Lichtenstein type**.

COMMENT: The history of pain in the hip is a typical presenting complaint because the disease in the polyostotic form often affects the femoral neck, which becomes weakened and subject to weight-bearing pathologic fracture. Also, the café au lait skin pigmentations with an irregular outline are associated with this type. Last, the patient's last name J-L was a clue... did you miss that one? It is also for these reasons that this would **not** be a case of craniofacial fibrous dysplasia, which only affects the maxilla and facial bones with no other stigmata.

3. The lesions in the jaws demonstrate **the full range of densities seen in fibrous dysplasia:**
   - **Radiolucent,** lower right quadrant
   - **Mixed radiolucent-radiopaque**, lower left quadrant
   - **Radiopaque ground-glass pattern** with areas of increased density, upper right quadrant
   - **Radiopaque-hyperostotic pattern**, upper left quadrant
4. If you thought this is the ghost image of the spine caused by slumping of the patient, you would have made a good effort. Actually, this is standard on the old **Panorex-brand machine,** in which the radiation was turned off so the patient would receive less radiation while the chair shifted for the other half of the exposure.

CASE 11-35

1. Radiographic pattern: **Pericoronal radiolucency with radiopaque flecks.**
2. Differential diagnosis:
   - **Calcifying epithelial odontogenic tumor (Pindborg tumor)**
   - **Calcifying odontogenic cyst (Gorlin cyst)**
   - **Ameloblastic fibro-odontoma**
   - **Ameloblastic odontoma**
   - **Odontoameloblastoma**
   - **Adenomatoid odontogenic tumor**
3. Diagnosis: **Calcifying epithelial odontogenic tumor.**

COMMENT: The features of Pindborg tumor demonstrated in this case include: an expansion pattern in the occlusal view characterized by buttress formation—that is, the expanded margin is thicker toward the distal, suggesting a solid lesion; the associated tooth is a molar that is not usually impacted; there is occlusal or coronal clustering of the calcified material also seen in the Gorlin cyst; there is a knife-edge pattern of root resorption sometimes seen in the Pindborg tumor; the impacted tooth has been pushed down into the inferior cortex, a characteristic of the Pindborg tumor; possibly the calcified material can be seen to be small, smoothly rounded clumps corresponding to the calcified amyloid.

The Gorlin cyst shows a hydraulic effect at the expanded margin—that is, the expanded bone is the same thickness throughout and meets the bone at an equal angle both mesially and distally. The Gorlin cyst is rarely associated with an unerupted molar. The root resorption in Gorlin cyst is not of the knife-edge pattern.

CASE 11-36

1. Radiographic appearance: **interradicular multilocular radiolucency.**
2. Differential diagnosis:
   - **Botryoid odontogenic cyst (botryoid lateral periodontal cyst)**
   - **Odontogenic keratocyst**
   - **Ameloblastoma**
   - **Central giant cell granuloma**
3. Diagnosis: **Botryoid odontogenic cyst.**
4. **Surgical excision. Recurrence 8-10 years after excision** is possible. Thus long-term radiographic follow-up is in order.

COMMENT: The developmental lateral periodontal cyst has three subtypes. First is the soft tissue variant called the *gingival cyst* of the adult and can erode the outer cortex and present as a faintly

radiolucent lesion with trabeculation in the lumen. Second is the *lateral periodontal cyst.* Third is the *botryoid odontogenic cyst,* which is grossly like a cluster of grapes and often but not always multilocular radiologically. All three variants may present as interradicular radiolucencies in the lower canine-premolar area. All three are similar histologically and are characterized by the presence of epithelial plaques on the cyst wall.

CASE 11-37

1. Diagnosis: If you said **nasopalatine duct cyst** (incisive canal cyst)... great!
2. Radiographically, we can see the **corticated margin** is quite a bit thicker than what we see in a normal cyst. This is reactive bone secondary to infection, which may occur when there is a connection to the mouth and explains the salty taste and discomfort. Second, there is **no inferior corticated margin** at all; this is a characteristic sign of a nasopalatine duct cyst when the duct diameter is relatively wide as compared with the cyst.
3. Anatomic structure: **Incisive foramen.** It is radiolucent but without a corticated margin; its maximum diameter is 5-6 mm.
4. Several old tooth-colored **restorations**; old because for the past 10-15 years these restorative materials are radiopaque. Second, **orthodontic treatment** with excessive force as noted by the shortening and blunting of the root tips of the laterals; in addition, they seem to have rotated back to the classic position in a class 2, division 1 malocclusion.
5. This radiograph (Figure 11-37, *B*) is a **sagittal linear tomogram**. It demonstrates the presence of the **lesion** and the radiolucent **incisive canal** extending from the superior border to the floor of the nose. Look carefully and you will see this feature.

CASE 11-38

1. Diagnosis: **Condensing osteitis** (focal sclerosing osteomyelitis). **Pulp tests** consisting of hot, cold, percussion, electrical, or a test preparation with the handpiece (with no anesthesia as routine pulp tests are difficult with crowns and large deep restorations) would indicate the **tooth is non-vital**.
2. **Root canal therapy or tooth extraction.** Approximately 75% of the cases **will regress** to a normal appearance, and they **will not progress** with successful treatment. (Progression may be an indicator of unsuccessful treatment or, more important, a

misdiagnosis. See the next case). In cases that do not regress (but have healed), the remaining periapical radiopacity is referred to as **bone scar.**
3. Lower 3rd molar caries: **Occlusal caries that need restoration**.

CASE 11-39

1. Diagnosis: **Idiopathic osteosclerosis**. Though there is no caries, **pulp testing** might still reveal the tooth to be non-vital as a result of trauma, factitial exposure of the pulp caused by excessive tooth brushing or a cracked tooth. In idiopathic osteosclerosis the **tooth is vital**.
2. **No treatment** is needed. Once discovered, the condition **does not tend to progress or regress**.
3. Lower 3rd molar caries: There is **probably root caries on the distal of the 2nd molar**. This is a common sequel of food impaction and chronic infection associated with this type of 3rd molar impaction. Rule out eburnation (cervical burnout) by confirming the presence of root caries with a bitewing radiograph and clinical probing. The impaction according to the **classification** in this text: **mesioangular** (tooth orientation), **class I** (space from distal of 2nd molar to ramus is equal or larger than the mesiodistal diameter of the 3rd molar), **position A** (the most superior aspect of the 3rd molar is level with or above the occlusal plane of the 2nd molar).

CASE 11-40

1. Diagnostic impression: **Malignant disease** either **primary** to the site **or metastatic** such as breast cancer.
   • **Signs of malignancy** include widened periodontal membrane space along one side of a tooth, in this case the mesial of the 2nd premolar and 1st molar; bone-like material extending beyond the normal crestal height of the alveolar bone; and the clumping effect as seen on the occlusal image.
   • **Signs of slow growth** (unusual for a malignant disease) include mesio-distal displacement of teeth and lingual displacement of the 2nd premolar. The 1-year-old bridge occludes with the lingually displaced 2nd premolar.
   • **Features indicating the nature of the abnormal radiopaque tissue** can best be seen in the periapical radiograph. Benign cartilaginous lesions demonstrate a pattern

of small round dots, referred to as *calcific foci,* which appear to be interconnected with fine trabecula-like lines to give an overall pattern of a snowflake. Malignant cartilaginous disease can be similar or so bizarre as to be unrecognizable. In this case you could easily make out the rounded, flocculent, calcific foci, and with a little imagination one or two snowflakes can be seen. This indicated the malignant tissue might be pretty well differentiated cartilaginous tissue.

- Ultimately a biopsy of the area was taken and proved to be well-differentiated **chondrosarcoma,** which can be slow growing and was the radiologic diagnostic impression. Ultimately the patient's toothache, the alert oral and maxillofacial radiologist, and the skilled surgical team may have greatly extended the patient's life as she is still alive today.

2. The 2nd premolar is not being pushed up by the tumor. It is projected upward because of its **lingual position within the layer** and the negative (–4 to –7 degrees) projection angle of the panoramic beam.

CASE 11-41

1. Diagnosis: **Dentigerous cyst** (follicular cyst).

   COMMENT: Note how the cyst has pushed the floor of the maxillary sinus in a superior direction. This folding-back phenomenon can be seen at the apex of the 1st premolar and corresponds to the thin black line in the CT image of the left sinus. This is all that remains of the original sinus space. The remainder of the sinus is occupied by the cyst and with the 3rd molar in the center.

2. The **3rd molar is positioned lingual** to the center of the layer of the panoramic radiograph; therefore it is projected upward with respect to other structures in the center of the layer or buccal to this position.

CASE 11-42

1. Diagnosis: **Osteopetrosis, malignant infantile form.** The "bone in a bone" feature and generalized increased bone density producing an amorphous structureless apppearance are highly suggestive. In fact, osteopetrosis is frequently a radiologic diagnosis.

   COMMENT: The *"petros"* part of the disease nomenclature is from the Greek word meaning "rock" or "stone," reflecting the rock-like increased density of the bone. This is caused by a failure of osteoclastic resorption of bone with a resulting imbalance between bone formation and bone resorption. Thus the name *Peter,* which also means

"rock." One of the synonyms for Peter is *Rock.* Did you get the clue?

2. Case management: In a nutshell, these patients have **difficulty with any bone infection,** mostly because the marrow, which is the source of the blood cells necessary to fight the infection, is greatly reduced or obliterated by the excessive deposition of bone. Thus this child must have the very best preventive dentistry the profession can offer. Also, these patients are more prone to bone fractures. **Jaw fractures** from boisterous play can be very troublesome to manage.

CASE 11-43

1. There is an **increased density** of the right mandibular body. The lower 1st molar demonstrates an **increase in the width of the periodontal membrane space along one side (mesial) of the root**; there is also a class 2 furcal involvement, possibly as a result of the increased mobility. Notice the **pathologic fracture** of the mandible just distal to the 3rd molar. In the occlusal view there is a **"sunburst" periosteal reaction**.

2. Diagnosis: **Osteosarcoma** (osteogenic sarcoma). This case is classic for the disease, though in the jaws many patients are around 20 years of age. If you saw the features and got it right, Bravo!

CASE 11-44

1. Diagnosis: **Florid cemento-osseous dysplasia complicated by multiple traumatic cysts.**

   COMMENT: In this case the one cyst previously operated on filled in with abnormal-appearing bone. The middle radiolucency may be an extension of the mesial traumatic cyst, which enlarged after surgery, and the most distal corticated traumatic cyst appears to be the most recent. This is the typical behavior of the most severe manifestation of this complication of florid osseous dysplasia. Remember that the other complication was local infection and sequestration of the cemento-osseous mass and the reminder about the traumatic cysts with that case . . . oh, NOW you remember!

2. Management consists of **thorough curettage of the traumatic cyst cavities** and the removal of all the cemento-osseous material; **several re-treatments** may be necessary to induce healing.

CASE 11-45

1. Radiographic pattern: **Floating tooth.**

   COMMENT: As soon as you say "floating tooth," you must then determine if it is of the

benign type caused by periodontal disease or the malignant type caused by primary or metastatic disease.

2. The **radiolucent lesion surrounds the root** of the left central incisor; throughout the lesion, **trabecular remnants** can be seen; though well demarcated, there is **no evidence of reactive bone at the periphery.**

3. Diagnosis: If you said **malignant disease,** that would be as good as you can do because the hot spot on the technetium scan does not help us in this case. The inflammation of a periodontally involved floating tooth would also give a similar hot spot. So it's back to the radiograph, and the findings as described in answer 2 are classic for the malignant type of floating tooth pattern, especially the trabecular remnants whereby the bone destruction is so rapid that some bone is left behind.

Final diagnosis: **Metastatic adenocarcinoma of the lung,** which did show up on the lung scan.

CASE 11-46

1. Radiologic pattern: **Multilocular radiolucency.**

2. On the panoramic radiograph alone the lesion resembles many of the multilocular radiolucencies. However, when the axial CT image is added, we see minimal expansion, which significantly reduces our choices. So now the radiologic pattern must be modified to **multilocular radiolucency with minimal expansion.**

3. Differential diagnosis: The author can think of only one lesion that is multilocular but without appreciable expansion and that is **odontogenic keratocyst.**

4. Diagnosis: Odontogenic keratocyst.

COMMENT: Feel bad? . . . Don't . . . The author was given a variation of a case like this to present as an unknown to the rest of the radiologists at the 2002 annual meeting and guess what? I blew it!

CASE 11-47

1. Radiographic findings: There is **a geographic area** of bone destruction within which **permeative changes** consisting of small punctate radiolucencies without a radiopaque margin can be seen. In **the CT, note the demineralization of the buccal cortex and slight expansion.**

2. Diagnosis: Permeative change within a larger area of geographic bone destruction is always **malignant.** If you got this far, then you get almost full points. However, the slight expansion would make the malignant lesion slow growing, since expansion is not a feature of malignant disease. One malignant central

lesion in this area of the mandible that behaves this way is central mucoepidermoid carcinoma. Though there is nothing pathognomonic about this lesion in this location, remember that this is a favorite location for central mucoepidermoid carcinoma.

Final Diagnosis: **Central mucoepidermoid carcinoma.**

CASE 11-48

Jaw lesions:

1. Diagnosis: **Multiple odontogenic keratocysts.** Odontogenic keratocysts (OKCs) are known to imitate many other cysts, such as dentigerous, lateral periodontal, residual, periapical, and "globulomaxillary"; in this case they resemble dentigerous cysts because of their association with unerupted displaced teeth.

2. Radiopaque material: **Desquamated keratin,** which gives the "cloudy lumen" appearance of some OKCs and is the whitish, cheesy, curd-like material noted at surgery or upon aspiration.

3. Management: **Surgical removal** of the cysts and close **follow-up, because recurrence is high**—up to sixty percent 3 to 5 years after enucleation. In fact, two of these OKCs recurred. However, because of the close follow-up, they were noted as small 1-2 cm lesions and were easily removed.

Ribs:

4. Rib deformities:
   - **Bifid rib just below the right clavicle.**
   - **Bridging of ribs between the bifid rib and the one superior to it.**
   - **Hypoplastic ribs affecting the two ribs inferior to the bifid rib.**

Skin lesions:

5. **Basal cell nevi** (basal cell skin carcinomas).

Diagnostic impression:

6. **Nevoid basal cell carcinoma syndrome** (Gorlin or Gorlin-Goltz syndrome).
   Other features include a broad bridge of the nose and hypertelorism, palmar and plantar pits, calcification of the falx cerebri, and multiple other anomalies, especially skeletal problems like kyphoscoliosis and spina bifida occulta.

Bonus questions:

Forget about the details of this case for a moment. What if in another patient the skeletal finding was hypoplastic or missing clavicles:

7. Name of condition: **Cleidocranial dysplasia.**

8. In the jaws look for **numerous unerupted permanent teeth** with retained or missing primary teeth.

CASE 11-49

1. Radiology: Within a broad geographic area of bone effacement, small, punctate permeative changes can be seen. There are two radiopaque lesions at the apices of the 2nd premolar and mesial root of the 1st molar.
2. Diagnosis so far: Permeative changes are ominous and indicate **rapidly destructive malignant disease**. Note the similarity to vascular channels; however, permeative changes are not well-rounded, the margins can be blending, and there is no well-defined cortical margin. The radiopaque areas may in this case represent blastic malignant disease.
3. In *B*, you can see **"hot spots"** in the neck, superior cranial vault, and mandible. These correspond to **sites of metastasis to bone**. Lesser hot spots can be seen in the frontal and maxillary sinuses and probably are caused by sinus infection (sinusitis).
4. Diagnosis: **Metastatic prostate carcinoma**.

CASE 11-50

1. Radiology: In the maxillary posterior regions there are **multiple radiopaque masses surrounded by a variable radiolucent zone**. In the anterior maxilla, especially on the right side, the alveolar bone appears less dense, somewhat amorphous (lacking morphology or details) possibly corresponding to a **ground-glass** pattern, within which small radiopaque foci can be seen. Several teeth display a **widened periodontal membrane space,** and the **lamina dura appears absent** throughout the maxilla. The **mandible appears normal** and lacks all of the features seen in the maxilla.
2. Diagnosis: **Paget's disease of bone** (involvement of the maxilla only is the clue if you called this florid cemento-osseous dysplasia, plus this patient is white).
3. Dental anomaly: **Generalized hypercementosis**.
4. Removable partial denture loosens over time? **Possibly; however,** Paget's disease is slowly progressive and typically, like the hat size, dentures become too tight. In a partial denture, the base area may become too tight; however, the teeth may make poor abutments and loosen because of the bone disease.
5. Long term: A few patients may develop **osteosarcoma** and both **benign and malignant giant cell lesions** (central giant cell granuloma in the jaws and giant cell tumor in the remainder of the skeleton) in the bones affected by the disease.

CASE 11-51

1. Panoramic radiology (*A*): There is a **generalized demineralization** of the alveolar bone, creating a **ground-glass pattern** with a generalized **loss of the lamina dura**. There is a **loss of cortication** outlining the inferior alveolar canal bilaterally. Associated with the left 3rd molar is a more circumscribed radiolucent area with displacement of the 3rd molar into the mid-ramus, thought to be consistent with a **"brown tumor."**
2. Skull (*B*): There is a **generalized demineralization** of the skull, complete **effacement of the outer table**, **demineralization and thinning of the inner table,** and a **granular appearance** of the rest of the skull. In the frontal area there is a 1-cm, round, radiolucent area thought to represent a **"brown tumor."**
3. Hands (*C*): In this disease the characteristic very early finding is **subperiosteal erosion along the radial margin (toward the thumb) of the middle phalanges.** (The three bones in each of the fingers consist of distal, middle, and proximal phalanges; next are the metacarpals, then the carpals, and the bigger radius and smaller ulna on the side of the little finger.) In this case of more advanced disease, **all of the phalanges** are affected.
4. Diagnosis: **Hyperparathyroidism secondary to renal disease** (renal osteodystrophy).
5. Tetrad of features:
   - **Bones (demineralization, brown tumors)**
   - **Stones (kidney stones)**
   - **Abdominal groans (nausea, vomiting, anorexia, stomach ulcers, pancreatitis)**
   - **Psychic moans with fatigue overtones (mild personality change to severe psychosis; weak muscles)**
6. Management: **Dietary factors** such as low-phosphate diet and vitamin D supplements; however, **renal transplant** brings about resolution and regression of the signs and symptoms. **Delay orthodontic treatment** until after complete resolution, and remember that the cyclosporin anti-rejection drug suppresses the immune system; therefore immaculate home care will be needed.

COMMENT 1: Differential diagnosis for ground glass and loss of lamina dura:
   - Fibrous dysplasia
   - Paget's disease of bone
   - Hyperparathyroidism

COMMENT 2: Upon resolution, what happens to the brown tumors that are histologically identi-

cal to central giant cell granulomas? They generally fill in with dense sclerotic bone, especially in the skull.

FINAL COMMENT: Remember the name Rene P and the clue of organ (renal or kidney) and gland (parathyroids)? Did you catch that one? This is how some students develop that syndrome characterized by hunched shoulders and a flat forehead... you know, when asked a question, the student hunches the shoulders and says "I don't know" and when told the answer responds by palm-slapping the forehead saying "I knew that!" Okay, back to work!

CASE 11-52

1. There are **multiple radiopacities** consistent with **endosteal and periosteal osteomas**. There are several **unerupted and displaced teeth.** Some of the unerupted teeth may be **supernumerary teeth**; no **odontomas** can be seen in this case.
2. Diagnosis: **Gardner's syndrome.**
3. Malignant intestinal polyposis is associated with this syndrome. It usually begins at age 30, and by age 50 most patients are affected. Resection of the colon and rectum is the only way to survive.

COMMENT: Did you get the clue? How does your garden grow? Yes, Mary was a "gardener!"

CASE 11-53

1. Jaws (*A*): In the right ramus in and below the coronoid process and in the upper left ramus there are **multilocular radiolucent lesions with apparent cortication at the margins.** The remainder of the mandible demonstrates diffuse **osteoporotic** change. (These are typical features of jaw involvement.)
2. Skull (*B*): **Multiple "punched out" radiolucent lesions.** (These are classic and almost pathognomonic.)
3. Diagnosis: **Multiple myeloma.**

CASE 11-54

1. Panoramic radiograph (*A*): The mandibular **left 1st molar is impacted,** and the **distal root of the primary 2nd molar has been resorbed**. Surrounding much of the impacted 1st molar is a **radiolucent area** bounded inferiorly by a thin but distinct **radiopaque line**. There may be slight posterior displacement of the developing 2nd molar and resorption of the mesial occlusal portion of the bony crypt wall. A slightly more radiopaque area can be seen at the bifurcation of the 1st molar and may

represent a **cervical enamel extension** with which this lesion is believed to be associated in some cases.
2. Eruptive potential: The 1st molar **can still erupt** because the apices are open; however, as root length begins to exceed crown length, the eruptive potential diminishes.
3. Occlusal radiograph (*B*): There is **lingual displacement of the roots of the 1st molar** and a burnt-out radiolucent area buccal to this tooth corresponding to the lesion. The presence of a periosteal reaction cannot be determined from this occlusal though the radiopaque line in the panoramic view may suggest the presence of this reaction, which is sometimes present.
4. Differential diagnosis:
   - **Buccal bifurcation cyst (inflammatory paradental cyst)**
   - **Eruption cyst**
   - **Ameloblastic fibroma**
   - **Unicystic ameloblastoma**
5. Diagnosis: **Buccal bifurcation cyst.**

COMMENT: The unerupted 1st molar, possible cervical enamel extension, and various features of this case, especially the lingual displacement of the involved tooth, are typical. The lesion seems to be well recognized in Canada and Europe because many of the reports come from there.
6. Treatment: **Extract the 2nd primary molar, curette out the cyst** and associated granulation tissue, **smooth off the enamel extension,** and observe the tooth for eruption. If the tooth does not erupt within a month or two, initiate orthodontic traction. In either case, **maintain the position of the 1st molar** after eruption and until the premolars have erupted.

CASE 11-55

1. A **radiolucent area extends from the right 1st molar to the left 2nd molar**. Within this area there are multiple non-corticated and several corticated foramen-**like radiolucent areas.** Within the radiolucent area and beyond it into the left ramus, fine radiopaque striae are arranged in a parallel fashion to form **straight and curved canal-like structures,** some of which have the foramen-like areas interspersed. The left inferior alveolar canal cannot be seen, and the **right canal appears to first widen in the molar area** and then become indistinct with the appearance of the multiple smaller canals. There is associated resorption of the inferior cortex, especially on the left side, and resorption of several root tips and root displacement on the left side. It is not known

whether the most distal left mandibular tooth is a 2nd or 3rd molar. If, however, it is the 3rd molar, its position and development as compared with the other 3rd molars are significant. However, where did the 2nd molar go? It is rarely congenitally missing, and the author cannot answer this. Faster development and advanced eruption can be seen in teeth developing in the presence of a central vascular lesion.

2. Diagnostic impression: **Central vascular lesion of bone.**

    COMMENT: Nowadays most central vascular lesions seen in the jaws are believed to represent **arterial or venous malformations,** and probably the diagnosis of a central "hemangioma" is inappropriate for some pathologists.

    Preoperative recognition of a vascular lesion is important because there have been reports of a dozen or more deaths in association with the treatment of central vascular lesions, even when the nature of the lesion was known preoperatively. The patient seen here did not survive the procedure though all possible precautions were taken before and during the surgery.

    Simple extraction of a tooth associated with a central vascular lesion can lead to exsanguination of the patient before the bleeding can be stopped.

    Compressibility or pulsation of a tooth in the socket and perisulcular bleeding are further signs of an underlying vascular lesion.

CASE 11-56

1. Diagnosis: **Calcified acne scars.**

    COMMENT: Similar lesions include miliary osteomas and small phleboliths.

CASE 11-57

1. Diagnosis: The original diagnosis was cementifying fibroma. Currently this diagnosis would be **ossifying fibroma.** The "coiled worm" pattern, though rare, is suggestive and should be distinguished from the "fingerprint" pattern we saw for fibrous dysplasia.

CASE 11-58

1. First molar pattern: **Floating tooth;** this is either malignant disease like gingival carcinoma or advanced periodontitis.

2. The floating tooth appears to have developed from the long-standing open contact on the mesial. Calculus can be seen on the mesial root. The distal root is fractured and may be a contributing factor. The floor of the maxillary sinus appears inverted in the apical region of the tooth. The sinus is cloudy, indicating a sinusitis probably of reactive odontogenic origin. There are also small radiopacities within the radiolucent zone different from trabecular remnants but noteworthy just the same. This case appears inflammatory in origin and represents advanced chronic periodontitis. It is possible that the tiny radiopaque flecks represent dystrophic calcification much like those seen within long-standing residual radicular cysts.

3. The unerupted tooth is the 2nd premolar. It appears to have migrated mesially. There appears to be internal resorption within this tooth. There may be an additional pulpitis resulting from exposure of the apex to the periodontal defect.

4. Management involves extraction of the molar and the impacted premolar, followed by keen observation of healing. In this situation it is appropriate for the dentist to treat the sinusitis with an antibiotic, such as amoxicillin, and a decongestant.

CASE 11-59

1. The 1st premolar exhibits distal drift, the root apex appears resorbed with hypercementosis, and there is redecay beneath the amalgam restoration.

2. The 2nd molar is impacted and appears to be associated with a pericoronal radiolucency containing a radiopacity consisting probably of a complex odontoma but possibly a calcifying odontogenic cyst or a calcifying epithelial odontogenic tumor.

3. Immediately above this area there is a thickening of the sinus mucosa that may be of odontogenic origin, but the cause is not obvious in this radiograph.

Part **2,** Section **1** Answers

1. C		56. D	
2. B		57. E	
3. B		58. D	
4. D		59. B	
5. A		60. B	
6. C		61. B	
7. C		62. C	
8. E		63. B	
9. A		64. B	
10. B		65. C	
11. C		66. C	
12. D		67. C	
13. A		68. D	
14. A		69. B	
15. D		70. D	
16. B		71. C	
17. C		72. E	
18. B		73. A	
19. D		74. E	
20. A		75. A	
21. B		76. B	
22. D		77. A	
23. D		78. A	
24. C		79. B	
25. D		80. E	
26. D		81. C	
27. B		82. C	
28. D		83. D	
29. B		84. B	
30. C		85. C	
31. A		86. D	
32. D		87. C	
33. C		88. B	
34. B		89. D	
35. D		90. D	
36. E		91. B	
37. B		92. C	
38. C		93. D	
39. C		94. E	
40. C		95. B	
41. A		96. D	
42. B		97. B	
43. A		98. E	
44. D		99. E	
45. B		100. B	
46. B		101. B	
47. B		102. B	
48. C		103. C	
49. C		104. D	
50. E		105. E	
51. D		106. A	
52. A		107. C	
53. A		108. C	
54. D		109. C	
55. C		110. B	
		111. C	
		112. C	

113. B	170. A
114. D	171. B
115. C	172. D
116. A	173. D
117. C	174. D
118. A	175. A
119. E	176. B
120. A	177. A
121. C	178. E
122. A	179. D
123. B	180. C
124. D	181. D
125. B	182. D
126. B	183. D
127. C	184. A
128. C	185. C
129. B	186. D
130. B	187. C
131. A	188. B
132. A	189. E
133. D	190. A
134. A	191. A
135. A	192. D
136. A	193. A
137. D	194. D
138. A	195. B
139. D	196. A
140. B	197. C
141. D	198. D
142. D	199. B
143. C	200. E
144. C	201. A
145. A	202. A
146. A	203. D
147. B	204. A
148. A	205. D
149. D	206. E
150. A	207. D
151. B	208. E
152. D	209. E
153. A	210. B
154. A	211. C
155. C	212. E
156. D	213. C
157. C	214. A
158. C	215. B
159. E	216. C
160. B	217. A
161. D	218. C
162. A	219. A
163. A	220. D
164. C	221. C
165. D	222. C
166. D	223. E
167. C	224. C
168. A	225. B
169. A	226. B

227. D
228. E
229. C
230. D
231. B
232. E
233. C
234. C
235. A
236. E
237. C
238. A
239. E
240. D
241. B
242. A
243. B
244. D
245. E
246. B
247. A
248. A
249. B
250. A
251. E
252. E
253. B
254. B
255. B
256. D
257. C
258. D
259. A
260. B
261. A
262. D
263. B
264. D
265. D
266. E
267. A
268. D
269. B
270. B
271. D
272. C
273. A
274. D
275. B
276. C
277. D
278. B
279. D
280. A
281. D
282. B
283. C

284. D
285. E
286. A
287. A
288. B
289. E
290. E
291. D
292. C
293. D
294. D
295. D
296. C
297. B
298. A
299. E
300. C

Part 2, Section 2 Answers

301. C
302. A
303. D
304. D
305. B
306. D
307. C
308. A
309. D
310. C
311. D
312. A
313. C
314. C
315. B
316. D
317. B
318. A
319. D
320. D
321. C
322. A
323. E
324. D
325. B
326. D
327. D
328. D
329. D
330. B
331. A
332. A
333. C
334. D
335. A
336. B

337. B		394. C	
338. C		395. A	
339. D		396. D	
340. A		397. B	
341. A		398. D	
342. C		399. D	
343. D		400. D	
344. D		401. C	
345. A		402. B	
346. C		403. E	
347. B		404. E	
348. C		405. E	
349. D		406. D	
350. B		407. C	
351. D		408. D	
352. B		409. A	
353. D		410. E	
354. A		411. C	
355. C		412. A	
356. C		413. E	
357. D		414. B	
358. A		415. A	
359. D		416. D	
360. D		417. B	
361. A		418. C	
362. B		419. C	
363. C		420. C	
364. C		421. B	
365. C		422. A	
366. A		423. C	
367. B		424. C	
368. D		425. D	
369. D		426. B	
370. E		427. C	
371. B		428. A	
372. A		429. B	
373. C		430. C	
374. B		431. D	
375. D		432. C	
376. C		433. B	
377. D		434. A	
378. B		435. C	
379. B		436. A	
380. A		437. D	
381. B		438. C	
382. C		439. A	
383. B		440. B	
384. C		441. A	
385. A		442. C	
386. D		443. A	
387. C		444. D	
388. A		445. C	
389. D		446. C	
390. B		447. D	
391. A		448. B	
392. D		449. A	
393. C		450. E	

451. C
452. A
453. D
454. D
455. E
456. B
457. E
458. C
459. E
460. A
461. B
462. C
463. E
464. D

465. E
466. A
467. B
468. D
469. B
470. A
471. E
472. D
473. A
474. D
475. A

Index

Note: *Page numbers (1) in italics indicate intraoral radiographs, (2) in **boldface** indicate panoramic radiographs, (3) followed by i indicate diagrams or photographs; t, tables, (4) in regular font indicate regular text.*